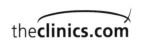

SURGICAL CLINICS
OF NORTH AMERICA

Biliary Tract Surgery

GUEST EDITOR
J. Lawrence Munson, MD

CONSULTING EDITOR
Ronald F. Martin, MD

December 2008 • Volume 88 • Number 6

SAUNDERS

An Imprint of Elsevier, Inc.
PHILADELPHIA   LONDON   TORONTO   MONTREAL   SYDNEY   TOKYO

W.B. SAUNDERS COMPANY

A Division of Elsevier Inc.

1600 John F. Kennedy Blvd., Suite 1800, Philadelphia, PA 19103-2899

http://www.theclinics.com

SURGICAL CLINICS OF NORTH AMERICA
December 2008
Editor: Catherine Bewick

Volume 88, Numb
ISSN 0039–
ISBN-10: 1-4160-63
ISBN-13: 978-1-4160-63

Surgical Clinics of North America (ISSN 0039–6109) is published bimonthly by Elsevier Inc., 360 Park Avenue South, N
York, NY 10010-1710. Months of publication are February, April, June, August, October, and December. Business and E
torial Offices: 1600 John F. Kennedy Blvd., Suite 1800, Philadelphia, PA 19103-2899. Customer Service Office: 6277 Sea H
bor Drive, Orlando, FL 32887-4800. Periodicals postage paid at New York, NY and additional mailing offices. Subscript
prices are $269.00 per year for US individuals, $432.00 per year for US institutions, $134.00 per year for US students a
residents, $330.00 per year for Canadian individuals, $537.00 per year for Canadian institutions, $371.00 for internatio
individuals, $537.00 per year for international institutions and $185.00 per year for Canadian and foreign students/re
dents. To receive student/resident rate, orders must be accompanied by name of affiliated institution, date of term, a
the *signature* of program/residency coordinator on institution letterhead. Orders will be billed at individual rate until pr
of status is received. Foreign air speed delivery is included in all *Clinics* subscription prices. All prices are subject to chan
without notice. POSTMASTER: Send address changes to *Surgical Clinics*, Elsevier Periodicals Customer Service, 118
Westline Industrial Drive, St. Louis, MO 63146. **Customer Service: 1-800-654-2452 (US). From outside of the Unit
States, call 1-314-453-7041. Fax: 1-314-453-5170.** E-mail: JournalsCustomerService-usa@elsevier.com (for print suppor
journalsonlinesupport-usa@elsevier.com (for online support).

Reprints. For copies of 100 or more of articles in this publication, please contact the commercial Reprints Department, Elsevier In
360 Park Avenue South, New York, New York 10010-1710; Tel. (212) 633-3812, Fax: (212) 462-1935, E-mail: reprints@elsevier.co

The Surgical Clinics of North America is also published in Spanish by McGraw-Hill Interamericana Editores S.A., P.O. B
5-237 06500 Mexico D.F. Mexico; and in Portuguese by Interlivros Edicoes Ltda., Rua Comandante Coelho 1085, CE
21250, Rio de Janeiro, Brazil; and in Greek by Paschalidis Medical Publications, Athens Greece.

The Surgical Clinics of North America is covered in *MEDLINE/PubMed (Index Medicus), EMBASE/Excerpta Medica, Curre
Contents/Clinical Medicine, Current Contents/Life Sciences, Science Citation Index*, and *ISI/BIOMED*.

Printed in the United States of America.

CONSULTING EDITOR

RONALD F. MARTIN, MD, Staff Surgeon, Marshfield Clinic, Marshfield; and Clinical Associate Professor, University of Wisconsin School of Medicine and Public Health, Madison, Wisconsin; Lieutenant Colonel, Medical Corps, United States Army Reserve

GUEST EDITOR

J. LAWRENCE MUNSON, MD, Senior Staff Surgeon, Lahey Clinic Medical Center, Burlington, Massachusetts

CONTRIBUTORS

MOHAMED AKOAD, MD, FACS, Senior Staff Surgeon, Division of Hepatobiliary and Liver Transplantation, Lahey Clinic Medical Center, Burlington, Massachusetts

DESMOND H. BIRKETT, MB, BS, FACS, Chairman, Clinical Professor of Surgery, Department of General Surgery, Lahey Clinic Medical Center, Tufts University School of Medicine, Burlington, Massachusetts

MITCHELL A. CAHAN, MD, Assistant Professor of Surgery, Director of Acute Care Surgery, Department of Surgery, The University of Massachusetts Medical School, Worcester, Massachusetts

CARLOS FERNÁNDEZ-DEL CASTILLO, MD, Department of Surgery, Massachusetts General Hospital, Wang Ambulatory Care Center, Boston, Massachusetts

DANIEL J. DEZIEL, MD, Professor of Surgery, Department of General Surgery, Rush Medical College, Rush University Medical Center, Chicago, Illinois

DAVID R. ELWOOD, MD, Attending Surgeon, Surgical Associates of Marietta and Kennestone Hospital, Marietta, Georgia

SEBASTIAN FLACKE, MD, PhD, Associate Professor of Radiology, Department of Radiology, Tufts University Medical School, Boston; and Department of Radiology, Lahey Clinic Medical Center, Burlington, Massachusetts

FREDRIC D. GORDON, MD, Lahey Clinic Medical Center, Hepatobiliary and Liver Transplantation, Burlington, Massachusetts

FREDERICK W. HEISS, MD, Assistant Professor of Medicine, Tufts Medical School; and Staff Physician, Department of Gastroenterology, Lahey Clinic, Burlington, Massachusetts

STEPHEN J. HELLER, MD, Director of Endoscopy, Department of Gastroenterology, Lahey Clinic, Burlington, Massachusetts

ROGER JENKINS, MD, FACS, Professor of Surgery, Tufts University School of Medicine; Chairman, Division of Surgery, Lahey Clinic Medical Center, Burlington, Massachusetts

ANN MARIE JOYCE, MD, Assistant Professor of Medicine, Tufts Medical School; and Staff Physician, Department of Gastroenterology, Lahey Clinic, Burlington, Massachusetts

STEPHANIE LAMBOU-GIANOUKOS, MD, MPH, Resident, Department of Medicine, Tufts Medical Center, Boston, Massachusetts

WILLIAM S. LAYCOCK, MD, MSc, Associate Professor of Surgery, Director, Department of General Surgery, Chief, Division of Minimally Invasive Surgery, Program Director, Minimally Invasive Fellowship, Dartmouth-Hitchcock Medical Center, Lebanon, New Hampshire

DEMETRIUS E.M. LITWIN, MD, Harry M. Haidak Distinguished Professor and Chairman, Department of Surgery, The University of Massachusetts Medical School; and Chief of Surgery, Department of Surgery, University of Massachusetts Memorial Medical Center, Worcester, Massachusetts

DAVID McANENY, MD, FACS, Associate Professor of Surgery, Section of Surgical Oncology, Boston University School of Medicine, Boston Medical Center, Boston, Massachusetts

KENNETH J. McPARTLAND, MD, Fellow, Division of Hepatobiliary Surgery and Liver Transplantation, Lahey Clinic Medical Center, Burlington; and Clinical Instructor of Surgery, Tufts University School of Medicine, Boston, Massachusetts

MARC MESLEH, MD, Department of General Surgery, Rush Medical College, Rush University Medical Center, Chicago, Illinois

J. LAWRENCE MUNSON, MD, Senior Staff Surgeon, Lahey Clinic Medical Center, Burlington, Massachusetts

EDWARD PINKUS, MD, Assistant Professor of Radiology, Department of Radiology, Tufts University Medical School, Boston; and Department of Radiology, Lahey Clinic Medical Center, Burlington, Massachusetts

ELIZABETH A. POMFRET, MD, PhD, FACS, Department of Hepatobiliary Surgery and Liver Transplantation, Lahey Clinic, Burlington; Associate Professor, Tufts University School of Medicine, Boston; and Director, Living Donor Liver Transplantation, Lahey Clinic, Burlington, Massachusetts

JAMES J. POMPOSELLI, MD, PhD, Division of Hepatobiliary Surgery and Liver Transplantation, Lahey Clinic Medical Center, Burlington; and Associate Professor of Surgery, Tufts University School of Medicine, Boston, Massachusetts

FRANCIS J. SCHOLZ, MD, FACR, Clinical Professor of Radiology, Department of Radiology, Tufts University Medical School, Boston; and Department of Radiology, Lahey Clinic Medical Center, Burlington, Massachusetts

KHASHAYAR VAKILI, MD, Department of Hepatobiliary Surgery and Liver Transplantation, Lahey Clinic, Burlington; and Clinical Instructor, Tufts University School of Medicine, Boston, Massachusetts

MELINA C. VASSILIOU, MD, MEd, Instructor of Surgery, Department of General Surgery, Division of Minimally Invasive Surgery, Dartmouth-Hitchcock Medical Center, Lebanon, New Hampshire

GREGORY VEILLETTE, MD, Department of Surgery, Massachusetts General Hospital, Boston, Massachusetts

JENNIFER E. VERBESEY, MD, Chief Resident, Clinical Associate, Department of General Surgery, Lahey Clinic Medical Center, Tufts University School of Medicine, Burlington, Massachusetts

CHRISTOPH WALD, MD, PhD, Assistant Professor of Radiology, Department of Radiology, Tufts University Medical School, Boston; and Vice Chairman, Department of Radiology, Lahey Clinic Medical Center, Burlington, Massachusetts

ROBERT E. WISE, MD, FACR, Chairman Emeritus, Department of Radiology, Lahey Clinic Medical Center, Burlington, Massachusetts

JILL ZALIEKAS, MD, Clinical Instructor in Surgery, Department of General Surgery, Lahey Clinic Medical Center, Tufts University Medical School, Burlington, Massachusetts

CONTENTS

> The anatomy of the biliary tree is variable and at times complex, thus posing great challenges for diagnosis and treatment of its many pathologic states. This article reviews the basic embryology of the bile ducts and the anatomy of the biliary system and its variations. We have analyzed three-dimensional CT reconstructions of CT images from 178 healthy potential living liver donors and report the most common anatomic patterns of the intrahepatic and extrahepatic biliary systems.

> Gallstone disease exacts a considerable financial and social burden worldwide leading to frequent physician visits and hospitalizations. Based on their composition, gallstones are categorized as cholesterol, black pigment, and brown pigment, with each category having a unique structural, epidemiologic, and risk factor profile. Cholesterol crystal formation requires the presence of one or more of the following: (a) cholesterol supersaturation, (b) accelerated nucleation, or (c) gallbladder hypomotility/bile stasis. Some risk factors for cholesterol stones include age, gender, genetics, obesity, rapid weight loss, and ileal disease. Generally, pigment stones are formed by the precipitation of bilirubin in bile, with black stones associated with chronic hemolytic states, cirrhosis, Gilbert syndrome, or cystic fibrosis, and brown stones associated with chronic bacterial or parasitic infections.

for diagnosis remains manometry, with basal biliary or pancreatic sphincter pressures measuring greater than 40 mm Hg. Patients who have increased pressures may benefit from endoscopic sphincterotomy.

Open Cholecystectomy

David McAneny

Open cholecystectomy is employed most commonly when severe inflammation precludes identification of critical anatomy during laparoscopic cholecystectomy. Several other situations, however, still require a laparotomy to remove the gallbladder. A current challenge is to teach young surgeons how to safely manage complex gallbladder disease, when there is minimal experience with open biliary surgery during residency.

Laparoscopic Cholecystectomy

Demetrius E.M. Litwin and Mitchell A. Cahan

Laparoscopic cholecystectomy (LC) has supplanted open chole-cystectomy for most gallbladder pathology. Experience has allowed the development of now well-established technical nuances, and training has raised the level of performance so that safe LC is possible. If safe cholecystectomy cannot be performed because of acute inflammation, LC tube placement should occur. A systematic approach in every case to open a window beyond the triangle of Calot, well up onto the liver bed, is essential for the safe completion of the operation.

Common Bile Duct Exploration for Choledocholithiasis

Jennifer E. Verbesey and Desmond H. Birkett

Laparoscopic common bile duct exploration has a high success rate, with rates reported from 83% to 96% in recent years. The morbidity rate has been reported to be approximately 10% Mortality rates are very low, at less than 1%.

Iatrogenic Biliary Injuries: Classification, Identification, and Management

Kenneth J. McPartland and James J. Pomposelli

Iatrogenic biliary injuries most commonly occur during laparo-scopic cholecystectomy. Biliary injuries are complex problems requiring a multidisciplinary approach with surgeons, radiologists, and gastroenterologists knowledgeable in hepatobiliary disease. Mismanagement can result in lifelong disability and chronic liver disease. Given the unforgiving nature of the biliary tree, favorable outcome requires a well–thought-out strategy and attention to detail.

cholangiocarcinoma remains to be defined in light of the recent promising results.

Distal cholangiocarcinoma (malignancy in the common bile duct from the cystic duct to the ampulla) remains a rare diagnosis. Most of these lesions are adenocarcinomas, and typically present with painless jaundice. If suspected, a high-quality CT scan and endoscopic retrograde cholangiopancreatography are required for diagnosis and staging. In addition, identification of risk factors, use of tumor markers, and advanced molecular testing may enhance diagnostic and prognostic capabilities. The treatment of choice for resectable disease is pancreaticoduodenectomy and the overall 5-year survival for resected distal cholangiocarcinoma remains 20% to 30%.

FORTHCOMING ISSUES

RECENT ISSUES

The Clinics are now available online!

www.theclinics.com

Foreword

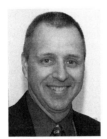

Ronald F. Martin, MD
Consulting Editor

There are many reasons to present an issue of the *Surgical Clinics of North America* on surgery of the biliary tract, and many of them are contradictory at some level. Nearly all general surgeons perform biliary tract surgery to some degree, and progressively fewer general surgeons seem comfortable with all aspects of biliary surgery. The historic progression of this "comfort dissociation" is fairly easy to trace but, in my opinion, difficult to completely understand. And, sadly, it may reflect a disturbing trend in our industry.

There are three main influences that have drastically altered the scope and distribution of biliary surgical practice: (1) the advent and wide distribution of available and competent flexible fiber optic endoscopic retrograde cholangiopancreatography (ERCP), (2) the rapid and nearly complete technical shift to laparoscopic cholecystectomy, and (3) the Wizard of Oz factor.

Although ERCP was developed in the 1970s, several years passed before it became widely available, and it remains readily available in far fewer facilities than laparoscopic cholecystectomy. ERCP is increasingly being performed by gastroenterologists or surgeons with advanced training beyond conventional residencies or fellowships. The clinical capability of advanced practice endoscopists has altered the conventional practice of biliary surgery in two major ways. First, it has provided a nonoperative solution to many problems that in the past were predominantly managed by surgeons. Second, it has created a patient geographic dislocation in that even in patients in whom endoscopic procedures do not resolve their problem, it is highly

doi:10.1016/j.suc.2008.09.008   *surgical.theclinics.com*

unlikely that they will be transferred back to the referring institution rather than stay at the "higher echelon" referral center.

The development of laparoscopic cholecystectomy has undoubtedly benefited untold numbers of patients. I will not insult the reader's intelligence by trying to enumerate the many positive aspects of laparoscopic cholecystectomy here; however, there are a few drawbacks to the development of laparoscopic cholecystectomy. The first, and probably most significant, is that a perception has developed among many that developing technique is more important than improving understanding of disease. This has led to the idea that the main issue confronting the patient and surgeon is how to avoid an "open" operation, rather than how to best solve the clinical problem. A second unavoidable drawback is the loss of a frequently performed operation that provided excellent training for fundamental open surgical skills for resident surgeon education. The conversion of primarily open cholecystectomy to laparoscopic cholecystectomy is beyond reproach, but it has led to a near extinction of exposure of surgical residents to open gallbladder operations, common bile duct explorations, and, in many cases, operative cholangiography. As of the 2009–2010 academic year, graduating surgical residents will have to demonstrate satisfactory completion of a Fundamentals of Laparoscopic Surgery course to sit for the American Board of Surgery Qualifying Examination. No Fundamentals of Open Surgery course exists to my knowledge.

All of the above has led to a Wizard of Oz factor. The decreasing comfort of many surgeons to deal with open biliary procedures, combined with an increasing perception that conversion to an open procedure from a laparoscopic starting point is a personal failure, has led to an increased willingness to transfer patients to the "wizard," who will either deal with complex problems with more sophisticated endoscopic equipment, laparoscopic equipment, or (coming soon, if not already, to a referral center near you) natural orifice transluminal endoscopic surgery (NOTES) equipment and techniques. It is not only the referring physicians who drive this "wizard" phenomenon—it is mightily reinforced by the wizards themselves. Those of us who take on these patient referrals have encouraged the notion, wittingly or otherwise, that we are somehow different: better equipped, better staffed, better trained, more experienced, and, as such, better suited to handle these problems. In some cases we are right, but certainly not in all cases.

There are many forces at play that drive the above-mentioned paradigm—not the least of which is economics. There is only so much time an individual surgeon with more constrained resources can apply to complicated problems before it becomes a marginal return on investment in the short run. In addition, those of us who make our living off of referrals stand to lose out economically by convincing would-be referring physicians that we are not the great and mighty Oz. So the question becomes: Are we serving the public by finding ways to better project capability to the furthest reaches of the "system" (something patients state they want, though the willingness to fund that proposal has not been warmly embraced), or is it better to find ways to concentrate certain procedures in the hands of the few in the hopes of decreasing adverse outcomes? You, dear reader, will have to decide this one for yourself.

Regardless of how one views the questions posed above, one thing remains reasonably certain: nearly all general surgeons will be responsible for patients with disorders of the biliary tract for some time to come. Whether that exposure is limited to cholecystectomy or includes complex intrahepatic biliary reconstruction, there is much to know and with which to be familiar. Dr. Munson and his colleagues have generated an outstanding collection of reviews that should place anyone in an excellent position to decide where she or he should be comfortable within the spectrum of care.

As always, I encourage reader feedback on this or any other topic in this series. We look forward to your comments on how we can better serve your needs for information, whether it relates to the content or the method of delivery and accessibility. Your interest in this series is deeply appreciated by all involved in its production.

Ronald F. Martin, MD
Department of Surgery
Marshfield Clinic
1000 North Oak Avenue
Marshfield, WI 54449, USA

E-mail address: martin.ronald@marshfieldclinic.org

ELSEVIER
SAUNDERS

Surg Clin N Am 88 (2008) xvii–xviii

SURGICAL
CLINICS OF
NORTH AMERICA

Preface

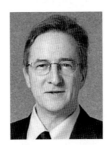

J. Lawrence Munson, MD
Guest Editor

In 1981, the *Surgical Clinics of North America* published an issue entitled "Biliary Tract Disease" [1]. This predated any of our attempts at laparoscopic biliary surgery and was state-of-the-art. In 1994, the *Clinics* published "Biliary Tract Injuries Revisited," straddling the era of "all open" biliary surgery and emerging laparoscopic surgery [2]. This was a trying time for practicing surgeons to learn new techniques, and exciting for residents in training who were becoming competent in the new technology. The experience with referral centers, such as the Lahey Clinic, was a five-fold increase in biliary injuries referred from laparoscopic procedures. Since the introduction of laparoscopic cholecystectomy by Mouret in 1987, an entire generation has grown up with the expectation that biliary surgery is predominantly a minimally invasive procedure. Four "generations" of surgical residents training for 5 years have witnessed this evolution. However, evolution has come with a price. Since Deziel [3] reported a national average of 0.6% common duct injuries, (about a five-fold increase) with laparoscopic cholecystectomy in 1993, this most dreaded biliary complication has never returned to pre-laparoscopic levels.

Surgeons in training now receive fewer opportunities for open operations in the right upper quadrant. Graduating chief residents performed an average of only one open common bile duct exploration in the ACGME logs of 2007 [4]. The fears expressed by Rossi and Pitt [2] that we are turning out fewer residents with the skills necessary for complex biliary surgery or open conversion of laparoscopic cases have not been resolved. We cannot reverse the progression of laparoscopic surgery, but we can strive to train our

0039-6109/08/$ - see front matter © 2008 Elsevier Inc. All rights reserved.
doi:10.1016/j.suc.2008.09.009   *surgical.theclinics.com*

residents in the principles of safe laparoscopy and provide them with the knowledge and skills to perform open surgery when necessary.

This issue of the *Surgical Clinics of North America* will try to add on to the traditions of biliary surgery set forth in previous issues. We have learned much about the mechanisms and prevention of laparoscopic bile duct injuries in the last 20 years, and a review of pertinent anatomy and operative techniques will be presented. Diagnosis, palliation, and surgical management of injuries and pathology of the biliary tract have advanced logarithmically. Radiologic techniques are emerging that provide three-dimensional reconstructions of complex biliary anatomy. Endoscopic imaging and treatment options are evolving as rapidly as laparoscopic instrumentation. All of these new technologies are leading to safer, more effective management of proximal and distal biliary malignancy, biliary reconstruction, and preoperative planning for all biliary surgery. We hope that this issue will prove a useful tool both for surgeons just beginning their practice and more senior surgeons whose careers (sometimes anxiously) have bridged the eras of open and laparoscopic surgery.

I wish to thank Dr. Ronald Martin, Consulting Editor, for offering me this opportunity to contribute to the *Surgical Clinics of North America*. I would also like to acknowledge the mentorship of Drs. John Braasch and Ricardo Rossi at the Lahey Clinic, both of whom have taught generations of surgeons to tread cautiously about the right upper quadrant. Finally, I would like to thank our editor, Catherine Bewick, at Elsevier for her invaluable assistance in making this issue come to fruition.

J. Lawrence Munson, MD
Department of General Surgery
Lahey Clinic Medical Center
41 Mall Road
Burlington, MA 01805, USA

E-mail address: john.l.munson@lahey.org

References

[1] Matolo NM, editor. Biliary tract disease. Surg Clin North Am 1981;61(4).
[2] Rossi RL, editor. Biliary tract injuries revisited. Surg Clin North Am 1994;74(4).
[3] Deziel DJ, Millikan KW, Economou SG, et al. Complications of laparoscopic cholecystectomy: a national survey of 4,292 hospitals and an analysis of 77,604 cases. Am J Surg 1993; 165:9–14.
[4] ACGME General Surgery Case Logs, 2007.

SURGICAL
CLINICS OF
NORTH AMERICA

Surg Clin N Am 88 (2008) 1159–1174

Biliary Anatomy and Embryology

Khashayar Vakili, MD[a,b],
Elizabeth A. Pomfret, MD, PhD, FACS[a,b,c],*

[a]*Department of Hepatobiliary Surgery and Liver Transplantation, Lahey Clinic,
41 Mall Road, Burlington, MA 01805, USA*
[b]*Tufts University School of Medicine, 145 Harrison Avenue, Boston, MA 02111, USA*
[c]*Live Donor Liver Transplantation, Lahey Clinic, 41 Mall Road, Burlington, MA 01805, USA*

Biliary tract pathology is commonly encountered and it can also present significant diagnostic and therapeutic challenges to the practitioner. One of the main challenges is attributable to the variability in the anatomy of the biliary system. The development of the liver and biliary system is a complex process that can lead to numerous anatomic variations. A thorough knowledge of this anatomy is essential in radiologic, endoscopic, and surgical approaches to the biliary system.

This article briefly describes the basic embryology of the biliary system but the main focus is on its anatomic variations. The current descriptions of the biliary anatomy are based on studies using cadaver dissection, resin casts, direct surgical observations, or radiologic contrast studies.

Couinaud's [1] description and classification of the biliary tree pattern is widely used. As part of our preoperative planning for living donor liver transplantation, potential donors undergo helical CT scanning of the liver with subsequent three-dimensional (3D) reconstruction of the hepatic vasculature and biliary system. The axial images are processed at MeVis Medical Solutions (Bremen, Germany). Preoperative knowledge of the biliary and vascular anatomy greatly enhances the efficiency and safety of the donor hepatectomy operation. Our operative experience has shown that the 3D reconstructions have proved to be extremely accurate. We have reviewed the 3D biliary reconstructions of 178 healthy potential living liver donors to study anatomy and to assess the frequency of normal variation. This article includes representative reconstruction images from the most commonly encountered biliary anatomic variations. The advantage of using

* Corresponding author. Department of Hepatobiliary Surgery and Liver Transplantation, Lahey Clinic, 41 Mall Road, Burlington, MA 01805.
E-mail address: elizabeth.a.pomfret@lahey.org (E.A. Pomfret).

0039-6109/08/$ - see front matter © 2008 Elsevier Inc. All rights reserved.
doi:10.1016/j.suc.2008.07.001
surgical.theclinics.com

these images is that they are an accurate representation of what is encountered surgically. Furthermore, the topographic relationship between the vascular and biliary anatomy can be better appreciated with the 3D images.

Embryology of the biliary system

The biliary system and liver originate from the embryonic foregut. Initially, at week four, a diverticulum arises from the ventral surface of the foregut (later duodenum) cephalad to the yolk sac wall and caudad to the dilation that will later form the stomach. The development of the liver involves an interplay between an endodermal evagination of the foregut and the mesenchymal cells from the septum transversum. The liver diverticulum initially separates into a caudal and cranial portion. The caudal portion gives rise to the cystic duct and gallbladder and the cranial portion gives rise to the intrahepatic and hilar bile ducts. As the cranial diverticulum extends into the septum transversum mesenchyme, it promotes formation of endothelium and blood cells from the mesenchymal cells. The endodermal cells differentiate into cords of hepatic cells and also form the epithelial lining of the intrahepatic bile ducts (Fig. 1) [2–4].

The ductal cells follow the development of the connective tissues around the portal vein branches. This developmental process results in the similarity seen between the portal vein branching pattern and the bile duct pattern. At

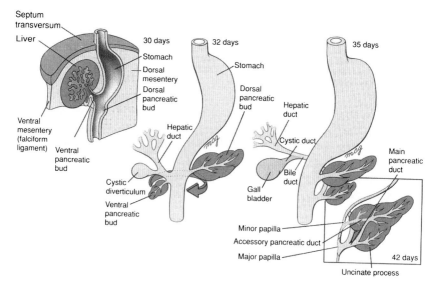

Fig. 1. Development of the liver, gallbladder, bile ducts, and pancreas. The liver bud begins to expand into the ventral mesentery during the fourth week. (*From* Larsen W. Development of the gastrointestinal tract. In: Larsen W, editor. Human embryology. Hong Kong (China): Churchill Livingstone; 1997. p. 237; with permission.)

first, the bile duct precursors are discontinuous but eventually they join one another and then connect with the extrahepatic bile ducts.

The extrahepatic biliary system is initially occluded with epithelial cells but later it canalizes as cells degenerate. The stalk that connects the hepatic and cystic ducts to the duodenum differentiates into the common bile duct (CBD). Initially the duct is attached to the ventral aspect of the duodenum but when the duodenum undergoes rotation later on in development, there is repositioning of the CBD to the dorsal aspect of the duodenal wall [4].

Overview of the liver and the biliary system

Hepatocytes secrete bile into the bile canaliculi. Hepatocytes are surrounded by canaliculi on all sides except for the side adjacent to a sinusoid. The bile canaliculi are actually formed by the walls of the hepatocytes. Bile that is secreted by the hepatocytes flows through the canaliculi toward the center of the hepatic cords and drains into hepatic ductules that are lined by epithelial cells. The ductules then coalesce and drain into successively larger ducts. The segments of the liver are based on its biliary drainage. In the late 1940s, Hjortsjö [5] proposed the idea that bile ducts follow a segmental pattern. The liver terminology used in this article is based on the Brisbane 2000 terminology of liver anatomy and resections [6].

The right and left lobes of the liver are defined by the Cantlie line, which corresponds to an oblique line through the gallbladder fossa and the fossa of the inferior vena cava. Healey and Schroy [7] examined 100 hepatic casts and found that bile duct, hepatic artery, and portal vein branches never crossed the Cantlie line. The right lobe is divided into anterior (segments 5 and 8) and posterior sections (segments 6 and 7) [6]. Each section is then divided into superior (8 and 7) and inferior segments (5 and 6).

The left lobe is divided into medial (segment 4) and lateral (segments 2 and 3) sections, which are separated by the umbilical fissure. The bile ducts draining each segment are considered third-order ducts. The sectoral bile ducts are second-order ducts with the main right and left ducts referred to as the first-order ducts [7]. The hepatic ducts course along the portal vein and hepatic artery branches, which together constitute the portal triad (see Fig. 1). The extrahepatic relationship of these structures can be variable and is discussed later in this article.

Right lobe bile duct anatomy

The right hepatic duct (RHD) drains segments 5, 6, 7, and 8 of the liver. In the most common configuration, the union of posterior (6 and 7) and anterior (5 and 8) sectoral ducts forms the RHD (Fig. 2A). There is significant variation in the topographic configuration in which these sectoral ducts join one another. In addition, frequently one of the right sectoral ducts may

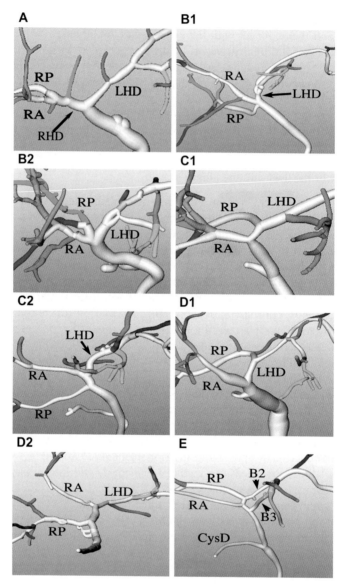

Fig. 2. Most common variations of the hepatic duct confluence. (*A*) Usual configuration of the confluence, (*B1, B2*) triple confluence, (*C1*) right posterior sectoral duct (RP) draining into LHD, (*C2, D2*) RP draining into CBD, (*D1*) RP draining into LHD more peripherally than in C1, (*E*) absence of hepatic duct confluence.

drain into the left hepatic duct (LHD) (Fig. 2C1, D1). The right posterior sectoral duct is generally oriented in a horizontal direction as opposed to the right anterior sectoral duct, which runs in a vertical direction. The posterior sectoral duct is typically more superior and longer than the anterior duct (Fig. 3A). In most cases, the anterior sectoral duct drains segments 8 and 5; however, in 20% of cases, segment 8 joins the right posterior sectoral duct [7]. In some instances, the anterior inferior duct (segment 5) may drain into the RHD (Fig. 3B), right posterior sectoral duct (Fig. 3D), or the CBD (Fig. 3C).

In a liver cast study, 34.5% of casts were found to have a subvesical duct, which was located in the gallbladder fossa and usually drained into the anterior sectoral duct or the RHD [7]. In some cases it drained into more segmental branches and in one case into the LHD. It was never shown to communicate with the gallbladder and was not accompanied by a portal vein branch.

The right sectoral branches coalesce anterior to the right portal vein branch (Fig. 4A) [8]. The right posterior duct generally runs posterior to the right portal vein or the anterior right portal vein before joining the right ductal confluence cephalad to the right portal vein [9]. There is significant variability at the confluence of the right hepatic bile ducts. When there is a true RHD, the length of the duct may range from 2 to 25 mm with an average length of 9 mm [7]. The absence of an RHD is a rare occurrence that may occur during development because of the persistent presence of the proximal portion of the left vitelline vein [10].

Left lobe bile duct anatomy

The left lobe is divided into left lateral and left medial sections that are separated by the umbilical fissure. The left lateral section is further divided into superior and inferior segments or segments 2 and 3, respectively (Fig. 5). Compared with the RHD, there is less anatomic variation of the LHD. There is significant variation in the anatomy of the bile ducts draining the left medial section, however, which is divided into superior (4a) and inferior (4b) segments. Usually the sectoral branches from the lateral and medial sections join each other within the umbilical fissure to form the LHD. The orientation of the LHD and left portal vein are typically horizontal at the hilum before entering the umbilical recess where they lie in a more vertical direction. The LHD courses horizontally at the base of segment 4 superior to the left portal vein. It then joins the RHD anterior to the portal vein bifurcation to form the common hepatic duct.

Segment 3 bile duct (B3) is usually larger than the segment 2 duct (B2) and runs in a concave fashion. B2 has an oblique course toward the porta hepatis and may join the B3 branch either posterior to the umbilical portion of the left portal vein (42.7%), left of the fissure (41.7%), or to the right of the fissure (15.6%) [11]. Fig. 5C illustrates a case in which B2 and B3 join to the right of the umbilical fissure and relatively close to the confluence of the main hepatic ducts. In most cases, the configuration of the B2 and B3 ducts are similar to those in Fig. 5A and B.

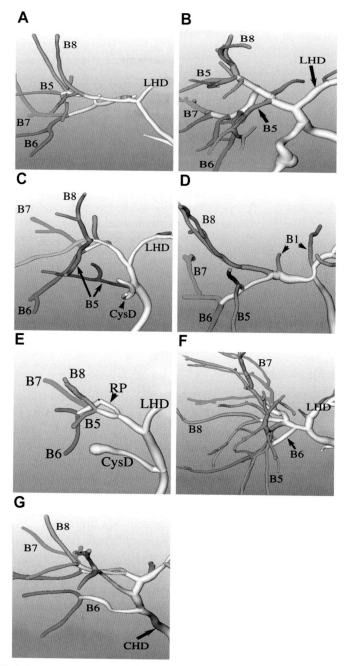

Fig. 3. Variations of the right intrahepatic segmental ductal system. (*A*) Anterior segments (B5 and B8) form the right anterior sectoral duct and join the posterior sectoral duct (formed by B6 and B7) to form the RHD, (*B*) ectopic drainage of segment 5 (B5), (*C*) ectopic drainage of B5 into CBD, (*D*) B5 draining into the right posterior duct, (*E*) long RHD, (*F*) absence of right posterior duct, (*G*) drainage of B6 into common hepatic duct (CHD).

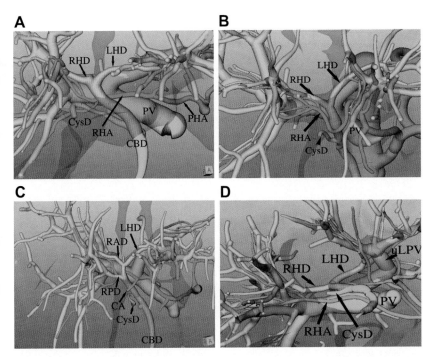

Fig. 4. Relationship of bile ducts, hepatic artery branches, and portal vein branches. (*A*) Right hepatic artery (RHA) courses posterior to common bile duct (CBD), (*B*) RHA anterior to the CBD, (*C*) right anterior bile duct (RAD) draining into LHD, (*D*) replaced RHA.

Segment 4 biliary drainage has a complex and variable pattern. Segment 4 is divided into a superior (4a) and inferior area (4b) with two ducts draining each area or subsegment. Healey and Schroy [7] categorized the drainage pattern of segment 4 into four types. Type I (60%) had all ducts joining to form a single medial sector duct (Fig. 6A). Type II (24%) had one of the subsegmental ducts with a separate drainage. In type III (10%), the inferior duct and superior duct had separate drainage sites (Fig. 6B), and in type IV (6%), two subsegmental ducts had a common duct and two drained separately into the LHD.

In the study by Onishi and colleagues [11] examining cadavers and liver casts they further classified the confluence patterns of segment 4 bile ducts (B4) based on the location of their drainage relative to the midpoint between the confluence of B2 and B3 and the LHD and RHD. Most frequently (54.6%), B4 joined the B2/B3 system on the peripheral side and in 35.5% of cases it joined on the hilar side. Usually, B4 takes a J-shaped course before joining the LHD. In 9.9% of the cases, there is drainage into both the peripheral and hilar sides of the B2/B3 systems [11]. It is extremely rare (1%) for B4 to drain into B2 and it was never observed to cross to the left side of the umbilical fissure [7]. During its horizontal course along the inferior portion of segment 4, the LHD may receive small branches from the left medial

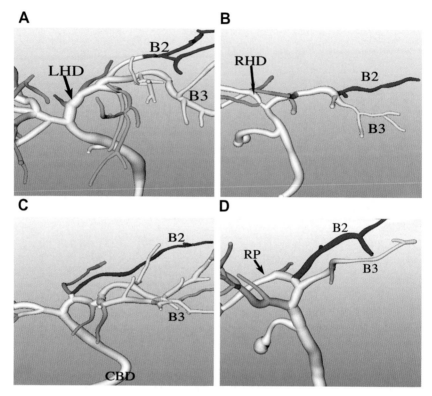

Fig. 5. Variations of segment 2 (B2) and segment 3 (B3) bile ducts. (*A–C*) Usual configuration with B2 and B3 joining each other at variable distances from the main confluence. (*D*) Non-union of B2 and B3 with right posterior duct draining into B2.

segment. The average distance between B2/B3 confluence and the main hepatic duct confluence is 3.25 cm with a range of 0.5 to 5.7 cm [11].

In our study, we found that B4 drainage had a single, common duct in 60% of cases (see Fig. 6A). In 12% of cases, we observed a separate drainage of the medial superior and inferior areas (see Fig. 6B). When the confluence of B2 and B3 is more toward the hilum as seen in 22% of the cases, B4 tends to join B3 (Fig. 6C). If B4a and B4b have separate drainages then B4b may drain into B3 (Fig. 6D). In accordance with the observations of others, we also found that on rare occasions (<2%) B4 may drain separately into the common hepatic duct (CHD) (Fig. 6E) or very close to the main hepatic ductal confluence (Fig. 6F).

Caudate lobe bile duct anatomy

The caudate lobe (segment 1) is divided into a caudate lobe proper, which is located between the inferior vena cava and the umbilical fissure, and the

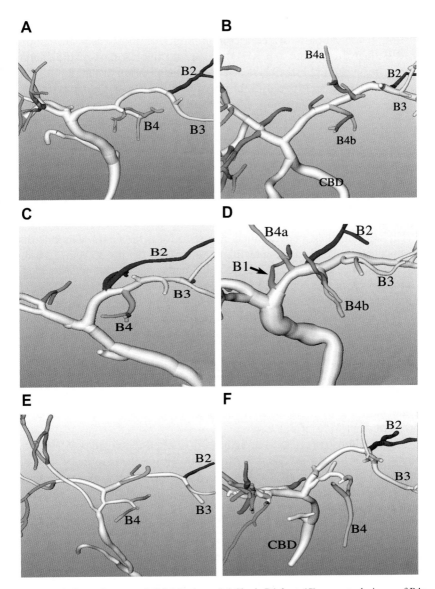

Fig. 6. Variations of segment 4 (B4) bile ducts. (*A*) Single B4 duct, (*B*) separate drainage of B4a and B4b, (*C*) drainage of B4 into B3 (note B2 and B3 join close to the main confluence), (*D*) separate drainages of B4a and B4b, and B4b drainage into B3, (*E*) absence of drainage of B4 into a true left system, (*F*) drainage of B4 into the main confluence.

caudate process, which connects the caudate lobe to the right hepatic lobe. Based on the biliary drainage of the caudate lobe, it cannot be designated as solely part of the either the right or the left lobe. The caudate lobe itself can be divided into right, left, and caudate process. Healey and Schroy [7] noted that in 44% of cases, three separate ducts drained each part of the caudate lobe. In 26% of cases, the caudate process duct and the duct from the right portion of the caudate formed a common duct. In most cases, the caudate process duct drains into the RHD (85%) and the left part of the caudate lobe drains into the LHD (93%). Because of the position of the right portion of the caudate lobe, it could drain into either the left or right systems.

Fig. 7 shows the commonly encountered drainage patterns of segment 1. There may be small branches from the caudate lobe that may not be represented because of the resolution of the scan. The major branching patterns that are more likely clinically relevant are similar to those described by others [7].

Bile duct confluence and common hepatic duct anatomy

The left and right hepatic ducts merge to form the CHD. The bile duct confluence is located in the hilar plate anterior to the portal vein. Extrahepatically, a sheath covers the bile duct and hepatic artery branches, which is continuous with the hepatoduodenal ligament. Opening the connective tissue of the hilar plate inferior to segment 4 of the liver exposes the LHD and the confluence of hepatic duct. The intrahepatic portion of the bile ducts is covered by the Glisson sheath except for the bile ducts of the left medial section [10].

The formation of the CHD can be variable. The most commonly encountered confluence pattern is where RHD and LHD merge to form the CHD (see Fig. 2A). Couinaud [1] reported this to be present in 57% of cases and Healey and Schroy [7] reported a 72% incidence. In our study, we observed this pattern in 57% of our cases.

The next most prevalent configuration is when the right posterior duct joins the LHD (see Fig. 2C1). We found this to be the case in 19% of our cases, which is comparable to Couinaud's reported 16%. As can be seen in Fig. 2D1, the right posterior duct may join the LHD more peripherally in 5% of cases.

In 11% of our cases, the LHD and the right anterior and posterior ducts formed a trifurcation. The relationship of the right posterior (RP) or right anterior (RA) ducts to one another at the trifurcation may vary as illustrated in Fig. 2B1, B2. It is about three times more likely for the RP hepatic duct to be superior to the RA duct (see Fig. 2B2).

Finally, 4.5% of our cohort had the RP hepatic duct join the CHD after the RA and LHD had merged. The point at which the RP joins may be close to the confluence of the RA and LHD (see Fig. 2C2) or more distal (see Fig. 2D2).

Common bile duct anatomy

The cystic duct drains into the common hepatic duct to form the CBD. The CBD is situated anterior to the portal vein along the right edge of

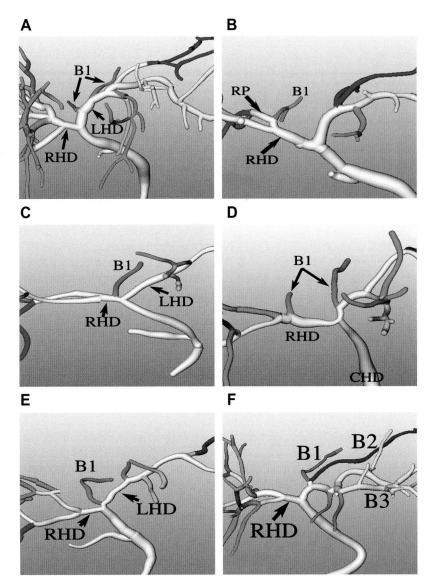

Fig. 7. Variations of segment 1 (B1) bile ducts. (*A*) Drainage of B1 into the LHD, (*B*) drainage of B1 into right posterior duct (RP), (*C*) B1 draining into RIID, (*D*) B1 draining into both the RHD and LHD, (*E*) B1 drainage at the main confluence, (*F*) B1 drainage into B2 (note the proximity of B2 and B3 union to the main confluence).

the lesser omentum. It courses caudad behind the first portion of the duodenum then runs in an oblique fashion on the dorsal aspect of the pancreas in the pancreatic groove. Most of the time, the CBD in the pancreatic groove is covered by pancreatic tissue or embedded within pancreatic tissue and in

12% of cases it has a posterior bare area [12]. CBD usually joins the pancreatic duct (70%) and they enter the second portion of the duodenum on its posteromedial wall at the major papilla [13]. The union of the CBD and the major pancreatic duct creates the ampulla of Vater. A sheath of circular smooth muscle fibers surrounds the ampulla and the intraduodenal portion of the CBD and the major pancreatic duct and is known as the sphincter of Oddi [14]. In some cases, the pancreatic duct and the CBD do not join and each enters the duodenum separately on the duodenal papilla. The site of entrance of the CBD into the duodenum has been studied by several groups and it was found that the CBD enters the descending portion of the duodenum in greater than 80% of the cases. Other sites of entrance of the CBD are the transverse duodenum and at the angle created by the junction between the descending and transverse duodenum [14].

Anatomic studies have shown the external diameter of the suprapancreatic CBD to range from 5 to 13 mm with a mean diameter of 9 mm. The internal diameter range is 4 to 12.5 mm with a mean diameter of 8 mm. The external diameter seems to remain fairly constant from the hepatic confluence to the papilla. The internal diameter decreases to a range of 1.5 to 7.5 mm with a mean of 4 mm near the duodenal papilla [12].

There are several anatomic variations in which sectoral ducts may enter the CBD directly. One example is shown in Fig. 3C. Although rare, if not recognized these variations can result in morbidity following biliary surgery.

Arterial blood supply of the biliary system

The extrahepatic bile ducts may receive their arterial blood supply from several different major arteries. Northover and Terblanche [15] conducted a resin cast study in human cadavers in which they described two major axial vessels that ran along the lateral borders of the supraduodenal CBD. They named these the 3 o'clock and 9 o'clock arteries. They reported an average of 8 small arteries with a diameter of 0.3 mm supplying the supraduodenal CBD. These arteries arise from below (posterior or anterior superior pancreaticoduodenal artery, gastroduodenal artery, retroportal artery) and above (right hepatic artery, cystic artery, left hepatic artery). In rare cases, there is nonaxial supply from the common hepatic artery [15].

The hilar ducts receive numerous arterial branches from the right and left hepatic arteries. These form a rich network around the ducts and are in continuity with the plexus around the CBD. In some cases, the 3 o'clock and 9 o'clock arteries may supply the hilar ducts. The retropancreatic portion of the CBD is usually supplied by multiple small branches from the posterior superior pancreaticoduodenal artery [15]. The various contributing arteries form an arterial plexus within the wall of the bile duct before giving rise to a capillary plexus. In the study by Northover and Terblanche [15], no end-arteries to the CBD were noted.

Gunji and colleagues [16] used cadaver dissection and corrosion casts to describe a communicating arcade between the right and left hepatic arteries. They identified small branches from the communicating arcade that supplied the hilar bile ducts. This arcade runs in the hilar plate and on the right side may branch from the right hepatic artery or the anterior right hepatic artery and on the left side it branches from the left hepatic artery or segment 4 artery. At the time of biliary surgery, attention to the preservation of the blood supply to the bile ducts is imperative in the assurance of anastomotic integrity and the prevention of strictures.

Venous drainage of the biliary system

A fine venous plexus that drains into marginal veins surrounds the surfaces of the extrahepatic and intrahepatic bile ducts [17]. The marginal veins run in the 3 o'clock and 9 o'clock positions similar to the arterial vessels. Inferiorly, the marginal veins drain into the pancreaticoduodenal venous plexus. Superiorly, the marginal vessels have been shown to enter the hepatic substance or join the hilar venous plexus, which eventually drains into branches of the portal vein [18]. The intrahepatic bile duct venous plexus drains into the adjacent portal vein. The veins of the gallbladder do not follow arterial branches and have direct drainage into the liver [19].

Gallbladder and cystic duct anatomy

The gallbladder is a piriform sac that is situated in the cystic fossa on the inferior and posterior aspect of the right lobe of the liver. On extremely rare occasions, the gallbladder has been found on the left side of the liver or intrahepatically where it is completely surrounded by liver tissue [20]. The gallbladder is separated from the liver parenchyma by the cystic plate, which is in continuity with the hilar plate. At times, it may be embedded deeply in the liver or it may have a mesentery [8].

The gallbladder is about 4 cm wide and 7 to 10 cm long in most adults. It is composed of a fundus, body, and neck. The fundus is the blind-ending portion that projects below the inferior edge of the liver where it is in contact with the anterior abdominal wall at the level of the ninth costal cartilage in about 50% of cases [2]. The body is the largest part of the gallbladder and is pointed up and to the left close to the right side of the porta. The body decreases in width and forms the infundibulum as it becomes the neck of the gallbladder with an average length of 5 to 7 mm. On the right side of the neck, sometimes as a result of chronic dilatation, there may be a recess that projects toward the duodenum called the Hartmann pouch.

The neck of the gallbladder is connected to the cystic duct, which is 3 to 4 cm long and courses inferiorly and to the left of the neck eventually joining the common hepatic duct to form the CBD. The cystic duct has 5 to 12 oblique folds, creating a spiral valve known as the valve of Heister [2]. In greater than 70% of cases, the cystic duct joins the right lateral edge of the common hepatic duct superior to the pancreas and about 2 cm inferior to the RHD and LHD confluence [21]. In the study by Moosman and Coller [21], the mean diameter of cystic duct was about 4 mm and its length ranged from 4 to 65 mm with a mean length of 30 mm. They also found a short cystic duct parallel to the CHD in 15% of cases and a long cystic duct in 4% of cases. In 10% of cases, the cystic duct joined the CHD on its anterior or posterior aspect. On rare occasions, the cystic duct may join the hepatic duct near the confluence of the RHD and the LHD creating a trifurcation. The union of the cystic duct with the CHD has been described as angular (75%), parallel (20%), or spiral (5%) [22].

The blood supply of the gallbladder is by way of the cystic artery, which usually branches from the right hepatic artery and courses superior to the cystic duct. The cystic artery reaches the superior aspect of the neck of the gallbladder where it divides into a superficial branch that runs on the inferior aspect of the gallbladder and a deep branch that is on the superior aspect between the gallbladder and the liver bed [2].

Some rare anatomic variations of the gallbladder include anomalies in its form and number. Agenesis of the gallbladder [23], multiple gallbladders [24], bilobed gallbladder [25], and double cystic duct [26] have been reported. In cases of a double gallbladder, each gallbladder may have its own cystic duct or the duct may join to form a common cystic duct before joining the common hepatic duct [27]. When the entire gallbladder is covered by peritoneum resulting in a true mesentery, it has been referred to as a floating gallbladder [28].

Relationship of extrahepatic bile ducts to vascular structures

An understanding of the relationship of various structures within the porta hepatis is critical in performing safe dissections in this region. Fig. 4 illustrates the relationship between the bile ducts and portal vein and hepatic artery branches. The CBD is invariably located slightly to the right and anterior to the portal vein. In most cases, the right hepatic artery that originates from the proper hepatic artery courses posterior to the CBD (see Fig. 4A). In 22% of cases, it is situated anterior to the CBD (see Fig. 4B). In 10% to 15% of cases, the blood supply to the right lobe of the liver is by way of a replaced right hepatic artery, which arises from the superior mesenteric artery and courses posterior to the portal vein and the CBD (see Fig. 4D).

In some cases, the right hepatic artery may project beyond the CHD and form a "knuckle," which at times may run along the cystic duct and the gallbladder neck [19]. In this situation, the cystic artery is likely to be very short. It is important to recognize this to avoid injury to the right hepatic artery during cholecystectomy.

Summary

The anatomy of the biliary tree is variable and at times complex, thus posing significant challenges for the diagnosis and treatment of its many pathologic states. Over the past 60 years, there have been a great number of pioneers who have elucidated our understanding of the complex liver and biliary anatomy through cadaver dissections and cast studies. This study used 3D reconstructions of CT images to analyze the biliary anatomy of 178 patients who underwent imaging studies in preparation for living donor hepatic lobectomy. Our results confirm earlier studies regarding the anatomy of the biliary system. We have found that preoperative assessment of the biliary and vascular anatomy by CT arteriography, venography, and cholangiography is of significant benefit during complex liver and biliary surgery.

Acknowledgment

We thank Carol Spencer, MSLS for her assistance in acquiring many of the journal articles and books used in the preparation of this manuscript.

References

[1] Couinaud C. Le foie, etudes anatomiques et chirurgicales. Paris: Masson & Cie; 1957.
[2] Bannister L. Alimentary system. In: Williams P, editor. Gray's anatomy. 38th edition. New York: Churchill Livingston; 1995. p. 1683–812.
[3] Larsen W. Development of the gastrointestinal tract. In: Larsen W, editor. Human embryology. Hong Kong (China): Churchill Livingstone; 1997. p. 229–59.
[4] Moore K, Persaud T. The digestive system. In: Moore K, Persaud T, editors. The developing human. Clinically oriented embryology. 6th edition. Philadelphia: W.B. Saunders Company; 1998. p. 271–302.
[5] Hjortsjö CH. The topography of the intrahepatic duct systems. Acta Anat (Basel) 1951;11: 599–615.
[6] Clavien A, Gadzijev E, et al. The Brisbane 2000 terminology of liver anatomy and resections. HPB 2000;2:333–9.
[7] Healey JE Jr, Schroy PC. Anatomy of the biliary ducts within the human liver; analysis of the prevailing pattern of branchings and the major variations of the biliary ducts. AMA Arch Surg 1953;66:599–616.
[8] Blumgart L, Hann L. Surgical and radiologic anatomy of the liver, biliary tract, and pancreas. In: Blumgart L, editor. Surgery of the liver, biliary tract, and pancreas, vol. 1. 4th edition Philadelphia: Saunders; 2006. p. 3–29.
[9] Ohkubo M, Nagino M, Kamiya J, et al. Surgical anatomy of the bile ducts at the hepatic hilum as applied to living donor liver transplantation. Ann Surg 2004;239:82–6.
[10] Kawarada Y, Das BC, Taoka H. Anatomy of the hepatic hilar area: the plate system. J Hepatobiliary Pancreat Surg 2000;7:580–6.
[11] Onishi H, Kawarada Y, Das BC, et al. Surgical anatomy of the medial segment (S4) of the liver with special reference to bile ducts and vessels. Hepatogastroenterology 2000;47: 143–50.
[12] Kune GA. Surgical anatomy of common bile duct. Arch Surg 1964;89:995–1004.

[13] Hollinshead WH. The lower part of the common bile duct: a review. Surg Clin North Am 1957;37:939–52.

[14] Lindner HH, Pena VA, Ruggeri RA. A clinical and anatomical study of anomalous terminations of the common bile duct into the duodenum. Ann Surg 1976;184:626–32.

[15] Northover JM, Terblanche J. A new look at the arterial supply of the bile duct in man and its surgical implications. Br J Surg 1979;66:379–84.

[16] Gunji H, Cho A, Tohma T, et al. The blood supply of the hilar bile duct and its relationship to the communicating arcade located between the right and left hepatic arteries. Am J Surg 2006;192:276–80.

[17] Saint JH. The epicholedochal venous plexus and its importance as a means of identifying the common duct during operations on the extrahepatic biliary tract. Br J Surg 1961;48: 489–98.

[18] Vellar ID. Preliminary study of the anatomy of the venous drainage of the intrahepatic and extrahepatic bile ducts and its relevance to the practice of hepatobiliary surgery. ANZ J Surg 2001;71:418–22.

[19] Hand BH. Anatomy and function of the extrahepatic biliary system. Clin Gastroenterol 1973;2:3–29.

[20] Newcombe J, Henley F. Left-sided gallbladder: a review of the literature and a report of a case associated with hepatic duct carcinoma. Arch Surg 1964;88:494–7.

[21] Moosman DA, Coller FA. Prevention of traumatic injury to the bile ducts: a study of the structures of the cystohepatic angle encountered in cholecystectomy and supraduodenal choledochostomy. Am J Surg 1951;82:132–43.

[22] Kune GA. The influence of structure and function in the surgery of the biliary tract. Ann R Coll Surg Engl 1970;47:78–91.

[23] Rogers AI, Crews RD, Kalser MH. Congenital absence of the gall bladder with choledocholithiasis. Literature review and discussion of mechanisms. Gastroenterology 1965;48:524–9.

[24] Harlaftis N, Gray S, Skandalakis J. Multiple gallbladder. Surg Gynecol Obstet 1977;145: 928–34.

[25] Hobby J. Bilobed gallbladder. Br J Surg 1970;57:870–2.

[26] Perelman H. Cystic duct reduplication. JAMA 1961;175:710–1.

[27] Gross R. Congenital abnormalities of the gallbladder: a review of 148 cases with report of a double gallbladder. Arch Surg 1936;32:131–62.

[28] McNamee E. Intrahepatic gallbladder. Am J Roentgenol Radium Ther Nucl Med 1935;33: 603–10.

SURGICAL
CLINICS OF
NORTH AMERICA

ELSEVIER
SAUNDERS

Surg Clin N Am 88 (2008) 1175–1194

Lithogenesis and Bile Metabolism

Stephanie Lambou-Gianoukos, MD, MPH[a],
Stephen J. Heller, MD[b],*

[a]Department of Medicine, Tufts Medical Center, 800 Washington Street,
Boston, MA 02111, USA
[b]Department of Medicine, Fox Chase Cancer Center, 333 Cottman Avenue, Philadelphia,
PA 19111, USA

Lithogenesis

Autopsies of Egyptian and Chinese mummies have demonstrated the existence of gallstones for at least 3500 years. Today, gallstones occur commonly, especially in the West and Westernized societies. Complications of gallstones include biliary colic, acute cholecystitis, choledocholithiasis, cholangitis, gallstone pancreatitis, and gallstone ileus.

Burden

Gallstone disease exacts a considerable amount of financial and social burden worldwide. Gallstones lead to frequent physician visits and hospitalizations. In 2000, more than 750,000 outpatient visits in the United States were because of gallstones. In the same year, gallstone disease (defined as cholelithiasis with acute cholecystitis) was the most common inpatient diagnosis among gastrointestinal disorders, with more than 250,000 hospitalizations, a median inpatient charge of $11,584, and an estimated annual cost of almost $6.5 billion [1]. Notably, cholecystectomy is the most common elective abdominal operation performed in the United States, with more than 700,000 performed annually [2].

Prevalence of gallstones

The first systematic studies of gallstone prevalence involved autopsies, but the emergence of diagnostic ultrasonography has allowed a more accurate and specific determination of the prevalence of gallstones in the general

---

* Corresponding author. Department of Medicine, Fox Chase Cancer Center, 333 Cottman Avenue, Philadelphia, PA 19111.
E-mail address: stephen.heller@fccc.edu (S.J. Heller).

0039-6109/08/$ - see front matter © 2008 Elsevier Inc. All rights reserved.
doi:10.1016/j.suc.2008.07.009   *surgical.theclinics.com*

population. It has been estimated that in the United States approximately 20 million people harbor gallstones. Gallstones, cholecystectomies, and gallbladder disease are more prevalent in women than men at all ages [2].

The prevalence of gallstones varies widely in different countries and among different ethnic groups living in the same country. The highest rates occur among American Indians, especially the Pima Indians of North America, Scandinavians, and Mexican-American women [3,4]. The lowest rates are seen among African Americans [5].

Although gallstones are less common in the non-Westernized world, the prevalence of cholelithiasis increased in African and Asian countries during the twentieth century [6,7]. For example, the prevalence of gallstones in Tokyo has more than doubled since the 1940s; a shift from pigment to cholesterol gallstones has also been observed. It has been theorized that this increase is attributable to nutritional and environmental changes, such as the Westernization of the diet (increased consumption of imported food, decreased fiber and protein intake, increased fat intake) and the decreased rate of chronic biliary infections.

The type of gallstone also varies among populations. For example, cholesterol stones (found primarily in the gallbladder) are more prevalent in developed countries, whereas pigment gallstones (found primarily in the bile ducts) are more common in developing countries of Africa and Asia.

Gallstone composition

All gallstones consist of poorly soluble components of bile that precipitate on a three-dimensional matrix of mucins and proteins. Precipitants include cholesterol, calcium bilirubinates, and calcium salts of phosphate, carbonate, or palmitate. The matrix consists of large, polymeric mucin glycoproteins and small polypeptides. Based on their composition, gallstones are categorized as cholesterol, black pigment, and brown pigment, with each category having a unique structural, epidemiologic, and risk factor profile. The pathogenesis of each type of stone is defined based on the physical-chemical properties of each stone and the differences among stones result mainly from changes in the lipid and lipopigment composition of gallbladder bile (Table 1). Gallstones usually take many years to form. The estimated growth rate of gallstones was found to be approximately 2 mm per year [8].

Bile metabolism

Bile production and composition

Bile is formed in hepatic lobules and is isotonic to plasma. It is then secreted into a complex network of canaliculi, small bile ductules, and larger bile ducts. These larger ducts run between the hepatic lobules (interlobular) and eventually coalesce to form the macroscopic hepatic ducts. Bile acids flow from the liver through these ducts to the gallbladder, where they are

Table 1
Comparison of the three major types of gallstones

Characteristic	Cholesterol stones	Black pigment stones	Brown pigment stones
Color	Yellow-white	Black–dark brown	Yellow brown–orange
Shape	Round or faceted	Faceted or spiky	Round or irregular
Number	Single or multiple	Multiple	Single or multiple
Location	Gallbladder	Gallbladder	Bile ducts
Composition	Cholesterol, Ca bilirubinate	Black pigment polymer, Ca bilirubinate, Ca phosphate	Ca bilirubinate, Ca palmitate, Cholesterol
Geography	West	West, Asia	Mostly Asia
Causes	Increased cholesterol secretion, Decreased bile salt secretion	Increased bilirubin excretion, Increased Ca excretion, Increased bile pH	Bacterial/parasitic infection, Hydrolysis of bilirubin conjugates and lecithins
Clinical correlations	Diabetes, obesity, pregnancy, weight loss, total parenteral nutrition, drugs	Chronic hemolysis, cirrhosis, Gilbert syndrome, ileal disease (Crohn)	Chronic bacterial infections, biliary parasitic infections, biliary strictures
Other factors	Age, female gender, Native Americans, relatives with gallstones	Age	Chronic cholangitis, Asians
Bile cultures	Sterile	Sterile	Infected (*Escherichia coli, Bacteroides, Ascaris*)
Recurrent stones	Rare	Rare	Frequent
Radiographic appearance	Radiopaque (usually)	Radiopaque	Radiolucent

stored for future use. The total solute concentration of bile from the liver is 3 to 4 g/dL and the total daily basal secretion is 500 to 600 mL.

The composition of bile in the gallbladder differs from that of hepatic bile because water and inorganic anions (chloride, bicarbonate) are reabsorbed across the gallbladder epithelium. As a result, the total solute concentration of bile in the gallbladder increases to 10 to 15 g/dL. The solute composition of bile in the gallbladder includes approximately 80% bile acids, 16% phospholipids (mostly lecithin), 4% unesterified cholesterol, and other compounds (conjugated bilirubin, proteins, electrolytes, mucus, rarely drugs and their metabolites). In lithogenic states, the percentage of unesterified cholesterol can reach 8% to 10% of the total solute composition.

Bile acid synthesis

Bile acids, which are synthesized in the liver, are the end products of cholesterol metabolism. Bile acid synthesis is the major mechanism of bodily excretion of excess cholesterol. Because hepatic synthesis can increase only four to five times its normal synthetic rate, this mechanism is not sufficient for the excretion of excess dietary cholesterol. On a daily basis, the liver processes more than 18 to 24 g of bile acid.

Primary bile acids are synthesized in the liver from cholesterol molecules. The most abundant primary bile acids in human bile are chenodeoxycholic acid (45% of total) and cholic acid (31%). The initial and rate-limiting step in the synthesis of bile acids is catalyzed by the enzyme 7α-hydroxylase (Fig. 1). The carboxyl group of the primary bile acids is then conjugated with the amino acid glycine or taurine to yield glycoconjugates and tauroconjugates, respectively (Fig. 2). These conjugated primary bile acids are then secreted into bile, stored in the gallbladder, and eventually secreted into the duodenum. Conjugation increases the bile acid water solubility, preventing passive reabsorption once bile is secreted into the small intestine, although some passive reabsorption of bile salts occurs. Around 85% to 90% of the total secreted amounts of conjugated bile acids that are not immediately reabsorbed in the small intestine pass to the distal ileum and colon. There, ileocolonic anaerobic bacteria enzymatically deconjugate (by removing the glycine and taurine residues) and dehydroxylate (by removing the 7α-hydroxy group) the primary bile acids, thus yielding the secondary bile acids deoxycholate (from cholic acid) and lithocholate (from chenodeoxycholic acid), which are eventually readily absorbed from the colon.

Bile acids are detergent-like molecules that can form micelles (molecular aggregates) in aqueous solutions if their concentration exceeds 2 mmol/L. As a result, they are able to solubilize hydrophobic molecules, such as cholesterol, or emulsify digested fats in the intestine. Specifically, bile acids perform the following major physiologic functions:

Solubilize cholesterol in the liver and facilitate its excretion into the intestine through bile. Bile acid synthesis from cholesterol and subsequent

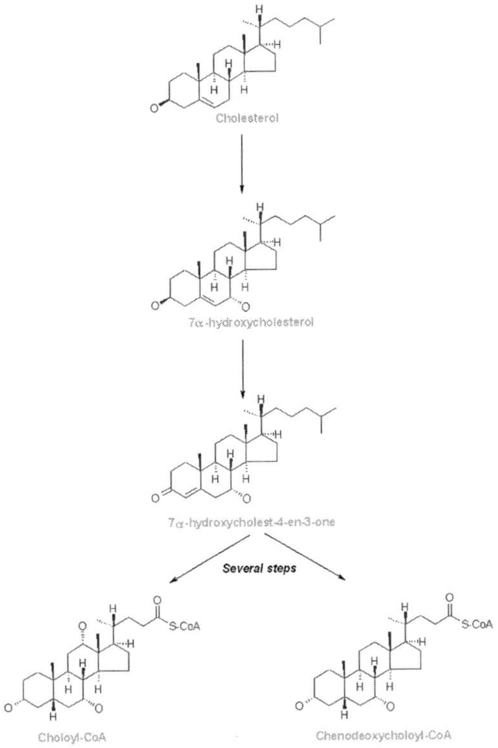

Fig. 1. Primary bile acid synthesis in the liver. The diagram demonstrates the synthesis of the two primary bile acids, cholic acid and chenodeoxycholic acid, from cholesterol. The reaction is catalyzed by the enzyme 7α-hydroxylase, which is the rate-limiting step in bile acid synthesis.

excretion in the stool is the most significant mechanism of eliminating excess cholesterol. In this way, bile acids also prevent cholesterol precipitation in the gallbladder during bile storage (phospholipids also play a role).

Emulsify intestinal dietary fats, such as triglycerols, thus rendering them accessible to pancreatic lipases.

Facilitate intestinal absorption of fat-soluble vitamins.

Regulation of bile salt synthesis is determined by multiple factors, such as the viability of hepatocytes, the availability of cholesterol (the precursor molecule), and the amount of bile salts returning to the liver by way of the enterohepatic circulation (feedback inhibition by dihydroxy bile salts).

Enterohepatic circulation

The ultimate fate of bile acids is secretion into the small intestine, where they aid in the emulsification of dietary lipids, promote the absorption of fat-soluble vitamins, and allow the fecal excretion of excess cholesterol.

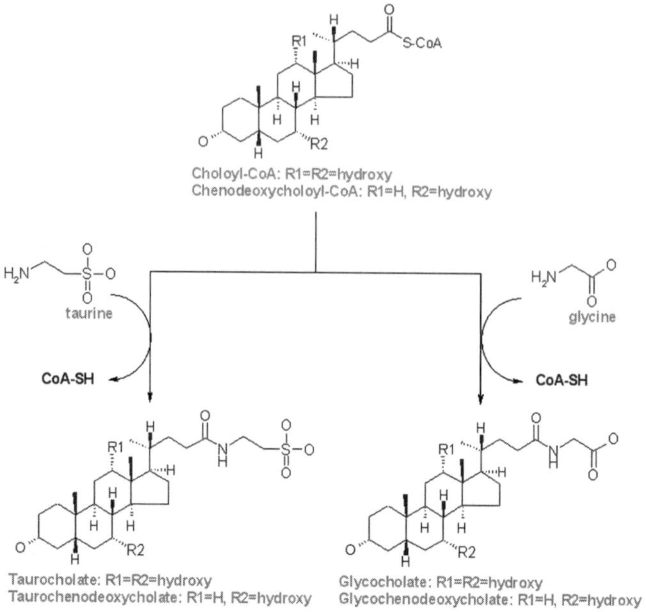

Choloyl-CoA: R1=R2=hydroxy
Chenodeoxycholoyl-CoA: R1=H, R2=hydroxy

taurine

CoA-SH

glycine

CoA-SH

Taurocholate: R1=R2=hydroxy
Taurochenodeoxycholate: R1=H, R2=hydroxy

Glycocholate: R1=R2=hydroxy
Glycochenodeoxycholate: R1=H, R2=hydroxy

Fig. 2. Conversion of primary bile acids to glycoconjugates and tauroconjugates. Before excretion into bile, the carboxyl group of the primary bile acids is conjugated with either glycine or taurine to yield glycoconjugates and tauroconjugates, respectively. In the large intestine, glycine and taurine residues are removed and the primary bile acids are converted to secondary bile acids by enteric bacteria.

A small amount of bile acid is excreted fecally, whereas most is reabsorbed in the large intestine and returned to the liver by way of the portal venous system. This process whereby bile is secreted from the liver, concentrated in the gallbladder, released into the duodenum, and finally reabsorbed in the ileum is termed the enterohepatic circulation.

Normally, a small amount of intestinally secreted bile acid is absorbed along the entire gut by passive diffusion, especially in the small bowel. Some 85% to 90% of the secreted bile acids, however, are actively reabsorbed in the distal ileum by way of the ATP-dependent intestinal bile acid transporter in the apical membrane of the ileal enterocytes. The remaining 10% to 15% of bile salts that reach the colon are deconjugated and dehydroxylated by anaerobic colonic bacteria. The resulting unconjugated bile acids are passively absorbed in the colon. In sum, approximately 95% of bile salts originally secreted into bile are reabsorbed into the portal circulation. Fecal loss of bile composes approximately 5% of intestinally secreted bile salts per cycle (about 0.3–0.6 g/dL).

The enterohepatic circulation occurs 6 to 10 times daily irrespective of eating, with additional cycles occurring during meals. The normal total body pool of bile salts (2–4 g) is maintained because the rate of hepatic de novo synthesis balances the rate of fecal loss. The bile acids that return to the liver inhibit the rate-limiting enzyme cholesterol 7α-hydroxylase, thus suppressing de novo hepatic synthesis of primary bile acids from cholesterol.

Cholesterol stones

Cholesterol stones are the most common type of gallstones, making up about 80% of gallstones in developed countries. They are composed purely of cholesterol or have cholesterol as their major constituent. Cholesterol gallstones are mainly composed of cholesterol monohydrate crystals (> 50%) and calcium salts, bile pigments, proteins, and fatty acids. Grossly, they may be large (up to 4.5 cm) and are yellowish-white in color. Microscopically, they appear as long, thin crystals that are bound together by a matrix of mucin glycoproteins. Cholesterol stones are typically found in the gallbladder in a sterile environment.

The sources of cholesterol in the body include dietary absorption and de novo hepatic synthesis from acylcoenzyme-A (acyl-CoA). Most of this pool is solubilized and secreted into bile or converted to bile acids. An association of gallstones with serum cholesterol has not been clearly defined, although gallstones have been associated with low serum HDL and elevated serum triglycerides [9,10].

Pathogenesis

Cholesterol is essentially insoluble in aqueous solution, such as bile. As a result, cholesterol in bile is transported either in unilamellar bilayered vesicles (cholesterol complexed with phospholipids, mostly lecithin) or in mixed multilamellar micelles (cholesterol complexed with phospholipids and bile acids). The total and relative proportions of cholesterol to phospholipids and bile salts determine the solubility of free cholesterol in bile.

When cholesterol concentration exceeds its solubility, cholesterol crystals can precipitate in bile, eventually giving rise to gallstones. Cholesterol crystal formation requires the presence of one or more of the following factors: (a) cholesterol supersaturation, (b) accelerated nucleation, or (c) gallbladder hypomotility/bile stasis (Fig. 3).

Supersaturation

Cholesterol solubility is a delicate balance of the relative concentrations of cholesterol, phospholipids, and bile acids. If there is an excess of cholesterol relative to phospholipids and bile acids, or if there is a shortage of phospholipids and bile acids, supersaturation of cholesterol in bile occurs. Although originally believed to be sufficient for gallstone formation, supersaturation is not sufficient by itself to produce cholesterol precipitation in vivo. In fact, supersaturated bile is secreted in most normal individuals who do not have gallstones.

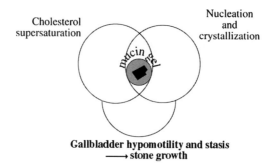

Fig. 3. Cholesterol gallstone formation. The Venn diagram illustrates how cholesterol gallstone formation requires the presence of at least one of three factors: cholesterol supersaturation, nucleation/crystallization, or gallbladder hypomotility/bile stasis. Cholesterol supersaturation occurs when there is an excess of cholesterol relative to phospholipids and bile acids, or if there is a shortage of phospholipids and bile acids. Nucleation refers to the initial process of aggregation of the submicroscopic cholesterol crystals (formed in supersaturated bile) into larger particles. After nucleation, crystallization creates the cholesterol monohydrate crystals that are the precursors to cholesterol gallstones. Gallbladder hypomotility leads to incomplete emptying of bile and the resulting biliary stasis facilitates the development of cholesterol crystals.

Several factors may play a role in causing supersaturation of bile with cholesterol. The most common mechanism is an increase in synthesis and secretion of cholesterol, which is associated with various environmental factors, such as obesity, aging, and drug effects. Genetic factors, such as mutations of the CYP7A1 and MDR3 genes, also play an important role. Finally, bile acid hyposecretion alone can also cause supersaturation. Bile acid hyposecretion can be caused by a decrease in bile acid production or by excessive intestinal losses.

Nucleation

Nucleation refers to the initial process of condensation and aggregation of the submicroscopic cholesterol crystals (formed in supersaturated bile) into larger particles. After nucleation, crystallization creates the cholesterol monohydrate crystals that are the precursors to cholesterol gallstones. The recent development of an assay that accurately measures crystal nucleation time has enabled researchers to study specific factors that may alter the rates of nucleation.

The most important pronucleating factor that has been identified is gallbladder mucin glycoprotein, which consists of a protein complex with a hydrophobic core that can bind cholesterol and provide a nidus for stone formation. Mucin glycoproteins are normally secreted continuously from the gallbladder, but have been shown to have increased secretory rates in lithogenic bile and thus accelerate cholesterol crystallization [11]. Antinucleating factors include apolipoproteins A-I, A-II, and biliary glycoprotein.

Gallbladder hypomotility

In a large proportion of patients who have gallstones, abnormalities in gallbladder emptying are observed. Decreased motility of the gallbladder leads to incomplete emptying of bile, as evidenced by larger fasting and residual volumes [11]. The resulting biliary stasis facilitates the development of cholesterol crystals within the gallbladder and the agglomeration of these crystals over time. A sluggish gallbladder is common in pregnancy, fasting, and during caloric restrictions, all conditions that have been linked to gallstone formation [12].

The exact mechanism of gallbladder hypomotility and cholesterol gallstone disease remains unknown. In patients who have cholesterol gallstones specifically, the degree of hypomotility increases in proportion to the cholesterol content of the gallbladder, even in healthy subjects [13]. In contrast, hypomotility has not been found to be a key factor in the pathogenesis of pigment gallstones. This discrepancy suggests that perhaps excess cholesterol molecules are myotoxic to the smooth muscles of the gallbladder wall. Additionally, the role of the autonomic system or of cholecystokinin, which is considered the most potent physiologic stimulator of gallbladder contraction, remains controversial.

Biliary sludge

Biliary sludge was first described in the 1970s with the widespread use of ultrasonography. It is also referred to as microlithiasis, pseudolithiasis, and microcrystalline disease. Sludge is a viscous fluid that is defined as a mixture of particulate matter and bile that occurs when solutes in bile precipitate. On ultrasound, sludge appears as low-level echoes that lack acoustic shadowing in the dependent portion of the gallbladder. On microscopy, which is considered the diagnostic gold standard for sludge, it is composed of cholesterol monohydrate crystals, lecithin-cholesterol crystals, and calcium bilirubinate granules, all embedded in mucin gel. Sludge can also contain undefined residue, protein-lipid complexes, and xenobiotics (such as ceftriaxone) [14].

The natural history of biliary sludge varies greatly and its course is unpredictable. Once sludge forms, it may resolve permanently, resolve and recur, or progress to gallstones. The presence of biliary sludge suggests an imbalance between mucin production and elimination and that the process of nucleation is already occurring. Complications of sludge include biliary colic, acute cholangitis, and acute pancreatitis, conditions that are also associated with gallstones.

It has been hypothesized that sludge may be the precursor of gallstones and that stones are generated from further precipitation of the sludge constituents [15]. This hypothesis does not fully explain, however, why in most patients sludge resolves spontaneously and why gallstones develop in only a small minority of people who have sludge. The few studies examining the natural history of sludge have been limited by inadequate follow-up and inconclusive evidence. Nevertheless, it has been shown that sludge can develop with disorders that cause gallbladder hypomotility or biliary stasis, such as rapid weight loss, pregnancy, prolonged fasting, and long-term administration of total parenteral nutrition (TPN) [16–19]. In patients who receive TPN, sludge resolves after reinstitution of oral feedings.

Risk factors for cholesterol gallstones

Many risk factors for the formation of gallstones have been identified and studied. These myriad risk factors underscore the multifactorial pathogenesis of gallstone formation.

Age

The cumulative prevalence of gallstones increases with age, with the highest incidence in the first four decades of life [20]. The incidence of gallstones increases by 1% to 3% per year.

Gender

Female gender is the most prominent and proven risk factor for gallstone formation, with most studies showing the incidence of gallstones increased two to threefold in females. This difference between men and women diminishes with increasing age, with incidence rates becoming essentially equal after the fifth decade of life [21].

Obesity

Obesity is a well-established risk factor for gallstone disease. It is independently associated with increased activity levels of HMG-CoA reductase, which is a rate-limiting enzyme in cholesterol synthesis. This increase in turn leads to elevated cholesterol production in the liver, thereby increasing cholesterol secretion into bile. In a large prospective cohort database from the Nurses Health Study, patients who had a body mass index (BMI) $> 45 \, \text{kg/m}^2$ had a sevenfold elevation in the development of gallstones compared with non-obese control subjects. The same study showed that the yearly rate of gallstone formation increased linearly with increasing BMI. Specifically, the group of women who had BMI greater than 45 presented with a 2% per year increase in incidence [22].

Weight loss

It has been shown that the incidence of gallstones increases with very low-calorie diets [23]. Possible physiologic mechanisms for the development of stones in this setting include increases in saturation of bile, gallbladder secretion of mucin and calcium, and concentration of prostaglandins and arachidonic acid [24–26]. Gallstone formation has also been demonstrated as a complication of rapid weight loss [27]. In a sample of morbidly obese patients who underwent gastric bypass surgery, nearly 40% developed gallstones within the first 6 months after the surgery, which coincided with the period of maximum weight loss [16].

Total parenteral nutrition

Pitt and colleagues [19] showed that patients on TPN had a significantly greater gallstone prevalence compared with controls that were not on TPN (45.7% versus 12.2%, respectively). Possible factors explaining the effect of TPN on gallstone formation include the increased occurrence of biliary stasis and sludge secondary to impaired gallbladder emptying, and the presence of an ileal disorder (such as Crohn disease or previous ileal resection), which can affect the enterohepatic circulation of bile acids.

Genetics

The considerable variation in gallstone disease in the population is complex and involves the interaction of genes with various environmental factors. Several epidemiologic and family studies have suggested a strong genetic component in the causation of gallstone disease. No single gene or gene family has been identified, however. A well-established predisposition for gallstones among certain ethnic groups, such as the Pima Indians, strongly supports the role of genetic factors. A study of biliary lipid composition in twins showed that monozygotic twins have very similar cholesterol saturation indices, which is a critical factor in gallstone formation [28]. Several ultrasound studies have also confirmed an increased prevalence of gallstones in first-degree family members of patients who have gallstone disease [29]. All mechanisms of the pathogenesis of cholesterol gallstone formation are under genetic control. It is theorized that genetics mostly influence the availability of cholesterol in bile, mainly by way of genetic polymorphisms in cholesterol-transporting lipoproteins, such as apoE, apoB, and apoA1. For example, individuals who have the E4/E4 alleles of apoE have statistically significant higher concentrations of serum cholesterol and LDL when compared with the E3/E3 alleles [30]. In fact, several reports have shown a higher E4 allele frequency in patients undergoing cholecystectomy compared with patients who were gallstone-free [31].

Pregnancy

Pregnancy is a risk factor for the development of biliary sludge and gallstones [17]. It is hypothesized that estrogen directly effects bile composition by promoting cholesterol secretion. It has also been proposed that pregnancy-induced smooth muscle relaxation resulting in gallbladder hypomotility can cause an increase in gallbladder volume and stasis. The lithogenicity of bile increases during pregnancy and in the early postpartum period [32]. Interestingly, sludge and gallstones are not always found repeatedly in serial ultrasounds of the same patients during pregnancy, illustrating the dynamic state of gallbladder contents during pregnancy [33]. After delivery, gallbladder motility and volume return to the prepregnancy state.

Diet

Investigators have studied several dietary factors in the pathogenesis of cholelithiasis, but the data are conflicting. Dietary studies are limited by inadequate dietary assessment tools, short follow-up periods, recall bias, and incomplete control of confounding factors. In addition, gallstones are most often asymptomatic, making it difficult to determine the precise time of onset. In theory, diet could explain some of the discrepancies in gallstone prevalence in different countries. Presently, it is believed that a diet high in calories, total fat, cholesterol, or refined carbohydrates is positively associated with the presence of gallstones; alternatively, dietary fiber, vitamin C, and moderate alcohol intake seem to be protective against gallstones [12].

Recently, there has been much interest in exploring the influence of different types of fat on bile lithogenicity and cholesterol gallstone formation, although the mechanism by which fats alter gallstone formation is still under investigation. Thus far, cis-unsaturated, monounsaturated, and polyunsaturated fats have been shown to reduce the risk for cholesterol gallstones (by 20% during 14 years of follow-up), presumably by improving insulin sensitivity [34]. One proposed mechanism for this effect comes from observations that hyperinsulinemia increases the activity of the rate-limiting enzyme of hepatic synthesis of cholesterol [35]; therefore, if the opposite is true, unsaturated fats can protect from cholesterol gallstone disease. Interestingly, in a large population-based, case-control study in Italy, Misciagna and colleagues [36] suggest that for women there may be factors other than saturated fat intake (ie, hormonal or metabolic) that are more powerful risk factors for gallstone formation. A recent large prospective study in men only indicated that a higher intake of trans-fatty acids is associated with a higher risk for gallstones, because trans fats have been shown to reduce serum plasma concentration of HDL and increase LDL and triglyceride concentration [37]. Last, in patients who have gallstones, dietary cholesterol intake increases the risk for gallstones by way of an increase in biliary cholesterol secretion and a decrease in the bile salt pool (both conditions that predispose to gallstones) [38]. This process does not occur in patients who do not have gallstones who are on high-cholesterol diets.

Ileal disease

The prevalence of gallstones in patients who have Crohn disease is consistently found to be higher than the general population. For example, it was found that 34% of patients who had terminal ileal Crohn disease had gallstones compared with 8% among healthy matched controls (prevalence is lower for patients who had colonic Crohn disease) [39]. In patients who have Crohn disease, age, disease site at diagnosis (higher risk with ileal disease), and history of resections are independently associated with gallstones. For many years, the pathogenesis of gallstones in these patients was attributed to bile acid malabsorption in the diseased or resected ileum (secondary to bile acid receptor loss), leading to excessive fecal bile salt excretion, a diminished bile acid pool, and hepatic excretion of cholesterol supersaturated bile. This theory, however, is no longer universally accepted because recent studies have found that the excretion of supersaturated bile is transient, and others have shown evidence of normal and even low-cholesterol bile saturation in these patients. It is possible that for those patients who have Crohn disease who undergo surgery, it is the prolonged fasting or TPN that explains the higher prevalence of gallstones [40]. Patients who have Crohn disease also have elevated bilirubin levels in bile, thus predisposing them to pigment gallstones also. It is postulated that the altered colonic bacterial flora may enhance the deconjugation of unconjugated bilirubin and lead to increased absorption [41].

Lipid profile

Hypertriglyceridemia and a low HDL are associated with gallstones [9,10]. Because triglycerides increase with BMI, it is not surprising that obese patients who have hypertriglyceridemia and a low HDL are at higher risk for developing stones. It has also been shown, however, that high total serum cholesterol does not increase the risk for gallstones [42].

Diabetes

Given the association of diabetes with hypertriglyceridemia and obesity, it is hypothesized that patients who have diabetes are prone to gallstones. No studies to date have shown a clear and statistically significant association between diabetes (as an independent risk factor) and gallstones. Furthermore, although it is believed that patients who have diabetes are at increased risk for serious complications from gallstones, it has been shown that the natural history of gallstones in people who have diabetes in fact follows the same pattern observed in patients who do not have diabetes. In the current literature, hypomotility of the gallbladder alone is regarded as the main cause of impaired gallbladder emptying in patients who have diabetes. The degree of hypomotility is directly proportional to the duration of the diabetes [43]. There is strong evidence that the microarterioles of patients who have diabetes are thickened by the deposition of periodic acid-Schiff-positive (PAS) material, thus leading to vascular stenosis and an impaired blood supply, which contribute to gallbladder hypomotility [44].

Drugs

Estrogen. Studies have shown that women, particularly women younger than 40 years old, on oral contraceptive steroids and estrogens have an increased risk for gallstone formation [45]. Physiologically, contraceptive hormones are believed to accelerate biliary cholesterol secretion by promoting de novo cholesterol synthesis or by increasing hepatic LDL receptor expression, which leads to additional LDL uptake in the liver.

Progesterone. Few studies have looked at the effect of progesterone alone on gallstone formation. In animal studies, progestins decrease the activity of the cholesterol 7α-hydroxylase enzyme and impair gallbladder emptying [46,47]. In humans, progesterone, a proven smooth muscle relaxant, can, in theory, inhibit gallbladder motility and cause larger residual volumes, like those seen in pregnancy [48].

Octreotide. As a long-acting somatostatin analog, octreotide is used as chronic therapy for acromegaly and various other gastrointestinal disorders. Approximately 30% of patients who have acromegaly develop gallstones within the first 2 years of octreotide therapy [49]. Octreotide decreases gallbladder motility and prolongs intestinal transit time. The increased amount of deoxycholic acid reabsorbed by the colon results in supersaturation of cholesterol.

Ceftriaxone. This third-generation cephalosporin is excreted in urine; as much as 40% of the drug is secreted unmetabolized into bile, reaching a concentration of 100 to 200 times higher than its concentration in serum [50]. Once the saturation level is exceeded, ceftriaxone complexes with calcium and forms an insoluble salt that precipitates. Biliary pseudolithiasis and sludge have been reported in patients who receive high-dose ceftriaxone therapy. Generally, stones and sludge disappear after treatment is withdrawn [51]. For the most part, the gallstones and sludge spontaneously disappear after treatment is withdrawn.

Pigment stones

Bilirubin and its metabolism

One cannot comprehend the pathogenesis of pigment stones without understanding the role of bilirubin and its metabolism in the liver. Bilirubin is the breakdown product of normal hemoglobin catabolism from destroyed erythrocytes. Like cholesterol, it is insoluble in water. In the liver, it is conjugated with glucuronic acid producing diglucuronides (75%–80%) and monoglucuronides (20%), which are soluble in water and can be secreted into bile. Normally, the remainder of the bilirubin that reaches the liver (about 3%) is hydrolyzed by β-glucuronidases and becomes unconjugated. Unconjugated bilirubin and its calcium salts are poorly soluble in water. In healthy individuals, pigment stones are not formed because the amount of unconjugated and thus insoluble bilirubin is not sufficient to promote stone formation. In abnormal states, though, the excessive amount of unconjugated bilirubin becomes an important factor in pigment gallstone pathogenesis.

Overview of pigment stones

In the United States, pigment stones make up approximately 20% of all gallstones, but this percentage is much higher in Asian populations. Pigment stones are subclassified into black and brown types, each with unique morphology, pathogenesis, and clinical associations. Generally, the prevalence of pigment stones increases with age and is higher in women.

As the name implies, pigment stones are formed by the precipitation of bilirubin in bile. This process can occur as a consequence of an increase in ionized calcium concentration (as in hyperparathyroidism) or an increase in unbound bilirubinate anions in bile. Causes of the latter include:

Increased secretion of conjugated bilirubin into bile, as in patients who have chronic hemolysis (ie, sickle cell disease, cirrhosis)

Increased synthesis of unconjugated bilirubin as a result of increased amount/activity of β-glucuronidase (which hydrolyzes conjugated bilirubin to create its unconjugated form) [52].

Black pigment stones

Black pigment stones are composed primarily of pure calcium bilirubinate, but they also contain calcium carbonate and calcium phosphate in polymer-like complexes with mucin glycoproteins. They are formed in the gallbladder in a bacterially sterile environment. Black stones are found in individuals who have chronic hemolytic states (ie, sickle cell disease, hereditary spherocytosis), liver cirrhosis, Gilbert syndrome, and cystic fibrosis (CF). Patients who have ileal disease (ie, Crohn disease) or ileal resections are also predisposed to pigment stones.

The pathogenesis of black stones involves two mechanisms: the hypersecretion of bilirubin conjugates and a defect in the acidification of bile. In the presence of chronic hemolysis, the concentration of bilirubin conjugates (especially monoglucuronides) increases tenfold from the action of the endogenous enzyme β-glucuronidase. The bilirubin conjugates are then unconjugated, form salts with calcium or phosphate, and eventually precipitate. The inability of an inflamed gallbladder mucosa to acidify bile may be an additional factor in pigment gallstone formation. By increasing the solubility of calcium carbonate, an acidic bile pH promotes the supersaturation of bile with calcium cations and allows the precipitation of calcium salts. To date, no defects in gallbladder motility have been found in patients who have black stones.

Risk factors for pigment gallstones

Chronic hemolytic states

Patients who have chronic hemolytic states frequently develop pigment gallstones as a result of recurrent episodes of hemolysis, which result in elevated bilirubin excretion and stone formation. Sickle cell disease is the most common hemolytic disorder associated with gallstone formation. It is also the most important cause of cholelithiasis in children. In fact, pigment stones form in 15% of children who have sickle cell disease who are younger than 10 years old and in greater than 50% by the age of 22 [53]. The most common complication of hereditary spherocytosis is black pigment gallstones, with as many as 50% of patients presenting with cholelithiasis [54]. In hereditary spherocytosis, the high biliary concentration of monoconjugated bilirubin acts as the source of unconjugated bilirubin, which can coprecipitate with calcium.

Cirrhosis

People who have advanced liver disease have a 30% increased risk for developing pigment stones compared with the general population [55]. Various mechanisms are responsible for the formation of gallstones in cirrhosis. Potential mechanisms include reduced hepatic synthesis and transport of bile salts, abnormal hemoglobin metabolism, and hyperestrogenemia.

Gilbert syndrome

This benign condition of decreased bilirubin conjugation is caused by the diminished activity of the conjugating enzyme uridine diphosphate-glucuronyl transferase (UGT1A1). Patients who have Gilbert syndrome have been shown to have an increased production of monoconjugated bilirubin [56]. As in hereditary spherocytosis, this form of bilirubin acts as a source of excess unconjugated bilirubin, which can bind to calcium and precipitate to form stones.

Cystic fibrosis

Patients who have CF have an increased prevalence of gallstones compared with healthy age-matched control counterparts (30% versus 5%, respectively) [57]. It was originally believed that because of the intestinal bile salt malabsorption and the steatorrhea in CF, these gallstones were cholesterol stones. It was later proved that the major component of gallstones in CF is calcium bilirubinate and not cholesterol [58]. The most recent proposed mechanism of the pathogenesis of gallstones in CF suggests that the leakage of bile salts from the small intestine to the colon promotes the resorption of large amounts of unconjugated bilirubin. The unconjugated bilirubin returns to the liver by way of the enterohepatic circulation and promotes the secretion of large amounts of conjugated bilirubin (hyperbilirubinbilia). After deconjugation in the more alkaline bile of patients who have CF, this excess bilirubin precipitates with calcium to form pigment stones.

Brown pigment stones

Brown pigment stones are composed of calcium salts of unconjugated bilirubin with varying amounts of cholesterol and protein. They are formed as the result of chronic bacterial infection of the bile and are almost always associated with colonization of bile by enteric organisms. The most common bacteria found in brown stones are *Escherichia coli*, *Bacteroides*, and

Clostridium. In populations that are prone to pigment stones, a clear shift to cholesterol gallstones has been observed. This shift has been attributed to a decline in chronic biliary infections. For example, the proportion of pigment stones in the Japanese population dropped from 60% to 24% since 1940 [59]. Unlike the other two types of stones, these stones are primarily found in the intrahepatic or extrahepatic bile ducts. Rarely, brown pigment stones are formed in the gallbladder as a consequence of acute cholecystitis.

Equally important is the association of certain parasitic infections with biliary stone formation that has been well documented in the literature (eg, *Opisthorchis veverrini* and *Clonorchis sinensis*, liver flukes prevalent in Thailand and China, respectively). Although the exact mechanism of how parasitic infections lead to pigment stone formation is not clearly understood, it is believed that the parasite worm or egg directly stimulates stone formation. The calcified overcoat of the parasite egg, for example, may serve as a nidus and enhance the precipitation of calcium bilirubinate [60].

Chemically, brown pigment stones are caused by an excess of unconjugated, insoluble bilirubin in bile that eventually forms stones. The pathogenesis of these stones is believed to involve stasis in the bile ducts and chronic anaerobic infection of bile [61]. Stasis facilitates the bacterial infection, which in turn promotes the accumulation of mucin and bacterial cytoskeletons in the bile ducts. The hydrogen ions in the bile are buffered by the mucin, resulting in a less acidic environment where calcium carbonate, phosphate, and bilirubin precipitate easily. The three bacterial compounds that play a key role in brown stone formation are β-glucuronidase (which produces unconjugated bilirubin), phospholipase A (which produces palmitic and stearic acids), and bile acid hydrolases (which produce unconjugated bile acids). The anionic counterparts of all three products form insoluble complexes with calcium and precipitate to form stones. The enlarging stone causes further ductal obstruction, which promotes more stasis and bacterial infection, thus perpetuating the cycle.

References

[1] Russo MW, Wei JT, Thiny MT, et al. Digestive and liver diseases statistics, 2004. Gastroenterology 2004;126:1448–53.

[2] Everhart JE, Khare M, Hill M, et al. Prevalence and ethnic differences in gallbladder disease in the United States. Gastroenterology 1999;117:632–9.

[3] Everhart JE. Gallstones. In: Johanson JF, editor. Gastrointestinal diseases: risk factors and prevention. Philadelphia: Lippincott-Raven; 1998. p. 145–72.

[4] Maurer KR, Everhart JE, Ezzati TM, et al. Prevalence of gallstone disease in Hispanic populations in the United States. Gastroenterology 1989;96:487–92.

[5] Sichieri R, Everhart JE, Roth H. A prospective study of the hospitalization with gallstone disease among women: role of dietary factors, fasting period, and dieting. Am J Public Health 1991;81:880–4.

[6] Adedeji A, Akande B, Olumide F. The changing pattern of cholelithiasis in Lagos. Scand J Gastroenterol Suppl 1986;21:63–6.

[7] Su CH, Lui WY, P'eng FK. Relative prevalence of gallstone diseases in Taiwan—a nation-wide cooperative study. Dig Dis Sci 1992;37:764–8.

[8] Paumgartner G, Sauerbruch T. Gallstones: pathogenesis. Lancet 1991;338:1117–21.

[9] Thornton J, Symes C, Heaton K. Moderate alcohol intake reduces bile cholesterol saturation and raises HDL cholesterol. Lancet 1983;2:819–22.

[10] Barbara L, Sama C, Moreselli Labate AM, et al. A population study on the prevalence of gallstone disease: the Sirmione study. Hepatology 1987;7:913–7.

[11] Lamont JT, Carey MC. Cholesterol gallstone formation. 2. Pathobiology and pathome-chanics. Prog Liver Dis 1992;10:165–91.

[12] Cuevas A, Miquel JF, Reyes MS, et al. Diet as a risk factor for cholesterol gallstone disease. J Am Coll Nutr 2004;23:187–96.

[13] van der Werf SD, van Berge Henegouwen GP, Palsma DM, et al. Motor function of the gallbladder and cholesterol saturation of duodenal bile. Neth J Med 1987;30:160–71.

[14] Ko CW, Murakami C, Sekijima JH, et al. Chemical composition of gallbladder sludge in patients after marrow transplantation. Am J Gastroenterol. 1996;91:1207–10.

[15] Ko CW, Sekijima JH, Lee SP. Biliary sludge. Ann Intern Med 1999;130:301–11.

[16] Shiffman ML, Sugerman HJ, Kellum JM, et al. Gallstone formation after rapid weight loss: a prospective study in patients undergoing gastric bypass surgery for treatment of morbid obesity. Am J Gastroenterol 1991;86:1000–5.

[17] Maringhini A, Ciambra M, Baccelliere P, et al. Biliary sludge and gallstones in pregnancy: incidence, risk factors, and natural history. Ann Intern Med 1993;119:116–20.

[18] Bolondi L, Gaiani S, Testa S, et al. Gallbladder sludge formation during prolonged fasting after gastrointestinal tract surgery. Gut 1985;26:734–8.

[19] Pitt HA, King W, Mann LL, et al. Increased risk of cholelithiasis with prolonged total parenteral nutrition. Am J Surg 1983;145:106–12.

[20] Attili AF, Capocaccia R, Carulli D, et al. Factors associated with gallstone disease in the MICOL experience. Hepatology 1997;26:809–18.

[21] Jensen KH, Jorgensen T. Incidence of gallstones in a Danish population. Gastroenterology 1991;100:790–4.

[22] Stampfer MJ, Maclure KM, Colditz GA, et al. Risk of symptomatic gallstones in women with severe obesity. Am J Clin Nutr 1992;55:652–8.

[23] Everhart JE. Contributions of obesity and weight loss to gallstone disease. Ann Intern Med 1993;119:1029–35.

[24] Festi D, Colecchia A, Larocca A, et al. Review: low caloric intake and gallbladder motor function. Aliment Pharmacol Ther 2000;14(Suppl 2):51–3.

[25] Shiffman ML, Shamburek RD, Schwartz CC, et al. Gallbladder mucin, arachidonic acid, and bile lipids in patients who develop gallstones during weight reduction. Gastroenterology 1993;105:1200–8.

[26] Shiffman ML, Sugerman HJ, Kellum JH, et al. Gallstones in patients with morbid obesity. Relationship to body weight, weight loss, and gallbladder bile cholesterol solubility. Int J Obes Relat Metab Disord 1993;17:153–8.

[27] Jorgensen T. Gallstones in a Danish population: fertility period, pregnancies, and exogenous female sex hormones. Gut 1988;29:433–9.

[28] Kesaniemi A, Koskenvuo M, Vuoristo M, et al. Biliary lipid composition in monozygotic and dizygotic pairs of twins. Gut 1989;30:1750–6.

[29] Sarin SK, Negi VS, Dewarn R, et al. High familial prevalence of gallstones in the first-degree relatives of gallstone patients. Hepatology 1995;22:138–41.

[30] Sing CF, Devignon J. Role of apolipoprotein E polymorphism in determining normal plasma lipid and lipoprotein variation. Am J Hum Genet 1985;37:268–85.

[31] Bertomeu A, Ros E, Zambon D, et al. Apolipoprotein E polymorphism and gallstones. Gastroenterology 1996;111:1603–10.

[32] Valdivieso V, Covarrubias C, Siegel F, et al. Pregnancy and cholelithiasis: pathogenesis and natural course of gallstones diagnosed in early puerperium. Hepatology 1993;17:1–4.

[33] van Bodegraven AA, Bohmer CJ, Manoliu RA, et al. Gallbladder contents and fasting gall-bladder volumes during and after pregnancy. Scand J Gastroenterol 1998;33:993–7.

[34] Tsai CH, Leitzman MF, Willett WC, et al. The effect of long-term intake of cis-unsaturated fats on the risk for gallstone disease in men. Ann Intern Med 2004;141:514–22.

[35] Chait A, Bierman EL, Albers JJ. Low-density lipoprotein receptor activity in cultured human skin fibroblasts. Mechanism of insulin-induced stimulation. J Clin Invest 1979;64:1309–19.

[36] Misciagna G, Centonze S, Leoci C, et al. Diet, physical activity, and gallstones—a population based, case control study in southern Italy. Am J Clin Nutr 1999;69:120–6.

[37] Tsai CJ, Leitzman MF, Willett WC, et al. Long-term intake of trans-fatty acids and risk of gallstone disease in men. Arch Intern Med 2005;165:1011–5.

[38] Kern F. Effects of dietary cholesterol on cholesterol and bile acid homeostasis in patients with cholesterol gallstones. J Clin Invest 1994;93:1186–94.

[39] Whorwell PJ, Hawkins R, Debury K, et al. Ultrasound survey of gallstones and other hepato-biliary disorders in patients with Crohn's disease. Dig Dis Sci 1984;29:930–3.

[40] Hutchinson R, Tyrrell PN, Kumar D, et al. Pathogenesis of gallstones in Crohn's disease: an alternative explanation. Gut 1994;35:94–7.

[41] Lapidus A, Akerlund JE, Einarsson C. Gallbladder bile composition in patients with Crohn's disease. World J Gastroenterol 2006;12:70–4.

[42] The Rome group for epidemiology and prevention of cholelithiasis (GREPCP). The epidemiology of gallstone disease in Rome, Italy: part II. Factors associated with the disease. Hepatology 1988;8:907–13.

[43] Fraquelli M, Pagliarulo M, Colucci A, et al. Gallbladder hypomotility in obesity, diabetes mellitus, and celiac disease. Dig Liver Dis 2003;35:12–6.

[44] Ding X, Gong JP, Lu CY, et al. Relation of abnormal gallbladder arterioles to gallbladder emptying in patients with gallstones and diabetes mellitus. Hepatobiliary Pancreat Dis Int 2004;3:275–8.

[45] Khan MK, Jalil MA, Khan MS. Oral contraceptives in gall stone diseases. Mymensingh Med J 2007;16:40–5.

[46] Gilloteaux J, Karkare S, Don AQ, et al. Cholelithiasis induced in the Syrian hamster: evidence for an intramucinous nucleating process and down regulation of cholesterol 7-alpha-hydroxylase (CYP7) gene by medroxyprogesterone. Microsc Res Tech 1997;39: 56–70.

[47] Smith JJ, Pomaranc MM, Ivy AC. The influence of pregnancy and sex hormones on gall-bladder motility in the guinea pig. Am J Phys 1941;132:129–40.

[48] Kern F, Everson GT. Contraceptive steroids increase cholesterol in bile: mechanisms of action. J Lipid Res 1987;28:828–39.

[49] Montini M, Gianola D, Pagani MD, et al. Cholelithiasis and acromegaly: therapeutic strategies. Clin Endocrinol 1994;40:401–6.

[50] Arvidsson A, Alvan G, Angelin B, et al. Renal and biliary excretion and effect on the colon microflora. J Antimicrob Chemother 1982;10:207–15.

[51] Lopez AJ, O'Keefe P, Morrissey M, et al. Ceftriaxone-induced cholelithiasis. Ann Intern Med 1991;115:712–4.

[52] Carey MC. Pathogenesis of gallstones. Am J Surg 1993;165:410–9.

[53] Suell MN, Horton TI, DisiIop MK, et al. Outcomes for children with gallbladder abnormalities and sickle cell disease. J Pediatr 2004;145:617–21.

[54] Guidice EM, Perrotta S, Nobili B, et al. Coinheritance of Gilbert syndrome increases the risk of developing gallstones in patients with hereditary spherocytosis. Blood 1999;94:2259–62.

[55] Acalovschi M, Badea R, Pascu M. Incidence of gallstones in liver cirrhosis. Am J Gastroenterol 1991;86:1179–81.

[56] Fevery J, Blanckaert N, Leroy P, et al. Analysis of bilirubins in biological fluids by extraction and thin-layer chromatography of the intact tetrapyrroles: application to bile of patients with Gilbert's syndrome, hemolysis, or cholelithiasis. Hepatology 1983;3:177–83.

[57] Wasmuth HE, Keppeler H, Herrmann U, et al. Coinheritance of Gilbert syndrome-associated UGT1A1 mutation increases gallstone risk in cystic fibrosis. Hepatology 2006;43:738–41.
[58] Angelico M, Gandin C, Canuzzi P, et al. Gallstones in cystic fibrosis: a critical reappraisal. Hepatology 1991;14:768–75.
[59] Nagase M, Hikasa Y, Soloway RD, et al. Gallstones in Western Japan: factors affecting the prevalence of intrahepatic gallstones. Gastroenterology 1980;78:684–90.
[60] Sripa B, Kanla P, Sinawat P, et al. Opisthorchiasis-associated biliary stones: light and scanning electron microscopy study. World J Gastroenterol 2004;10:3318–21.
[61] Cahalane MJ, Neubrand MW, Carey MC. Physical-chemical pathogenesis of pigment gallstones. Semin Liver Dis 1988;8:317–28.

ELSEVIER
SAUNDERS

SURGICAL
CLINICS OF
NORTH AMERICA

Surg Clin N Am 88 (2008) 1195–1220

An Update on Biliary Imaging

Christoph Wald, MD, PhD[a,b],*,
Francis J. Scholz, MD, FACR[a,b],
Edward Pinkus, MD[a,b],
Robert E. Wise, MD, FACR[b],
Sebastian Flacke, MD, PhD[a,b]

[a]Tufts University Medical School, 136 Harrison Avenue, Boston, MA 02111, USA
[b]Department of Radiology, Lahey Clinic Medical Center, 41 Mall Road,
Burlington, MA 01805, USA

This article provides an overview of the gamut of biliary imaging techniques currently available to the clinician. We provide a brief history of biliary imaging, particularly intravenous (IV) cholangiography, including most commonly used contrast agents. This history is followed by a detailed discussion of modern-day practice modalities, including fluoroscopic and barium cholangiography, CT cholangiography, and magnetic resonance cholangiopancreatography (MRCP).

Overview of current biliary imaging techniques

Conventional (tomographic) oral or intravenous cholangiography

Cholangiography after administration of either oral or IV iodinated biliary contrast agents is no longer used routinely in most countries.

Fluoroscopic cholangiography and barium cholangiography

Fluoroscopic cholangiography uses percutaneously or surgically placed biliary catheters, mostly in postoperative patients or in conjunction with percutaneous biliary interventions. Barium cholangiography can be attempted when (postsurgical) anatomy prevents endoscopic access and there are contraindications to either CT cholangiography or MRCP.

---

* Corresponding author. Department of Radiology, Lahey Clinic Medical Center, 41 Mall Road, Burlington, MA 01805.
  E-mail address: christoph.wald@lahey.org (C. Wald).

0039-6109/08/$ - see front matter © 2008 Elsevier Inc. All rights reserved.
doi:10.1016/j.suc.2008.07.007   *surgical.theclinics.com*

Ultrasonography

Ultrasonography (US) is an inexpensive and noninvasive way of assessing for the presence of gallstones and intra- and extrahepatic ductal dilation. The additional benefit of hepatic parenchymal and Doppler vascular evaluation can be important in patients who have coexisting chronic liver disease. The limited field of view and dependence on a suitable acoustic window and individual examiner skill limits this modality. Extrahepatic and peripheral intrahepatic ductal pathology may be difficult to evaluate.

Endoscopic retrograde cholangiography

Endoscopic retrograde cholangiography (ERC) is discussed in depth subsequently. This powerful combined diagnostic and therapeutic tool is an invasive technique with a well-documented small but real risk for serious adverse effects. As many as 25% of patients who undergo ERC have a postprocedural increase in serum amylase levels. In addition, the prevalence of clinical pancreatitis following diagnostic and therapeutic ERC is approximately 3% and 7%, respectively [1]. Cumulative major complication rates after ERC reported in the literature vary from 1.4% to 3.2% [2,3]. At times, endoscopic access may be difficult or impossible under certain conditions, such as prior Roux-en-Y biliointestinal anastomoses and occlusive ampullary pathology.

CT cholangiography

CT cholangiography has significantly evolved in recent years. Modern multidetector CT scanners are capable of acquiring single breath hold contiguous scans at submillimeter spatial resolution, which lend themselves to multiplanar and three-dimensional (3D) reconstruction. CT cholangiography involves the use of ionizing radiation and (in most cases) administration of biliary contrast agents with a small risk for adverse reactions. CT cholangiography provides some functional information about hepatocyte excretion, and, if there is normal excretion, affords excellent depiction of small, nondilated peripheral biliary radicles.

Magnetic resonance cholangiopancreatography

MRCP gained wide acceptance in the last 2 decades as magnetic resonance (MR) scanners became more available and scanning technique became more robust, enabling imaging with better spatial resolution and shorter breath-hold techniques. MRCP does not involve ionizing radiation. Recently, the addition of hepatocyte-specific contrast agents has provided additional tools for functional and anatomic hepatobiliary assessment.

Nuclear medical hepatobiliary evaluation

The most common indication for nuclear hepatobiliary imaging is to determine if a patient has acute cholecystitis. Less commonly, the study is ordered to evaluate for a bile leak. Rarely, the study is requested to determine the patency of the common bile duct (CBD) in an adult patient. Hepatobiliary imaging with gallbladder ejection fraction measurement is indicated in patients who have chronic abdominal pain that may be attributable to biliary dyskinesia or chronic cholecystitis. In infants who have neonatal jaundice, hepatobiliary imaging is useful to distinguish biliary atresia from neonatal hepatitis and can identify choledochal cysts. ^{99m}Tc iminodiacetic acid derivatives are normally rapidly taken up by hepatocytes and excreted unconjugated into the biliary tree. The gallbladder is normally seen within 30 minutes of injection and the small bowel is seen within 60 minutes. In most patients who have acute cholecystitis, the cystic duct is obstructed and thus the gallbladder never fills with the radiopharmaceutical. In the proper clinical setting, nonfilling of the gallbladder is highly suggestive of acute cholecystitis, but nonfilling of the gallbladder alone is a nonspecific finding. In patients who have an active bile leak because of trauma or surgery, the radiopharmaceutical accumulates in an abnormal location. Hepatobiliary imaging can demonstrate that the leak is continuing and can assess the magnitude of the leak. Because of limited spatial resolution and because this study depicts where bile accumulates, hepatobiliary imaging is rarely useful in locating the exact site of the leak. Hepatobiliary imaging can be helpful in assessing patients who have acute complete or nearly complete CBD obstruction. Jaundice attributable to partial CBD obstruction can usually not be distinguished from that caused by parenchymal liver disease. With acute complete or near-complete obstruction of the CBD, little or no bowel activity is seen, even on delayed images, despite relatively rapid uptake of the radiopharmaceutical agent by hepatocytes. Nonvisualization of the gallbladder has many causes. The most common causes are eating, prolonged fasting, acute or chronic cholecystitis, and severe liver disease.

Intravenous cholangiography and iodinated biliary contrast agents

History

It was not until 1924 that Graham and Cole [4] developed cholecystography. This development was a major step forward in imaging of the gallbladder and nonopaque gallstones. The common duct was only rarely visualized, however, and this faintly at best. Use of this technique continued until about 1940 when iodoalphionic acid was introduced in Germany, which resulted in the improvement of the image quality of the cholecystogram and, equally important, the increased safety of this technique. Iopanoic acid and triiodoethionic acid were introduced in 1951 and 1953, respectively.

The introduction of Biligrafin (sodium iodipamide) in Germany in 1953 opened an entirely new field for investigation of the physiology and pathology of the biliary tract. Among the initial papers appearing in 1954 were those by Bell, Jutars, Orloff, Glenn, Wise, O'Brien and respective coauthors

[5–9]. These early reports indicated that the CBD could be visualized in the postcholecystectomy state with satisfactory regularity [10,11]. Minor reactions occurred, but no fatalities were reported.

In 1955 iodipamide methylglucamine became available in the United States. The product in use here today and known as Cholografin (specifically designated "not for intrathecal use—for intravenous use only") is manufactured by Bracco Diagnostics, Inc., Princeton, New Jersey.

Further pharmacologic developments

Newer biliary contrast agents were developed during the second half of the 1970s, examples of which are meglumine iotroxate (Biliscopin, Schering AG, Berlin) and iodoxamate (Endobil, Bracco SpA, Milan). In a double-blind comparison of the newer agents in 400 cases published by Taenzer and Volkhardt [12] the authors reported equal imaging characteristics but a more favorable side effect frequency (by a factor of two) in iotroxate compared with iodoxamate. The agents continue to be used in many European CT cholangiographic studies today, although they never became available in the United States.

Adverse reactions of most commonly used compounds

Iodipamide meglumine (Cholografin)

In the group of 2034 injections performed during traditional IV cholangiography over a period of 8 years we experienced no anaphylactic reactions. From this study, it became apparent that the single most important factor influencing reactions is the speed of injection. A definite increase in rate, but not necessarily in severity, of minor adverse reactions, such as nausea and vomiting, followed rapid administration of the compound.

Mild adverse reactions to iodipamide meglumine may be as low as 4.1%, as suggested in a review by Ott and Gelfand [13], if the dose is kept to 20 mL, administered slowly, and the patient is not dehydrated. Maglinte [14] also found a low adverse reaction rate of 0.9% administration in his series of 113 consecutive patients undergoing IV cholangiography.

Meglumine iotroxate (Biliscopin)

The newer compound meglumine iotroxate found an overall rate of mild adverse reactions of 2.3% in 80 patients at one institution [15]. Breen and coworkers [16] reported 2 minor adverse reactions out of a total of 300 CT cholangiograms with IV injection of meglumine iotroxate. In a larger review, Sacharias reported 11 minor and moderate adverse reaction that occurred during a total of 1061 Biliscopin [17] infusions, a rate of approximately 1%. Nilsson performed a combined prospective study (on 196 patients) and retrospective review of the literature covering the period from 1975 to 1985 and found a cumulative adverse reaction rate to iotroxate compounds of 3.5%; however, this included iotroxate in various formulations and rates reported in the individual papers were diverse [18]. A large series of IV cholangiography in 1000 patients performed between 1991 and 1995 reported by Lindsey [19] found an overall minor adverse reaction rate of 0.7%.

Cholangiography and serum bilirubin

Robbins and colleagues [20] suggested that IV cholangiography with me-glumine iodoxamate may be feasible even in patients who have higher serum bilirubin levels. Other authors found that exclusion of patients who had a se-rum bilirubin level of 3 mg/dL or more would have resulted in a rate of un-successful examinations as low as 0.9% [15], whereas a higher level resulted in a larger number of nondiagnostic studies. In our own practice we use a se-rum bilirubin level of greater than 2 mg/dL as a relative contraindication for IV CT cholangiography. In desperate clinical situations we attempt the ex-amination in patients who have bilirubin as high as 5 mg/dL but we have had mixed success. Because of the exquisite image quality on current state-of-the-art multidetector computer tomography (MDCT) scanners (as compared with the equipment used in the aforementioned studies), even minimal excretion of biliary contrast may result in a diagnostic study.

The small but real risk for minor adverse reaction is in our view more than counterbalanced by the enormous benefit of gaining accurate preoper-ative information about the pertinent biliary anatomy, especially in context with live liver donation or complex biliary surgery. Administration of Chol-ografin and assessment of these patients who have 3D IV CT cholangiogra-phy has become part of our routine preoperative workup. The resulting images can be fused with vascular models derived from other CT scan phases obtained during the same session, which is discussed in more detail later in this article.

The Lahey Clinic experience with intravenous cholangiography

At the Lahey Clinic, one of the pioneering institutions for the use of IV cholangiography, the first IV cholangiogram was performed in April 1954. In the ensuing 5 years 2034 injections of Cholografin were given to 1829 in-dividuals. Of the 2034 injections, 609 were given to men and 1425 to women. Visualization of the bile ducts was achieved in 89.2% of injections. Only symptomatic patients were studied at Lahey Clinic during both pre- and postcholecystectomy injections.

Intravenous cholangiography in the early laparoscopic era

The value of traditional IV cholangiography in the detection of CBD stones has been shown in many series, but has become more significant dur-ing the laparoscopic cholecystectomy era. Lindsey and colleagues [19] found a sensitivity of 93.3% and a specificity of 99.3% for detection of CBD stones (compared with ERC in positive cases) in their large series. MRCP and ERC represent viable alternatives to this technique.

Fluoroscopic cholangiography and barium cholangiography

Examination of the biliary tree

In an ideal practice, radiologists would be able to contribute fluoroscopic imaging skills during endoscopic retrograde cholangiopancreatography (ERCP). Radiologists may be able to add diagnostic value by at least interpreting ERCP images obtained by the endoscopist. In the reality of many practices, a radiologist may never see an ERCP except in interdepartmental conferences. There are still fluoroscopic examinations performed to image the biliary tree, however. One is biliary tube cholangiography, performed following liver transplantation, segmental liver resections, or surgery on the bile duct. Indications may include (1) Biliary evaluation following percutaneous placement of transhepatic biliary catheters, to evaluate for bile leaks or presence of a stricture, and (2) prior cholecystostomy tube placement, to ensure full removal of gallbladder stones, patency of the cystic duct, and absence of common duct stones.

Barium cholangiography remains a rarely performed test but one that may yield critical information in patients who have biliary-jejunal anastomoses (BJA).

The surgeon must communicate the nature of the surgery to the radiologist so that accurate examinations can be performed to answer specific clinical questions.

Postoperative fluoroscopic cholangiography

T-tube cholangiography performed following cholecystectomy with common duct exploration was once a common procedure. The largest possible T-tube that would fit into the common duct was almost routinely left in place and a cholangiogram performed before the tube was removed. Now, following laparoscopic cholecystectomy with common duct exploration, the surgeon might leave either a small straight catheter or the smallest possible T-tube in place when there is suspicion of intraoperative trauma to the biliary tree or retained stones. Subsequent cholangiography may demonstrate injuries, such as a leak from small accessory right hepatic ductal branches directly communicating with the gallbladder lumen (Fig. 1).

Following cadaveric or living donor allotropic hepatic transplant, our surgeons typically leave a 5-French catheter in the biliary tree to mechanically support the fresh anastomosis and subsequently evaluate the anastomosis of the transplant biliary duct to the recipient's native duct or to a BJA. In patients who have a normal ampulla, contrast tends to freely flow into the duodenum rather than retrogradely into the intrahepatic ducts.

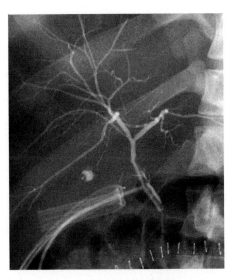

Fig. 1. Luschka duct leak. Image from a T-tube cholangiogram shows a leak from an intrahepatic radical draining into the gallbladder fossa following cholecystectomy. The astute surgeon recognized slight amount of bile weeping from the liver into the gallbladder bed. A T-tube was left in place to ensure maintenance of low biliary duct pressure and ease of follow-up examination. When a later repeat cholangiogram showed no further leak, the T-tube was removed.

If the anastomosis and the graft bile duct proximal to it cannot be visualized initially, the radiologist must attempt various maneuvers to define this anatomy. The basis for this is that radiographic contrast has a higher specific gravity than bile and thus tends to flow toward and settle in the dependent portions of the biliary system. During manual injection pressure should be carefully applied to minimize the risk for cholangitis.

During cadaveric liver transplant, the surgeon anastomoses the graft CBD to the recipient's CBD, usually just above the cystic duct [21]. A small catheter is usually inserted through the cystic duct stump. Following living related liver transplants, the right hepatic duct usually is anastomosed to a loop of jejunum. A small caliber catheter is usually placed just distal to the anastomosis inside the intrahepatic portion of the right hepatic duct. Following hepatic resections for tumor or after trauma, the surgeon makes anastomoses as indicated by the relationship of the remaining liver to the biliary tree and CBD. There may be one or multiple hepaticojejunostomies. After resection of a hilar cholangiocarcinoma there may be two or more hepatic duct–enteric anastomoses. Following resection of a CBD stricture or tumor, a choledocho-choledochal anastomosis, or a choledocho-jejunal anastomosis is fashioned, depending on the length of common duct that must be removed.

No matter what the nature of the surgery, the goal of the postoperative biliary catheter cholangiogram is to evaluate for stricture or leak [22].

Rarely a mechanical obstruction caused by kinking or inspissated sludge may be encountered It is critical to obtain a 10-minute delayed film to prove adequate drainage of contrast across and thus patency of the anastomosis. For this purpose it is necessary to tilt up the examination table to use gravity to induce sufficient contrast flow out of the intrahepatic bile ducts. Findings may include spidery appearance of ducts indicating nonspecific liver edema, vascular compromise, or possibly early rejection. At the conclusion of the examination, the biliary catheter must be flushed with at least 10 mL of sterile normal saline to prevent crystallization of contrast and subsequent occlusion of the tube.

Barium cholangiography

Just as the surgeon tailors each surgery to the specific problem of each patient, the radiologist must be prepared to modify each examination in evaluating the complex postoperative patient. Altered anatomy requires adaptation of examinations to fit the situation. One adapted examination is the barium cholangiogram (Fig. 2A, B) [23,24].

Patients who have had biliary-jejunal anastomoses created in the context of a Whipple procedure, or after repair of bile duct trauma or resection of tumor, can be difficult to evaluate. Air in the biliary tree may interfere with MR cholangiography. The length of the jejunal limb may prevent endoscopic retrograde cholangiography. Percutaneous cholangiography may define only one biliary segment and not be able to depict anatomy and adequacy of the BJA. Under these circumstances, barium cholangiography may be helpful.

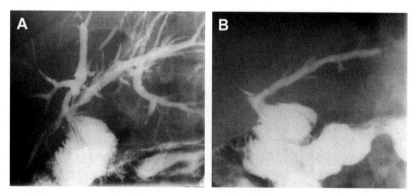

Fig. 2. (*A*) Sir Anthony Eden, then Britain's Foreign Secretary, was referred to and operated on at Lahey Clinic in 1953 following bile duct trauma during cholecystectomy. A follow-up barium cholangiogram performed in 1965 because of an episode of fever showed an intact anastomosis with slight distortion. (*B*) Onset of repeated febrile episodes in 1969 prompted a barium cholangiogram defining filling of only one major radical. This finding prompted revision of the anastomosis and the patient's symptoms abated. He eventually died of metastatic prostatic carcinoma in 1977.

This examination requires scrupulous adherence to technique by the performing radiologist and technologists. A routine upper gastrointestinal series is performed with barium to ensure that the esophagus, stomach, and duodenum are normal. During the remainder of the examination the most important concept is to work with gravity to move ingested barium toward and then across the biliointestinal anastomosis. Continuous, slow oral ingestion of barium by the patient in strict right lateral decubitus position is only interrupted by brief overhead upper abdominal radiographs approximately every 15 minutes. If and when there is barium evident in the ascending jejunal limb close to or (if the anastomoses are patent) in the bile ducts, the radiologist fluoroscopes the patient, carefully examining details of the biliary-jejunal anastomosis. Trendelenburg positioning may allow better definition of the BJA. Manual compression of the jejunal limb, which helps to push barium toward the liver, may fill the BJA. If there is barium within intrahepatic ducts but none seen across the anastomosis, slowly tilting the table upright may drain barium down from intrahepatic ducts across the BJA, at which point fluoroscopic exposures can be obtained in optimal projections. Failure to visualize the anastomosis does not prove it is abnormal. The chance for success of this examination visualization depends on the length of the jejunal limb.

The procedure may define biliary stones trapped above the anastomosis, anastomotic strictures, segmental intrahepatic strictures, or missing ducts (Fig. 3A–C). Knowledge of normal biliary ductal anatomy is critical, as is knowledge of the surgical procedure to appropriately recognize absence of filling of biliary radicals in a given patient.

CT cholangiography

History

Early attempts to use CT for biliary imaging included a study that involved oral administration of iopanoic acid followed by conventional CT and visualized bile ducts in 106 of 121 patients [25,26]. This older technique did not permit creation of contiguous datasets suitable for diagnosis of biliary disease and satisfactory (3D) visualization. The later advent of helical CT scanners introduced "volumetric" CT imaging for the first time, which in turn enabled improvements in CT biliary imaging. Better anatomic coverage could be obtained in a single breath hold contiguous scan.

Another factor driving interest in depiction of biliary anatomy was the rapidly increasing popularity of laparoscopic surgical techniques, especially laparoscopic cholecystectomy. The inherent limited field of view in this technique compared with open cholecystectomy explained the increasing interest of surgeons in better preoperative biliary imaging.

Several authors presented a technique of imaging the liver and biliary tree after IV contrast administration only and electronically extracting noncontrasted bile ducts on a workstation [27–29]. Although not suitable for

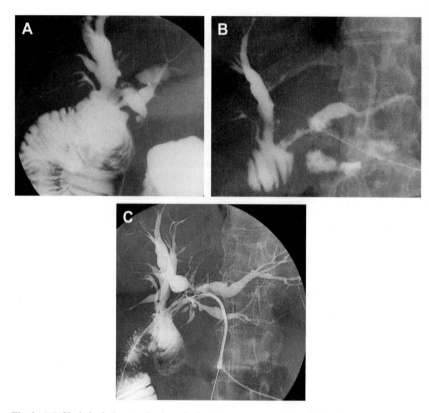

Fig. 3. (A) Choledochal cyst: a barium cholangiogram on a patient who had elevated liver function tests and an episode of fever who had a choledochal cyst removed 14 years earlier shows a dilated radical with no apparent communication to the hilum. The anastomosis and other radicals appear normal. (B) A percutaneous cholangiogram shows a narrowed irregular segment between the dilated duct and the hilar anastomotic region. This segment was brushed to exclude malignancy and was then presumed to be regional scarring. (C) Percutaneous dilatation was successfully performed to widen the narrowed segment. The patient improved and has remained asymptomatic for 5 years.

detection of stone disease and higher-order intrahepatic branches, this technique may serve as an adjunct to conventional contrast-enhanced CT imaging if the anatomy and branch pattern of the larger first-order central bile ducts are of interest, perhaps in context with surgical planning. It works particularly well and represents an interesting alternative for patients who have dilated (obstructed) bile ducts, who often have an elevated serum bilirubin and thus cannot receive IV biliary contrast anyway [30,31].

Later CT cholangiography after oral contrast administration (iopanoic acid) was revisited motivated by the low cost and simple oral route of administration [32–34]. Results are mixed; oral contrast needs to be administered many hours before the examination rendering this approach unsuitable for acute/subacute clinical situations and opacification of bile ducts and gallbladder was found to be less reliable than with IV contrast.

CT cholangiography in symptomatic patients

Klein and colleagues [35] compared conventional IV cholangiography with CT cholangiography and found depiction of the biliary tree to be superior on CT and 3D reconstructions of the pertinent biliary anatomy to be useful before laparoscopic cholecystectomy. Other investigators experimented with this innovative approach of creating 3D images of the biliary tree [36–41].

Stockberger and coworkers [42] compared CT cholangiography with ERCP in patients who had clinically suspected biliary disease. Diagnostic accuracy for choledocholithiasis correlated well with ERCP (7 of 8 positive cases). In a study of 80 symptomatic patients who had suspected choledocholithiasis, IV CT cholangiography was compared with ERCP [15]. CT cholangiography was found to have a sensitivity of 89% and a specificity of 98% for the detection of stones (which were present in 18/80 patients).

IV CT cholangiography was found to accurately depict the anatomy of the confluence of hepatic ducts and CBD in 100% and higher-order branches in 81% of patients in another study [43].

CT cholangiography compared well to ERC in identifying obstructive biliary disease; however, ERC was found to be superior in characterizing the exact length of strictures of higher-order intrahepatic branches [37].

Suggested indications

Symptomatic patients who have prior cholecystectomy (avoiding the risk for side effects associated with ERC) [42]

Before elective cholecystectomy (particularly for detection of anatomic variation), replacing any potential intraoperative imaging [14,39,44–46]

Failed ERC(P), which occurs in 5% to 10% of most series in gastroenterology literature [1]

Suspected choledocholithiasis, obstructive cholangiopathy [15,47–50]

Suspected biliary malignancy (should always be combined with vascular contrast-enhanced CT of the liver to detect extraluminal disease and increased overall sensitivity for detection of biliary malignancy [51,52])

Before complex reconstructive or curative (hilar) biliary surgery [53]

Evaluation of potential live liver donors [54,55]

Postoperative imaging of suspected biliary complications after liver transplantation [56–58]

May provide complimentary (functional) diagnostic information to non-contrast MRCP, especially in patients who have biliary air (attributable to sphincterotomy or prior biliointestinal anastomosis) [59]

Noninvasive imaging of biliary system in patients who have (relative) contraindications to MRCP, such as MR-incompatible ocular metal foreign bodies or cerebral aneurysm clips, prior pacemaker insertion, or claustrophobia

Biliary trauma (as part of comprehensive evaluation in conjunction with vascular contrast-enhanced CT) [41]

Examination technique

If there is a history of adverse reaction to iodinated contrast material, we follow our institutional allergy preparation policy: 1 vial (20 mL) of Cholografin [52% strength solution] mixed with 100 mL of normal saline is slowly infused intravenously over a period of 20 minutes. Once infusion is completed we wait 20 minutes and then image the patient on a 64-row multidetector CT scanner. Acquisition uses the smallest detector width, typically 0.6 mm, and the entire liver can typically be imaged in less than 10 seconds.

Images are reconstructed in an overlapping fashion into 1.2-mm slices, which are then transferred to a workstation for further image processing and 3D rendering. If there is an indication to obtain images of the upper abdomen with vascular contrast, we typically begin with that part of the examination and then perform the CT cholangiogram afterward.

If the patient has previously undergone partial hepatectomy and has one or several biliointestinal anastomoses, the patient is positioned so that the liver remnant is in the dependent part of the upper abdomen. We obtain one scan in that position and then turn the patient supine or even into the opposite direction followed by an immediate repeat image acquisition. This technique maximizes initial pooling of contrast in the dependent ducts and subsequently maximizes flow across the anastomoses to assess patency.

A recent publication by Breiman and coworkers [60] suggested that premedication of patients (in this specific case, normal potential liver donors) with IV morphine before CT cholangiography does not result in improved biliary ductal filling and visualization.

Image analysis

Electronic viewing on a PACS or workstation monitor greatly facilitates analysis of the many digital images created during the examination. Many different interactive display techniques may be helpful.

- Simple axial stacks as acquired (Fig. 4A) require interactive scrolling through the data set while viewing the images to comprehend the biliary anatomy.
- A 3D workstation enables image reconstruction, which allows for more intuitive evaluation of biliary anatomy, such as maximum intensity projection images (Fig. 4B).
- More advanced 3D processing using dedicated software can depict high-fidelity models of the entire biliary tree within the parenchymal liver volume (Fig. 4C) and furthermore allows fusion of vascular with biliary

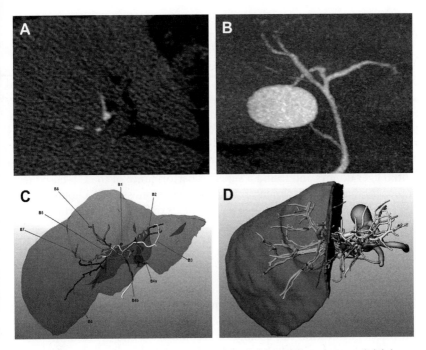

Fig. 4. (*A*) CT cholangiogram, axial image near hepatic hilum, biliary ducts are brightly contrasted. (*B*) Oblique coronal maximum intensity projection (MIP) CT cholangiographic image demonstrating gallbladder, cystic duct, proximal CBD, and intrahepatic ducts. (*C*) Volumetric reconstruction image of CT cholangiogram depicting liver and entire biliary tree labeled after Couinaud segmental scheme. (*D*) Composite 3D image for surgical planning derived by fusion of models from multiphasic CT with vascular contrast (arterial and portal phase) and CT cholangiogram. Demonstrates anticipated right lobe graft, hepatectomy resection line, and complex hilar anatomy.

images. The resulting high-fidelity images represent a powerful planning tool for the surgeon revealing the complex hepatic anatomy, including all intertwined portal, hepatic arterial, and venous vessels and biliary ducts in relationship to each other and to the planned resection plane (Fig. 4D)

When interpreting CT cholangiographic images one needs to remember that this technique does not opacify the biliary ducts with positive pressure. The rate of excretion of contrast is predicated on hepatocyte function, and even in patients who have normal hepatic function contrast flow is insufficient to judge whether a visible narrowing of a duct or anastomosis is truly flow limiting and thus functionally significant. Apparent short focal areas of narrowing at the biliointestinal anastomosis level are expected and often seen with no apparent functional consequence to the patient. On the other hand, segmental dilation of biliary ducts or even segmental lack of contrast excretion in the presence of normal segments in adjacent liver can corrobo-rate the diagnosis of a functionally significant anastomotic stricture.

One of the major advantages of IV CT cholangiography over traditional MRCP is the ability to depict even very small, nondilated biliary ducts be-cause of the active excretion of biliary contrast and the superb contrast and spatial resolution of modern CT scanners. This characteristic is particularly important when planning a left lateral hepatic segment adult-to-child dona-tion, because the peripheral biliary ducts in segments 2 and 3 are exceedingly small structures. Yeh and coworkers [55] compared IV CT cholangiography with conventional and excretory MRC in the depiction of bile ducts of po-tential liver donors and found a superior performance of the CT-based tech-nique. We have not experienced a single nondiagnostic CT cholangiogram in more than 200 preoperative liver donor examinations performed at our institution.

CT cholangiography in context with hepatic surgery and intervention

Occasionally we have used IV CT cholangiography in patients who have large hepatic primary or secondary tumors, typically for operative planning. As long as there is residual hepatocyte function in the affected liver segments, bile duct opacification can usually be accomplished and the resulting biliary images can be merged with the vascular 3D models. In patients who have (ma-lignant) biliary obstruction, percutaneous or internal drainage after stent placement should be performed first and then, when hepatic function has re-covered, CT cholangiography can be performed after a reasonable time period of 10 to 14 days, depending on the serum bilirubin level.

In a few instances, we have obtained CT cholangiograms in patients scheduled to undergo a percutaneous biliary access procedure in whom it was difficult to determine the best route of access (eg, in recipients of right lobe liver transplantation who have multiple biliointestinal anastomoses, some of which may be partially obstructed). 3D reconstructions of the bil-iary tree in these patients who have fused 3D images of the thoracic wall and other externally visible anatomic landmarks can be useful, identifying a safe route for percutaneous biliary access and decreasing procedure time.

Preoperative IV CT cholangiography versus intraoperative direct cholangiography in potential liver donors

The value and accuracy of preoperative biliary imaging in context with whole or partial organ transplantation of the liver is well documented [36,54–56].

In a small prospective series performed at Lahey Clinic with an Internal Review Board-approved protocol (Christoph Wald, MD, PhD, unpublished data, 2003) we compared preoperative IV CT with intraoperative direct cholangiography in right lobe donors undergoing live donor adult liver transplantation. CT correctly identified all biliary ducts compared with the time-consuming intraoperative imaging technique and provided the added advantage of fusion 3D imaging with contrast-enhanced vascular phase images. Since instituting this change, there has been no significant mismatch reported by our surgeons between preoperative biliary imaging findings and intraoperative findings in more than 70 patients who underwent right donor hepatectomy.

Direct injection CT cholangiography

This technique can be helpful in the depiction of multiple (overlapping) surgical biliointestinal anastomoses, suspected biliary stricture, complex postsurgical anatomy with multiple surgical clips, and the presence of metal stents. If the patient has previously undergone a percutaneous biliary procedure and a biliary drain or access tube is in place, this can be used to deliver contrast directly into the biliary system. Direct injection results in excellent ductal filling with the option of 3D rendering and fusion imaging with vascular phase CT images.

We use IV iodinated contrast, such as Omnipaque 300, diluted in 4 to 5 volume parts of sterile saline injected either under fluoroscopic guidance with subsequent transfer of the patient to the CT table or directly administered on the CT table. Imaging is performed in analogy to the previously described IV CT cholangiographic technique creating 3D reconstructions.

Resulting 3D images can often provide detailed spatially correct views of the biliary system as shown in this clinical example in a patient who had undergone a difficult cholecystectomy resulting in injury to two right-sided biliary ducts. Following referral, the patient underwent biliary reconstruction with three biliary-intestinal anastomoses. Subsequently, the clinical question of patency of the anastomoses arose. We injected diluted Omnipaque into the intestinal loop through one of the biliary catheters that had fallen into the loop. Contrast refluxed into all three ductal systems well demonstrated by 3D reconstruction showing patency of all three anastomoses (Fig. 5A, B).

In a small series by Kim and coworkers [61], findings on direct-injection CT cholangiography were compared with intraoperative and pathologic findings. The extent of malignant ductal involvement in 11 patients was correctly identified by this technique at all 11 primary and 18 out of 19 secondary biliary confluence levels and the authors concluded that this technique is accurate and feasible for defining the extent of ductal invasion by hilar cholangiocarcinoma, especially in patients who have prior external biliary drainage.

Magnetic resonance cholangiopancreatography

High diagnostic accuracy of MRCP has been demonstrated in context with various clinical conditions involving the biliary tree in the last decade [62–66]. Ductal dilatation, tumors, strictures, and stones can be readily

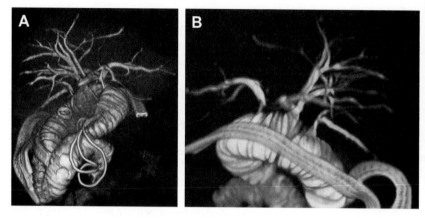

Fig. 5. (*A*) Frontal view of volume-rendered 3D CT image of liver, bile ducts, ascending intestinal loop in patient who had three biliointestinal anastomoses obtained after contrast injection through tube into jejunal lumen. (*B*) Detailed oblique posterior volume-rendered view clearly demonstrates three patent anastomoses.

demonstrated. Current indications to perform MRCP are similar to those for diagnostic ERCP, but also include those postoperative situations wherein access with the endoscope to the major papilla is not possible.

Technical considerations

In general there are two distinct approaches to visualize the biliary tree using MR. The first and more widely used method relies on the visualization of fluid-filled structures on heavily T2-weighted sequences. Fluid has a high signal on the resulting images based on its physical property of a long relaxation time. For this type of fluid imaging, two different technical approaches have been used: thick-slab (single shot fast spin echo) technique and multi-section thin-slab (single or multishot fast spin echo) techniques (Fig. 6A, B). For thick-slab techniques, 20- to 150-mm thickness oblique coronal slabs in various angles along the foot–head axis are acquired within a couple of seconds. This examination thus results in a set of images covering projections in 180° within approximately 1 minute of scan time. As this thick-slab technique readily generates a two-dimensional projection of all fluid-filled structures contained within the slab no further postprocessing is needed to appreciate the contiguous fluid-filled tubular structures of the biliary tree. Overlapping fluid-filled structures, such as the stomach, cystic liver lesions, or fluid-filled intestinal loops/colon potentially interfere with this type of imaging/display because they can obscure portions of the biliary tree on the derived projectional images. If necessary a commercially available iron-containing negative contrast agent can be administered, which renders the fluid within the stomach or duodenum dark. Alternatively, patients may ingest pineapple juice, which is cheaper and has a similar effect. The described

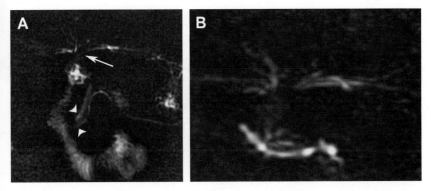

Fig. 6. A thick-slab image (*A*) of the biliary tree after right hemihepatectomy for cholangiocel-lular carcinoma and antecolic biliointestinal anastomosis (*arrow*) shows no gross abnormality of the biliary tree of the liver remnant. The remainder of the CBD and the main pancreatic duct are displayed (*arrowheads*). Postprocessed data of the thin-slab acquisition (*B*) are used to assess the biliary anastomosis and to better visualize the segmental branches within the liver remnant.

thick-slab technique is ideally suited to visualize and get an overview of the regional anatomy in a given patient. This method depends on patient compliance, however. Images may suffer from susceptibility artifacts because of the long time required for data acquisition, and visualization of small intraductal stones is often limited because of directly adjacent fluid. The presence of small intraductal lesions therefore needs to be confirmed with multisection thin-slab technique.

This second approach requires acquisition of individual multiple thin-section (2–5 mm thickness) images until a predetermined 3D volume of patient anatomy is covered. Each of these thin sections can be acquired in a single breath hold or during continuous shallow breathing, which is coregistered using a respiratory belt or a navigator pulse to later sort the acquired respiratory-gated data. This thin-slab method benefits from a higher spatial in plane resolution. Shorter echo times and shorter echo are rendering this technique more robust with regard to image artifacts. The acquisition of a 3D data set offers multiple options for postprocessing (Fig. 7A, B). This technique allows detection of small ductal filling defects and may visualize small tumors.

Recent studies investigated the significance of using IV secretin administration to stimulate pancreatic exocrine fluid excretion improving pancreatic duct visualization when focusing on pancreatic disorders. This approach allows assessment of the exocrine pancreatic secretion and the registration and analysis of flow dynamics, particularly in patients who have small ducts to better depict upstream duct detail within small branches [67,68]. This technique is helpful in the assessment of chronic pancreatitis, wherein subtle narrowing at the proximal side branch level together with mild dilatation of the side branch periphery may remain undetected without the secretory

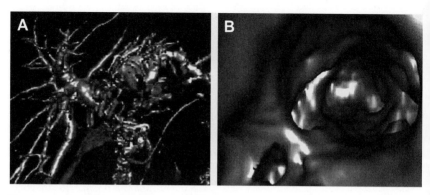

Fig. 7. A surface-rendered projection (*A*) and an endoluminal view of the biliary tree (*B*) can be generated from the thin-section acquisition. The usefulness of such image postprocessing still needs to be determined.

stimulus [69]. Already dilated ductal systems show no significant improvement in visualization after secretin administration. If secretin is administered repetitively over 10 minutes, pitfalls in imaging, such as the contraction of the sphincter of Oddi protruding into the distal CBD and thus mimicking a calculus, can usually be ruled out [70].

Both MRCP techniques described create images of the biliary tree based on the physical properties of the bile itself. Unlike retrograde or antegrade direct injection of contrast into the biliary tree during ERCP or percutaneous transhepatic cholangiography (PTC), MRCP using these heavily T2-weighted sequences is unable to image the flow-limiting character of a focal ductal narrowing. The functional impact of a bile duct stenosis or stricture may be suspected or deducted from the observed degree of anatomic narrowing and upstream ductal dilatation visualized on the MR images; however, prestenotic dilatation may fail to develop especially in transplanted livers despite the presence of significant ductal stenosis [60]. MRCP may provide complimentary information to ERCP in those patients in whom the retrogradely injected contrast could not pass a tight stenosis because MRCP allows imaging of all dilated prestenotic segments present [62,71]. The requirement for subsequent therapeutic segmental drainage of a segment not opacified during ERCP, the completeness of therapeutic drainage, and the overall extent of disease within the entire liver can be readily imaged because of the 3D character of data acquisition (Fig. 8A, B).

Magnetic resonance cholangiopancreatography enhanced with biliary magnetic resonance contrast agents

MR imaging of the biliary tree can be enhanced by the use of newer MR contrast agents that are actively secreted into the bile. This approach is less

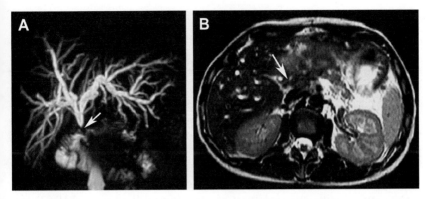

Fig. 8. (*A*) MRCP shows the abrupt stenosis of the biliary tree at the biliodigestive anastomosis after resection of a Klatskin tumor (*arrow*). The prestenotic dilatation of all segments is well appreciated and may guide further requirements for drainage. (*B*) The MR images acquired together with the MRCP show a soft tissue mass (*arrow*) at the anastomosis and confirm the diagnosis of tumor recurrence.

widely used primarily because of the limited availability of these contrast agents in some countries. A contrast agent that is actively secreted has the potential to illustrate the functional significance of a stenosis.

Currently one manganese-based agent (Mn-DPDP, Teslascan, licensed in the United States and Europe) and two gadolinium-based contrast agents are available, gadolinium-BOPTA (MultiHance, licensed in the United States and Europe) and gadolinium-EOB-DTPA (Primovist, licensed in Europe). After infusion, a small amount of manganese is excreted into bile and can be used to image the biliary tree [72]. The need for slow infusion and several unresolved mechanisms of manganese distribution within various organs limit its use for MRCP, however.

Both gadolinium-based chelated agents, which initially act as extracellular MRI contrast agents, are then actively transported into hepatocytes with a delay of 20 to 30 minutes because of their lipophilic character. These contrast agents shorten T1 relaxation times and are primarily used as a positive contrast agent to highlight hepatocytes. A fraction of the administered dose, approximately 10% of gadolinium-BOPTA and approximately 50% of gadolinium-EOB-DTPA, is actively secreted by hepatocytes into the bile and allows visualization of the biliary tree. This method fails if the secretory function of the hepatocytes is impaired. Even a small amount of contrast secreted by an intact hepatocyte allows visualization of enhanced bile on T1-weighted images. Both of these agents have already demonstrated their usefulness in the MR detection and characterization of liver lesions and showed potential to image hepatocyte function. Their definitive role in imaging of the biliary tree is still a matter of intensive investigation [73,74].

Normal anatomy and variants

The limited spatial resolution of MRCP compared with fluoroscopic images prohibits the visualization of the peripheral biliary tree in a healthy liver (with nondilated ducts) and the small distal intrapancreatic part of the pancreatic duct. Segmental and subsegmental branches of the liver and the entire extrahepatic biliary tree are readily imaged, however. Relevant anatomic variants, such an aberrant ostium of the right posterior segmental branch or a proximal or distal ostium of the cystic duct, are detected without difficulties.

Multiple saccular dilatations of the intrahepatic bile ducts are usually well defined on MRCP images. These congenital dilatations of the biliary system can be differentiated from smooth, round liver cysts. MRCP may fail to clearly define their connection with the biliary tree, however, unlike ERCP wherein injected contrast spreads from the tree into the biliary cysts. Additional information provided by the usual anatomic MR images customarily acquired in conjunction with the focused MRCP examination often leads to a more specific diagnosis. Caroli disease is typically associated with a dark (hypointense) center (a portal venous branch) surrounded by a bright (hyperintense) rim (dilated bile duct) seen on T2-weighted images, the so-called "central-dot sign" on MR images.

Inflammatory biliary disease

Findings in inflammatory biliary disease seen on MR are similar to those on ERCP. Stenoses in primary sclerosing cholangitis (PSC) are depicted as short segment cylindric narrowing attributable to the typically mild or absent prestenotic dilatation. Unlike ERCP, in which the distal branches of the biliary tree are distended by the injected contrast, MRCP often fails to show early pathologic alteration of the peripheral biliary tree because these small bile ducts are usually collapsed at the time of image acquisition. Later stages of the disease are characterized by multifocal biliary stenoses. Image findings of "pruned" appearance of bile ducts alternating with areas of segmental dilatation are seen on MRCP with the same diagnostic accuracy as ERCP. Because of the higher risk for complications during ERCP in patients who have PSC, MRCP should be considered the imaging modality of choice for primary evaluation in suspected PSC, for follow-up imaging of patients who have established PSC, and to rule out other reasons for extrahepatic cholestasis [75]. In addition, the use of MRCP is also more cost effective than ERCP in PSC [76].

Cholelithiasis/choledocholithiasis

If thin-slab technique MR imaging is used, small intraductal stones are depicted as biconcave signal voids in the lumen. Because of the limited resolution of MRCP, stones of less than 3 mm diameter may be missed, especially in an immediate preampullary position [77]. If small stones are not surrounded by bile they may be misinterpreted as strictures or stenosis. Physiologic narrowing of the CBD at the level of the porta hepatis attributable to a compression by the crossing hepatic artery or compression of the distal CBD by periampullary duodenal diverticula can usually be identified on the additional MRI sequences.

Benign and malignant strictures

Benign strictures are seen as smooth-walled tubular narrowing of the bile ducts, sometimes associated with mild displacement of the duct attributable to associated fibrosis [64,78]. The degree of stenosis is best depicted on thin-slab images. Thick-slab images and maximum intensity projection (MIP) tend to overestimate the degree of stenosis. MRCP is well suited for follow-up imaging of biliointestinal anastomoses because focal bile duct narrowing, stones, number of anastomoses, and associated segments are often well seen on the acquired images. PTC allows for a better delineation of bile duct narrowing in transplanted patients; however, because of its invasive character, it should be reserved for the symptomatic patients with the intention to treat by way of the percutaneous tract [58]. If the serum bilirubin level is less than 2 mg/dL, IV CT cholangiography can also be considered as a noninvasive imaging modality in these patients.

Abrupt stenoses with prestenotic dilatation often have a malignant cause [63]. In cholangiocarcinoma a diffuse increase in the periductal MR signal may be the only hint, because the endoluminal tumor growth is not reliably detected. This tumor tends to grow in a sheath-like fashion along and parallel to the bile ducts. MRCP may have advantages over ERCP for treatment planning if ERCP fails to opacify all segments of the biliary tree. Pancreatic head carcinoma can also cause a focal isolated stenosis of the CBD often associated with a stenosis of the pancreatic duct leading to the classic so-called "double duct sign." Ampullary carcinoma may lead to a similar pathologic configuration of the biliary and pancreatic duct. These tumors are best detected because of their typically hyperintense signal characteristics on T2-weighted MR images.

Gallbladder diseases

The assessment of the gallbladder is usually based on a combination of MRCP and MR images. Stones appear as a void within the lumen of the gallbladder on MRCP images if they are surrounded by bile. Sludge leads to mild homogenous signal decrease seen as a fluid level within the bright bile. If the gallbladder is not identified on MRCP images and cholecystectomy is excluded, the most likely diagnosis is complete obstruction with concretion or postinflammatory shrinkage. Congenitally absent gallbladder is a rare condition with an incidence of less than 0.4%. The combined assessment on MRCP and MR images may lead to the correct diagnosis in cases of complete gallbladder obstruction attributable to primary gallbladder cancer [79].

Imaging of the sphincter complex

Imaging of the sphincter complex may benefit from secretin stimulation of pancreatic excretion described earlier and serial imaging over several minutes. This approach also allows visualization of changes in the shape of the sphincter because of contractions, which occur about four to five times per minute. ERCP is better suited to assess for the presence of a papillary stenosis because MRCP cannot evaluate its functional significance. Furthermore, endoscopy also provides the therapeutic option of sphincterotomy, treatment of choice for fixed anatomic stenosis, and tissue sampling. After sphincterotomy or in conjunction with a periampullary duodenal diverticulum the ampulla may appear irregular and enlarged without the presence of any concerning pathology. Images obtained in this context should be interpreted carefully.

Summary

- Current MRCP techniques are based on imaging of bile-filled ducts with heavily T2-weighted sequences. As an alternative, contrast agents that are actively secreted by hepatocytes may be used to visualize the biliary tree.
- Data acquisition can be performed in thick or thin slabs, with the former being the faster imaging technique and the latter having a higher spatial resolution allowing detection of small intraluminal abnormalities and additional image postprocessing because of the inherent 3D character of data acquisition.
- Indication for MRCP includes all indications for diagnostic ERCP and PTC. MRCP reaches similar diagnostic accuracy for most biliary conditions. In conjunction with the MR images usually acquired during the same examination, the diagnostic yield may exceed that of ERCP and PTC.
- The ability to image anatomy proximal to a stenotic biliary segment MRCP provides complimentary information to ERCP if complete opacification of the biliary tree cannot be achieved in retrograde fashion.

References

[1] Sherman S, Lehman GA. ERCP- and endoscopic sphincterotomy-induced pancreatitis. Pancreas 1991;6:350.
[2] Loperfido S, Angelini G, Benedetti G, et al. Major early complications from diagnostic and therapeutic ERCP: a prospective multicenter study. Gastrointest Endosc 1998;48:1.

[3] Masci E, Toti G, Mariani A, et al. Complications of diagnostic and therapeutic ERCP: a prospective multicenter study. Am J Gastroenterol 2001;96:417.

[4] Graham EA, Cole WH. Roentgenologic examination of the gallbladder, new method utilizing intravenous injection of tetrabromophenolphthalein. JAMA 1924;82:613.

[5] Bell AL, Immerman LL, Arcomano JP, et al. Intravenous cholangiography: a preliminary study. Am J Surg 1954;88:248.

[6] Glenn F, Evans J, Hill M, et al. Intravenous cholangiography. Ann Surg 1954;140:600.

[7] Jutras A. [Intravenous cholegraphy; new aspects of biliary physiology; floating calculi]. Union Med Can 1954;83:1349 [in French].

[8] Orloff TL, Sklaroff DM, Cohn EM, et al. Intravenous choledochography with a new contrast medium, Cholografin. Radiology 1954;62:868.

[9] Wise RE, O'Brien RG. Intravenous cholangiography: a preliminary report. Lahey Clin Bull 1954;9:52.

[10] Wise RE, Johnston DO, Salzman FA. The intravenous cholangiographic diagnosis of partial obstruction of the common bile duct. Radiology 1957;68:507.

[11] Wise RE, Twaddle JA. Choledocholithiasis: postcholecystectomy diagnosis by intravenous cholangiography. Surg Clin North Am 1958;38:673.

[12] Taenzer V, Volkhardt V. Double blind comparison of meglumine iotroxate (Biliscopin), meglumine iodoxamate (Endobile), and meglumine ioglycamate (Biligram). AJR Am J Roentgenol 1979;132:55.

[13] Ott DJ, Gelfand DW. Complications of gastrointestinal radiologic procedures: II. Complications related to biliary tract studies. Gastrointest Radiol 1981;6:47.

[14] Maglinte DD, Dorenbusch MJ. Intravenous infusion cholangiography: an assessment of its role relevant to laparoscopic cholecystectomy. Radiol Diagn 1993;34:91.

[15] Takahashi M, Saida Y, Itai Y, et al. Reevaluation of spiral CT cholangiography: basic considerations and reliability for detecting choledocholithiasis in 80 patients. J Comput Assist Tomogr 2000;24:859.

[16] Breen DJ, Nicholson AA. The clinical utility of spiral CT cholangiography. Clin Radiol 2000;55:733.

[17] Sacharias N. Safety of Biliscopin. Australas Radiol 1995;39:101.

[18] Nilsson U. Adverse reactions to iotroxate at intravenous cholangiography. A prospective clinical investigation and review of the literature. Acta Radiol 1987;28:571.

[19] Lindsey I, Nottle PD, Sacharias N. Preoperative screening for common bile duct stones with infusion cholangiography: review of 1000 patients. Ann Surg 1997;226:174–8.

[20] Robbins AH, Earampamoorthy S, Koff RS, et al. Successful intravenous cholecystocholangiography in the jaundiced patient using meglumine iodoxamate (Cholovue). AJR Am J Roentgenol 1976;126:70.

[21] Keogan MT, McDermott VG, Price SK, et al. The role of imaging in the diagnosis and management of biliary complications after liver transplantation. AJR Am J Roentgenol 1999;173:215.

[22] Kapoor V, Baron RL, Peterson MS. Bile leaks after surgery. AJR Am J Roentgenol 2004; 182:451.

[23] Braasch JW. Anthony Eden's (Lord Avon) biliary tract saga. Ann Surg 2003;238:772.

[24] Lucas CE, Kurtzman R, Read RC. Barium cholangiography. Surg Forum 1965;16:384.

[25] Greenberg M, Greenberg BM, Rubin JM, et al. Computed-tomographic cholangiography: a new technique for evaluating the head of the pancreas and distal biliary tree. Radiology 1982;144:363.

[26] Greenberg M, Rubin JM, Greenberg BM. Appearance of the gallbladder and biliary tree by CT cholangiography. J Comput Assist Tomogr 1983;7:788.

[27] Park SJ, Han JK, Kim TK, et al. Three-dimensional spiral CT cholangiography with minimum intensity projection in patients with suspected obstructive biliary disease: comparison with percutaneous transhepatic cholangiography. Abdom Imaging 2001;26:281.

[28] Zandrino F, Benzi L, Ferretti ML, et al. Multislice CT cholangiography without biliary contrast agent: technique and initial clinical results in the assessment of patients with biliary obstruction. Eur Radiol 2002;12:1155.

[29] Zeman RK, Berman PM, Silverman PM, et al. Biliary tract: three-dimensional helical CT without cholangiographic contrast material. Radiology 1995;196:865.

[30] Kielar A, Toa H, Sekar A, et al. Comparison of CT duodeno-cholangiopancreatography to ERCP for assessing biliary obstruction. J Comput Assist Tomogr 2005;29:596.

[31] Kim HC, Park SJ, Park SI, et al. Multislice CT cholangiography using thin-slab minimum intensity projection and multiplanar reformation in the evaluation of patients with suspected biliary obstruction: preliminary experience. Clin Imaging 2005;29:46.

[32] Caoili EM, Paulson EK, Heyneman LE, et al. Helical CT cholangiography with three-dimensional volume rendering using an oral biliary contrast agent: feasibility of a novel technique. AJR Am J Roentgenol 2000;174:487.

[33] Chopra S, Chintapalli KN, Ramakrishna K, et al. Helical CT cholangiography with oral cholecystographic contrast material. Radiology 2000;214:596.

[34] Soto JA, Velez SM, Guzman J. Choledocholithiasis: diagnosis with oral-contrast-enhanced CT cholangiography. AJR Am J Roentgenol 1999;172:943.

[35] Klein HM, Wein B, Truong S, et al. Computed tomographic cholangiography using spiral scanning and 3D image processing. Br J Radiol 1993;66:762.

[36] Cheng YF, Lee TY, Chen CL, et al. Three-dimensional helical computed tomographic cholangiography: application to living related hepatic transplantation. Clin Transplant 1997;11:209.

[37] Fleischmann D, Ringl H, Schofl R, et al. Three-dimensional spiral CT cholangiography in patients with suspected obstructive biliary disease: comparison with endoscopic retrograde cholangiography. Radiology 1996;198:861.

[38] Gillams A, Gardener J, Richards R, et al. Three-dimensional computed tomography cholangiography: a new technique for biliary tract imaging. Br J Radiol 1994;67:445.

[39] Kwon AH, Uetsuji S, Ogura T, et al. Spiral computed tomography scanning after intravenous infusion cholangiography for biliary duct anomalies. Am J Surg 1997;174:396.

[40] Kwon M, Uetsuji S, Boku T, et al. [Three dimensional cholangiography with spiral CT for analysis of biliary tract: preliminary report]. Nippon Geka Gakkai Zasshi 1993;94:658 [in Japanese].

[41] Wicky S, Gudinchet F, Barghouth G, et al. Three-dimensional cholangio-spiral CT demonstration of a post-traumatic bile leak in a child. Eur Radiol 1999;9:99.

[42] Stockberger SM, Wass JL, Sherman S, et al. Intravenous cholangiography with helical CT: comparison with endoscopic retrograde cholangiography. Radiology 1994;192:675.

[43] Van Beers BE, Lacrosse M, Trigaux JP, et al. Noninvasive imaging of the biliary tree before or after laparoscopic cholecystectomy: use of three-dimensional spiral CT cholangiography. AJR Am J Roentgenol 1994;162:1331.

[44] Huddy SP, Southam JA. Is intravenous cholangiography an alternative to the routine peroperative cholangiogram? Postgrad Med J 1989;65:896.

[45] Kitami M, Takase K, Murakami G, et al. Types and frequencies of biliary tract variations associated with a major portal venous anomaly: analysis with multi-detector row CT cholangiography. Radiology 2006;238:156.

[46] Murakami T, Kim T, Tomoda K, et al. Aberrant right posterior biliary duct: detection by intravenous cholangiography with helical CT. J Comput Assist Tomogr 1997;21:733.

[47] Cabada Giadas T, Sarria Octavio de Toledo L, Martinez-Berganza Asensio MT, et al. Helical CT cholangiography in the evaluation of the biliary tract: application to the diagnosis of choledocholithiasis. Abdom Imaging 2002;27:61.

[48] Persson A, Dahlstrom N, Smedby O, et al. Three-dimensional drip infusion CT cholangiography in patients with suspected obstructive biliary disease: a retrospective analysis of feasibility and adverse reaction to contrast material. BMC Med Imaging 2006;6:1.

[49] Persson A, Dahlstrom N, Smedby O, et al. Volume rendering of three-dimensional drip infusion CT cholangiography in patients with suspected obstructive biliary disease: a retrospective study. Br J Radiol 2005;78:1078.

[50] Zandrino F, Curone P, Benzi L, et al. MR versus multislice CT cholangiography in evaluating patients with obstruction of the biliary tract. Abdom Imaging 2005;30:77.

[51] Campbell WL, Ferris JV, Holbert BL, et al. Biliary tract carcinoma complicating primary sclerosing cholangitis: evaluation with CT, cholangiography, US, and MR imaging. Radiology 1998;207:41.

[52] Campbell WL, Peterson MS, Federle MP, et al. Using CT and cholangiography to diagnose biliary tract carcinoma complicating primary sclerosing cholangitis. AJR Am J Roentgenol 2001;177:1095.

[53] Hashimoto M, Itoh K, Takeda K, et al. Evaluation of biliary abnormalities with 64-channel multidetector CT. Radiographics 2008;28:119.

[54] Schroeder T, Malago M, Debatin JF, et al. Multidetector computed tomographic cholangiography in the evaluation of potential living liver donors. Transplantation 2002;73:1972.

[55] Yeh BM, Breiman RS, Taouli B, et al. Biliary tract depiction in living potential liver donors: comparison of conventional MR, mangafodipir trisodium-enhanced excretory MR, and multi-detector row CT cholangiography—initial experience. Radiology 2004;230:645.

[56] Miller GA, Yeh BM, Breiman RS, et al. Use of CT cholangiography to evaluate the biliary tract after liver transplantation: initial experience. Liver Transpl 2004;10:1065.

[57] Tello R, Jenkins R, McGinnes A, et al. Biliary tree necrosis in transplanted liver detected by spiral CT with three-dimensional reconstruction. Clin Imaging 1996;20:8.

[58] Zoepf T, Maldonado-Lopez EJ, Hilgard P, et al. Diagnosis of biliary strictures after liver transplantation: which is the best tool? World J Gastroenterol 2005;11:2945.

[59] Eracleous E, Genagritis M, Papanikolaou N, et al. Complementary role of helical CT cholangiography to MR cholangiography in the evaluation of biliary function and kinetics. Eur Radiol 2005;15:2130.

[60] Breiman RS, Coakley FV, Webb EM, et al. CT cholangiography in potential liver donors: effect of premedication with intravenous morphine on biliary caliber and visualization. Radiology 2008;247:733–7.

[61] Kim HJ, Kim AY, Hong SS, et al. Biliary ductal evaluation of hilar cholangiocarcinoma: three-dimensional direct multi-detector row CT cholangiographic findings versus surgical and pathologic results–feasibility study. Radiology 2006;238:300.

[62] Kaltenthaler EC, Walters SJ, Chilcott J, et al. MRCP compared to diagnostic ERCP for diagnosis when biliary obstruction is suspected: a systematic review. BMC Med Imaging 2006; 6:9.

[63] Kim HC, Yang DM, Jin W, et al. The various manifestations of ruptured hepatocellular carcinoma: CT imaging findings. Abdom Imaging 2008, in press.

[64] Kim JY, Lee JM, Han JK, et al. Contrast-enhanced MRI combined with MR cholangiopancreatography for the evaluation of patients with biliary strictures: differentiation of malignant from benign bile duct strictures. J Magn Reson Imaging 2007;26:304.

[65] Mofidi R, Lee AC, Madhavan KK, et al. The selective use of magnetic resonance cholangiopancreatography in the imaging of the axial biliary tree in patients with acute gallstone pancreatitis. Pancreatology 2008;8:55.

[66] Sakai Y, Tsuyuguchi T, Tsuchiya S, et al. Diagnostic value of MRCP and indications for ERCP. Hepatogastroenterology 2007;54:2212.

[67] Calculli L, Pezzilli R, Fiscaletti M, et al. Exocrine pancreatic function assessed by secretin cholangio-Wirsung magnetic resonance imaging. Hepatobiliary Pancreat Dis Int 2008;7:192.

[68] Gillams AR, Lees WR. Quantitative secretin MRCP (MRCPQ): results in 215 patients with known or suspected pancreatic pathology. Eur Radiol 2007;17:2984.

[69] Balci NC, Alkaade S, Magas L, et al. Suspected chronic pancreatitis with normal MRCP: findings on MRI in correlation with secretin MRCP. J Magn Reson Imaging 2008;27:125.

[70] Van Hoe L, Mermuys K, Vanhoenacker P. MRCP pitfalls. Abdom Imaging 2004;29:360.

[71] Vanderveen KA, Hussain HK. Magnetic resonance imaging of cholangiocarcinoma. Cancer Imaging 2004;4:104.

[72] Kamaoui I, Milot L, Durieux M, et al. [Value of MRCP with mangafodipir trisodium (Teslascan) injection in the diagnosis and management of bile leaks]. J Radiol 2007;88: 1881 [in French].

[73] Dahlstrom N, Persson A, Albiin N, et al. Contrast-enhanced magnetic resonance cholangi-ography with Gd-BOPTA and Gd-EOB-DTPA in healthy subjects. Acta Radiol 2007;48: 362.

[74] Holzapfel K, Breitwieser C, Prinz C, et al. [Contrast-enhanced magnetic resonance cholan-giography using gadolinium-EOB-DTPA. Preliminary experience and clinical applications]. Radiologe 2007;47:536.

[75] Textor HJ, Flacke S, Pauleit D, et al. Three-dimensional magnetic resonance cholangiopan-creatography with respiratory triggering in the diagnosis of primary sclerosing cholangitis: comparison with endoscopic retrograde cholangiography. Endoscopy 2002;34:984.

[76] Meagher S, Yusoff I, Kennedy W, et al. The roles of magnetic resonance and endoscopic ret-rograde cholangiopancreatography (MRCP and ERCP) in the diagnosis of patients with suspected sclerosing cholangitis: a cost-effectiveness analysis. Endoscopy 2007;39:222.

[77] Romagnuolo J, Bardou M, Rahme E, et al. Magnetic resonance cholangiopancreatography: a meta-analysis of test performance in suspected biliary disease. Ann Intern Med 2003;139: 547.

[78] Park MS, Kim TK, Kim KW, et al. Differentiation of extrahepatic bile duct cholangiocar-cinoma from benign stricture: findings at MRCP versus ERCP. Radiology 2004;233:234.

[79] Elsayes KM, Oliveira EP, Narra VR, et al. Magnetic resonance imaging of the gallbladder: spectrum of abnormalities. Acta Radiol 2007;48:476.

ELSEVIER
SAUNDERS

SURGICAL
CLINICS OF
NORTH AMERICA

Surg Clin N Am 88 (2008) 1221–1240

Endoscopic Evaluation and Therapies of Biliary Disorders

Ann Marie Joyce, MD[a,b,*], Frederick W. Heiss, MD[a,b]

[a]Tufts Medical School, Burlington, MA, USA
[b]Department of Gastroenterology, Lahey Clinic, 41 Mall Road, 6 Central Suite,
Burlington, MA 01805, USA

Therapeutic endoscopic retrograde cholangiopancreatography (ERCP) has flourished and continues to grow after its introduction with the first biliary spincterotomies in 1974 in Germany and Japan. The therapeutic biliary endoscopist contributes to the management of all biliary disorders and in many cases endoscopy is the preferable approach.

Biliary disorders were once only accessible by orthodox surgery but are now diagnosed and treated by multiple methods and specialists. The multispecialty team approach is critical to the best outcomes, owing to the complexity of these disorders, the variety of treatment options, the associated degrees of invasiveness, and to the patient's tolerance. New and rapidly advancing technology in radiologic imaging provides high quality depictions of biliary structures and intra-abdominal anatomy without risk or discomfort. Advances in diagnostic endoscopy also supply precise anatomic detail, give access for biopsy of more pathologic sites, and permit therapeutic opportunities with newer instruments, such as endoscopic ultrasound and the transendoscopic choledochoscope.

While interventional radiologists can access biliary structures percutaneously, ordinarily the endoscopic approach is preferred to avoid complications related to puncture of the liver capsule and vascular structures. Skilled endoscopists should be able to enter the bile duct via the papilla of Vater greater than 95% of the time, whether or not bile ducts are dilated, while successful percutaneous biliary entry is markedly reduced with normal ducts. Endoscopic access is preferable in the presence of cirrhosis, ascites, and abnormal coagulation. In addition, the endoscopist can see the

* Corresponding author. Department of Gastroenterology, Lahey Clinic, 41 Mall Road, 6 Central Suite, Burlington, MA 01805.
 E-mail address: annmarie.joyce@lahey.org (A.M. Joyce).

0039-6109/08/$ - see front matter © 2008 Elsevier Inc. All rights reserved.
doi:10.1016/j.suc.2008.07.015   surgical.theclinics.com

duodenum and papilla of Vater, occasionally the site of biliary obstruction. Moreover, in-dwelling percutaneous catheters are poorly tolerated by patients and can be difficult to maintain.

Nevertheless, percutaneous access is often the only avenue open to complex hilar lesions or intrahepatic structures or when there has been a prior bilo-enteric anastomosis or other surgery precluding endoscopic access. Novel access with laparoscopic assistance may be necessary in patients in whom gastric bypass surgery has been performed. A port can be created in the stomach through which a duodenoscope can be easily passed for a sphincterotomy and stone extractions. Using endoscopic ultrasound, needle puncture with guide-wire placement can give biliary access through puncture of the bile duct from the duodenum or the left lobe of the liver from the stomach. This may become the preferable alternative when initial ERCP has failed or is not possible [1].

Despite widespread use since its introduction almost 40 years ago, ERCP continues to be troubled by its technical difficulty and potential for severe complications. The success and safety of ERCP are closely related to the experience, training, and skill of the operator. Experts debate and set guidelines for minimal experience needed to qualify for privileges and to maintain competence [2]. Acute pancreatitis is the most dreaded and common complication of ERCP, with rates of 2% to 9% seen in most unselected prospective series, but much higher rates are seen in high-risk patients [3,4].

Numerous pharmacologic agents are available that act at various sites in the proposed mechanism of post-ERCP pancreatitis (Box 1). The predictable high incidence of post-ERCP pancreatitis and its potentially serious sequellae have offered an opportunity to study preventative measures prospectively. Despite hundreds of published trials over the last 30 years, a pharmacologic agent of proven benefit in the prevention of post ERCP pancreatitis, unfortunately, has not been found to be effective, practical or available [5].

There is now considerable evidence that pancreatic stent placement reduces the risk of post-ERCP pancreatitis in high-risk patients [2,5]. However, several issues with regard to stent use have not been resolved and include: who should be stented, what kind of stent and guide-wire are best, and what are the risks? Freeman [2] has recently reviewed this topic and made several recommendations:

Apancreatic stent is not warranted in most patients undergoing ERCP;
Pancreatic stents should be used in patients with increased risk, such as those with proven or suspected sphincter of Oddi dysfunction (SOD), independent of any manometric findings;
When cannulation was difficult, especially in patients with high risk profile;
When precut sphincterotomy was preformed in which the cut was started at the papillary orifice;

When there has been significant pancreatic injection or instrumentation;
When minor or major pancreatic sphincterotomy was performed;
When there has been an ampullectomy; and
When biliary balloon dilation of an intact papilla was performed for stone extraction.

Pancreatic duct stenting should also be considered in patients with a prior history of post-ERCP pancreatitis, patients undergoing pancreatic brush cytology or other tissue sampling, after pancreatoscopy, and after tissue ablation in the vicinity of the pancreatic duct orifice.

The surest way to prevent post ERCP pancreatitis is to avoid an ERCP unless clearly indicated. This strategy has become more feasible at a time when very satisfactory alternatives for a diagnostic study are available. Good quality cholangiopancreatograms are now routinely obtained with

---

Box 1. Pharmacologic agents tested for prevention of post-ERCP pancreatitis

Sphincter of Oddi relaxants
Nitrates
Botulinum toxin
Epinephrine

Hormones to suppress pancreatic secretion
Somatostatin and octreotide
Secretin
Glucagon
Calcitonin

Protease inhibitors
Gabexate
Aprotonin
C1-INH
Ulinastatin

Anti-inflammatory agents
Steroids
Interleukin-10
Nonsteroidal anti-inflammatory drugs
Heparin

Antioxidants
Allopurinol
N-acetyl cysteine
Beta-carotene

magnetic resonance cholangiopancreatography (MRCP) and CT. Endo-scopic ultrasound (EUS) in many settings can answer anatomic questions that formerly required ERCP; EUS has the additional advantage of permitting tissue sampling.

The therapeutic potential of ERCP was soon realized after it was first reported. In 1974, the first endoscopic biliary spincterotomies were performed independently by Classen and Demling [6] in Germany and Kawai and associates [7] in Japan. Thereafter, the field has flourished and continues to grow. Many biliary disorders are now managed effectively and preferentially. The following disorders are areas in which a major impact has been made.

Choledocholithiasis

Common bile duct (CBD) stones are found in up to 15% of patients with gallbladder stones [8]. Patients with CBD stones may present with biliary colic, jaundice, and cholangitis. A small number of patients are asymptomatic. Patients with obvious bile duct obstruction may go directly to ERCP, but some patients will need further imaging tests to confirm the diagnosis. A transabdominal ultrasound is usually the first test chosen. This ultrasound is readily available and safe. Patients with CBD stones may have a dilated CBD, but it is uncommon to detect choledocholithiasis on an abdominal ultrasound. If detected, however, the specificity is 95% [9]. If the diagnosis is still uncertain, a MRCP should be the next test. MRCP should generally replace diagnostic ERCP because of the latter's significant risk [10]. MRCP is deficient in detecting small (<5 mm) stones or biliary sludge. A meta-analysis of 67 studies revealed the pooled sensitivity and specificity for detecting biliary obstruction were 95% and 97%, respectively [11]. MRCP will be discussed in further detail in this issue (see article by Wald and colleagues). A more invasive procedure than abdominal ultrasound and MRCP, but with less risk than an ERCP, is an endoscopic ultrasound. From the duodenal bulb, the entire length of the CBD can be examined. The stone appears as a hyperechoic focus within the CBD with an acoustic shadowing (Fig. 1). EUS is more accurate than ERCP for detecting small stones.

Tse and colleagues [12] performed a meta-analysis of the prospective studies of the role of the EUS for the diagnosis of CBD stones. There were 2,673 patients in total of 27 studies. The overall pooled sensitivity was 94% with a specificity of 95%. There was no standard method in the studies to confirm CBD stones. The use of EUS in patients with a moderate or low clinical suspicion for CBD stones may prevent unnecessary ERCPs. In a study of 110 patients with suspected biliary obstruction from CBD stones but normal imaging, EUS prevented 30% of unnecessary ERCP [13]. EUS is not readily available, the results are operator-dependent, and the test chosen depends on the local expertise.

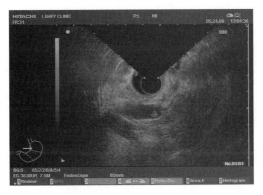

Fig. 1. EUS of CBD with hyperechoic focus and acoustic shadowing consistent with CBD stone.

Patients with a high clinical suspicion for a stone should be referred for ERCP. ERCP is effective for detecting CBD stones and relieving the obstruction (Fig. 2) [14]. The sensitivity of ERCP ranges from 90% to 95%. Smaller stones or sludge may not be seen during a cholangiogram. In patients with a high clinical suspicion for CBD stones, an ERCP is recommended before cholecystectomy. An intraoperative cholangiogram (IOC) may be considered in patients with moderate risk for CBD stones. Patients with moderate risk for CBD stones are defined as those with cholelithiasis, abnormal liver profile, and a normal CBD. If stones are detected on an IOC, then a postoperative ERCP or a CBD exploration is recommended. The procedure chosen is based on local expertise [15,16].

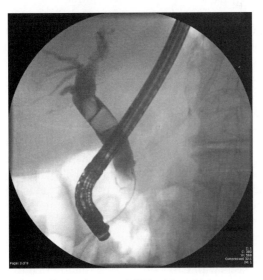

Fig. 2. Cholangiogram of CBD with multiple stones.

In the majority of cases, a sphincterotomy is performed to facilitate the removal of stones. In patients with a coagulopathy, a sphincterotomy is contraindicated. In this patient population, the sphincter may be dilated with a dilating balloon or a stent may be placed. A meta-analysis of eight studies involving over 1,000 patients revealed that there was a higher rate of pancreatitis with balloon dilation [17]. A United States-based multicenter trial of 237 patients was not included in this meta-analysis. The procedures were equally successful in the two groups. Pancreatitis occurred in 15.4% of patients with balloon dilation compared with 0.8% in the sphincterotomy group ($P < .001$) [18]. On the other hand, a Japanese study of 1,000 patients reported a pancreatitis rate of only 4.8% [19]. No explanation was given for this considerable difference in rate of pancreatitis. Therefore, balloon dilation is reserved for patients with a coagulopathy in most centers.

The majority of stones and sludge can be removed with a stone-retrieval balloon or Dormia basket after a sphincterotomy has been performed. Larger stones add to the challenge of an ERCP. It is important to perform a large sphincterotomy to remove larger stones. Biliary mechanical lithotripsy is one technique that is quite successful in crushing and removing stones. If the basket and stone cannot be removed then the stone can be crushed by advancement of a sheath. Mechanical lithotripsy is successful in the majority of cases [20]. Two factors that impact its success include size of the stone and stone impaction [21,22]. In selective centers, intraductal lithotripsy is used to break up stones. The laser lithotripsy uses an amplified light energy to shatter the stone. It is administered with a choledochoscope or with fluoroscopic guided catheters. The electrohydraulic lithotripsy has a power generator that releases power to a bipolar electrode, which generates a shock wave to shatter the stones. The intraductal lithotripsy is usually performed under direct visualization. Chen and Pleskow [23] reported the success of SpyGlass to assist with the treatment of stones in a small group of patients. The SpyGlass system is a single operator cholangiopancreatoscopy. Larger studies are needed to determine the role of the SpyGlass system in the management of the CBD stones.

In about 90% of cases, the ERCP is successful in that the CBD has been cleared of stones. In patients who are critically ill and cannot tolerate a prolonged procedure, patients with an edematous papilla, or those patients where the duct cannot be cleared out, a stent should be placed. Two types of stents include the nasobiliary drain and plastic biliary stent. The ERCP is usually repeated within 4 to 6 weeks and leaving the stent in place may help to fragment the stones. In elderly patients, the endoprosthesis may be used as a permanent treatment. This patient population can have high rate of late complications because stents can occlude after 3 months [24]. Close follow-up is suggested.

A cholecystectomy is recommended in most patients with CBD stones. A group of 120 subjects with CBD stones were randomized to "watchful waiting" or to have a cholecystectomy. There were recurrent symptoms in 47%

of the "watchful waiting" group as opposed to 2% in the cholecystectomy group in a 2-year period [25]. Patients who are not good surgical candidates should be treated expectantly.

Benign biliary strictures

Benign biliary strictures most commonly occur after surgery, during the course of sclerosing cholangitis, and as a result of acute and chronic pancreatitis. Other causes are numerous but rare. Postoperative bile duct injuries are seen following cholecystectomy and a biliary anastomosis during liver transplantation (Fig. 3). Although laparoscopic cholecystectomy has well-known advantages and now routinely replaces open cholecystectomy, the rate of bile duct injuries is higher than with the open procedure [26]. The approach to biliary strictures can be complex and should involve a number of specialists. Best outcomes require a team approach in an experienced referral center. High-quality radiology is required to accurately define the anatomy upon which corrective measures are contingent. The biliary surgeon, therapeutic endoscopist, and interventional radiologist must weigh the feasibility of available therapies and the medical status of the patient before a therapeutic decision is made, keeping in mind that an unsuccessful noninvasive approach does not preclude an alternative. Traditional surgical repair is usually successful but morbidity can be significant and recurring stricture rates can be high. Morbidity rates of approximately 18% to 51% and mortality rates of 4% to 13% have been reported [27]. Stricture recurrences of 10% to 30% are usual [28]. Endoscopic therapy, although not without

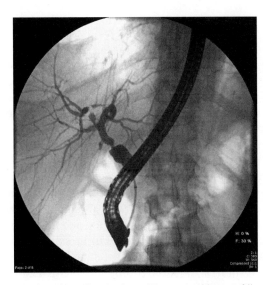

Fig. 3. Anastomotic stricture in a patient with a recent history of liver transplant.

drawbacks, enjoys significant advantage over orthodox surgery [29]. Being minimally invasive, it is less influenced by patient comorbidity.

The basic approach to strictures is to dilate and place stents to maintain patency over time. The expectation is that strictures will remodel in a patent configuration when healing takes place in the presence of stents. Once a stricture has been traversed with a guide-wire, it can be dilated with bilary dilating balloons or tapered passive plastic dilators in progressive dimensions. Balloon size for dilation is usually 1-mm to 2-mm larger than the downstream bile duct diameter. Clinical studies generally show that best outcomes are obtained when a larger number of stents are placed over a longer period of time. Ideally, two to four 10-F Amsterdam stents are placed after balloon dilation and are changed about every 3 months for a period of 1 year. With this approach, successful dilation has been reported in 74% to 90% of patients [27]. In a report by Bergman and colleagues [30], a group of 44 patients was followed for a median 9.1 years and recurrent stenosis developed in 20%, all occurring within 2 years of stent removal. Taking a more aggressive approach, Costamagna and colleagues [31] treated a group of 45 patients with increasing numbers of stents until complete disappearance of the biliary stricture in 89% was achieved. The mean number of stents used was 3.2 plus or minus 1.3 (range 1–6) with a mean follow-up of 48.8 months (range 2–11.3 years). There was no recurrence of symptoms caused by a relapsing stricture, although one patient sustained two episodes of cholangitis without stricture recurrence.

Endoscopic therapy is therefore an attractive alternative to orthodox surgery. All patients should be considered candidates for endoscopic management initially, except when there has been complete transection or ligation of the bile duct.

Stricture secondary to chronic pancreatitis

Strictures resulting from encasement of the distal bile duct by chronic pancreatitis are responsible for 10% of all common bile duct strictures. While they may be silent and only manifest themselves by abnormal liver tests, they can be responsible for serious morbidity [32]. Following an acute inflammatory relapse, a stricture may resolve spontaneously or after simple stenting. Dense fibrosis can make therapy and access difficult. A stricture often persists despite stenting and surgery may be needed. Surgery may be less than ideal because of comorbid illness, nutritional deficiency, associated liver disease, and thrombosis of the portal and splenic veins. Endoscopic therapeutic measures are therefore desirable alternatives despite limitations. Endoscopic therapy consists of balloon dilation and the use of single or multiple and serial stenting. Long-term studies using single stents show limited success, with only 10% to 28% of patients remaining free of obstruction after treatment [33,34]. In a 2004 study, subjects were treated with multiple simultaneous stents (group II) and compared with a group treated with single stents (group I). Treatment was for 14 and 12 months, respectively. Mean follow-up was for 4.2 years in group I and 3.9 years in group II. In group II, eight patients received four stents and four patients received five 10-F stents. Near normalization of biochemical tests of liver function was observed for all patients in group II, whereas only marginal benefit was noted in the single-stented patients. Four patients in group I had recurrent cholangitis, whereas none in group II had postprocedure cholangitis. In the patients with multiple stents, the distal common bile duct diameter increased from a mean of 1 mm to 3 mm after treatment; no change in diameter was observed in the single-stent group. The investigators concluded that multiple-stent therapy appears to be superior and may obviate the need for surgical diversion [39].

Biliary leaks

Biliary leaks are another disorder in which endoscopic therapy is very effective (Fig. 4). They occur in up to 1.1% of laparoscopic cholecystectomies and commonly (26% of cases) after cadaveric orthotopic liver transplantations [35]. The basic tenets of therapy are to percutaneously drain fluid collections (bilomas), to define the biliary anatomy, and to reduce the pressure gradient across the sphincter of Oddi, thereby providing preferential resistance free egress of the bile through the papilla of Vater [36]. Successful treatment has been achieved with numerous methods, including endoscopic sphincterotomy alone, endoscopic sphincterotomy and stent or nasal-biliary drain placement, and stent or nasal-biliary drain without preliminary endoscopic sphincterotomy. All methods have been effective in

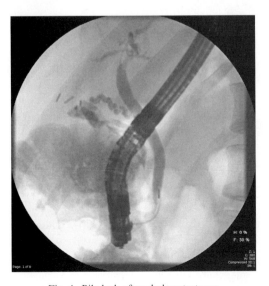

Fig. 4. Bile leak after cholecystectomy.

aiding closure of a fistula, but the ideal method has not been determined. In a recent large study from Toronto [37], the investigators classified bile leaks into low grade (leak identified only after intrahepatic opacification) or high grade (leak observed before intrahepatic opacification). Based on this distinction, low-grade leaks were treated with biliary sphincterotomy alone and high-grade leaks were treated with stent placement. Although the study was not randomized or controlled and the efficacy was not compared for sphincterotomy alone versus stent placement alone or stent placement with sphincterotomy, the value of a simplified system to guide therapy was confirmed.

Sclerosing cholangitis

Primary sclerosing cholangitis is a chronic cholestatic liver disease that is characterized by chronic inflammatory change and multiple fibrotic strictures of the intraheptic and extrahepatic biliary ducts (see Fig. 4; Fig. 5). The disease is progressive and results in liver cirrhosis and liver failure, and is complicated by cholangiocarcinoma in about 10% of cases. With the possible exception of ursodeoxycholic acid, there is no proven benefit of medical therapy. Orthotopic liver transplantation remains the only proven long-term treatment for primary sclerosing cholangitis and it is the fourth leading indication for liver transplantation in the United States [38]. Approximately 20% of patients with primary sclerosing cholangitis may have a dominant stricture during the course of their illness [39].

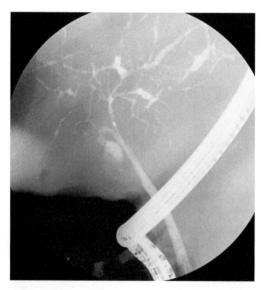

Fig. 5. Primary sclerosing cholangitis: diffuse strictures at the confluence, which are not amenable to endotherapy.

Clinically, these are suspected when there is significant worsening of laboratory parameters of cholestasis. Symptoms are pruritis, abdominal pain, fever, and chills (cholangitis). Surgical treatment for this complication is associated with substantial morbidity and mortality and increases the technical difficulty and risk of future liver transplantation [40]. Endoscopic biliary therapy, on the other hand, avoids the problems of surgery and published series have shown impressive success rates with therapeutic ERCP [38]. There is also evidence that endoscopic treatment has a favorable impact on survival [41].

The endoscopic therapy of primary sclerosing cholangitis consists of sphincterotomy, removal of stones, stricture dilation with balloons or graduated catheters, and placement of an endoprosthesis. Van Milligan deWit and colleagues [42] reviewed their experience with endotherapy following a policy of removing or changing stents electively after 2 to 3 months. They found it necessary to change stents sooner and attributable to occlusion in 50% of instances. In subsequent studies from the same unit [43], short-term stenting (1 week) was tested for symptomatic dominant strictures. Patients with a dominant stricture were treated with insertion of a 7-F or 10-F polyethylene endoprosthesis, which was extracted after a mean of 11 days (range 1–23 days). Short-term stenting was safe and effective and the beneficial effect was sustained for several years.

Malignant strictures

Malignant strictures of the bile duct arise from tumors within the duct or from extrinsic compression of the bile duct. Common causes of malignant strictures include ampullary carcinoma, pancreatic carcinoma, gallbladder carcinoma, cholangiocarcinoma, hepatocellular carcinoma, or metastases to the peri-hilar region or to the liver. Most of these patients present with painless jaundice. ERCP is indicated in patients that have pruritus or cholangitis.

The role of the ERCP is to obtain tissue and to relieve the obstruction. Tissue can be obtained through brushings and biopsy. Unfortunately, the yield of this tissue sampling is only 40% to 60% [44]. Harewood and colleagues [45] demonstrated that the yield was better when the pathologist was made aware of the clinical details. Dilating the stricture before brushing does not increase the yield of the cytology [46]. Fluoroscence in situ hybridization shows promising results to improve the sensitivity of CBD brushings [47]. EUS with fine needle aspiration has been shown to have a higher yield in certain pancreaticobiliary malignancies [48]. The EUS can be done at the time of the ERCP or as a separate procedure.

The next step is to relieve the obstruction. Plastic stents range in size from 7-F to 11.5-F in diameter with a variety of lengths. They are composed of Teflon, polyethylene, or polyurethane. The stents are straight, single pigtail, or double pigtail. There is a higher risk of stent occlusion if left in place for longer than 3 months. Stents become occluded because of the biofilm formation. The size of the stent is limited by the size of the accessory channel of the duodenoscope. For this reason, plastic stents are considered temporary. The alternative to plastic stents is self-expanding metal stents (SEMS). SEMS are used primarily for palliation of malignant biliary strictures. SEMS are available in larger diameters but are packaged in a small delivery device. Because of this larger diameter they have a longer duration of patency as compared with plastic stents. SEMS are more likely to become occluded by the ingrowth of tumor rather than biofilm. SEMS were compared with a plastic stent in a multicenter randomized study: the rate of stent occlusion was higher in the plastic stent group and those patients usually required more procedures [49].

When to choose plastic versus SEMS? In the authors' practice, if the diagnosis of malignancy is unclear, the patient will be having surgery, or the life expectancy is less than 6 months, then a plastic stent will be placed. This stent usually stays in place for about 3 months. Studies have shown that after 3 months the plastic stents seem to occlude. After the initial ERCP, most patients undergo more definitive treatment, such as surgery or chemoradiation. In patients that have surgery, the stent is removed at the time of the resection. If patients prove to have unresectable disease, then a more permanent stent is placed in the immediate postoperative time. In patients having chemoradiation, the stricture may decrease in size so a temporary stent is usually changed every three months. In patients not receiving further therapy, the stent may be exchanged for a more permanent stent immediately, left in place until it occludes, or changed every 3 months.

Distal common bile duct stricture

The most common cause of distal CBD strictures is pancreatic cancer (Fig. 6). Patients with lesions in the head of the pancreas most commonly present with painless jaundice. On cross-sectional imaging, they will have a dilated proximal CBD and dilated pancreatic duct, otherwise known as a "double duct" sign. In many cases, ERCP is the first procedure that will be done to relieve the obstruction and obtain a tissue diagnosis. ERCP has a sensitivity and specificity of 90% to 95% for diagnosing pancreatic cancer [50]. In some centers, an EUS and ERCP will be done in the same session. EUS can be helpful for staging and diagnosing pancreatic cancer. EUS is helpful to detect small (less than 2 cm) lesions as compared with CT and MRI scans [51]. EUS, CT, and MRI are complementary in regards to determining resectability [52]. EUS with fine needle aspiration has a sensitivity of 85% to 90% [53,54]. Biliary decompression is indicated for relief of pruritus and cholangitis. Patients generally feel better after the relief of jaundice [55,56]. Some oncologists and surgeons prefer relieving the

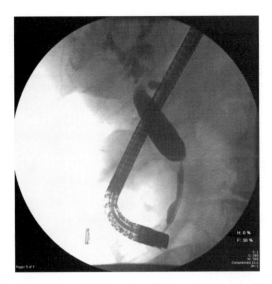

Fig. 6. Distal CBD stricture in the setting of a mass in the head of the pancreas.

obstruction before further treatment. In patients undergoing surgery within a short period of time, no benefit has been shown in relieving the biliary obstruction preoperatively [57]. The decision process of choosing plastic versus SEMS has previously been discussed. SEMS have been shown to be superior to plastic stents for the palliation of distal CBD strictures [49,58,59]. Covered stents were introduced to prevent tumor ingrowth. Multiple studies have been published that demonstrate minimal tumor ingrowth. The major concern is the higher rates of stent migration, cystic duct obstruction, and pancreatitis [60]. Covered stents are not recommended for use in hilar or intrahepatic ducts. Three prospective randomized studies compared surgical versus endoscopic palliation [61–63]. Ten French plastic stents were placed endoscopically; surgery was choledochojejunostomy, cholecystojejunostomy, or choledochoduodenstomy. Both methods were shown to effective for palliation. The endoscopic patients had fewer early complications and shorter hospitalizations but required more procedures as compared with surgery. The overall survival of the two groups did not differ. In a study of 66 patients with unresectable pancreatic cancer, endoscopic palliation proved to be more cost effective as compared with surgical bypass [64]. Surgery is considered in patients that do have not resectable disease at the time of exploratory laparoscopy or in patients with gastric outlet obstruction.

Proximal bile duct stricture

The majority of extrahepatic cholangiocarcinomas are located in the hilum (Fig. 7) [65]. Cholangiocarcinoma has a poor prognosis, and few

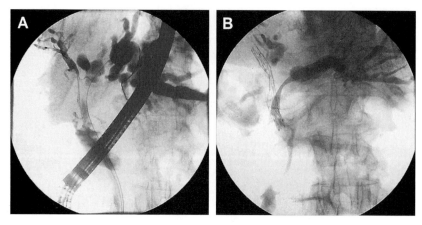

Fig. 7. Klatskin tumor. (A) Bilateral wire placement. (B) Bilateral SEMS placement.

patients are resectable at the time of diagnosis. Endoscopic palliation plays an important role in the management of these patients.

Endoscopic stenting of hilar strictures can be challenging. MRI scans are helpful for the diagnosis and staging of cholangiocarcinomas [66]. ERCP is useful for preoperative drainage and tissue diagnosis. Unfortunately, biliary cytology has a low yield because of the desmoplastic nature of the tumor. The use of brush biopsy and cytology increase the yield from 30% to between 40% and 70% [67]. Unilateral or bilateral stenting is dependent upon the location of the stricture and the degree of biliary contamination. About 25% to 33% of healthy liver needs to be drained to relieve jaundice. It is felt that stenting of one side should be adequate for palliation. In a prospective randomized trial, De Palma and colleagues [68] demonstrated a higher success rate of stent placement and drainage with a lower rate of early complications in the unilateral stent group. The patients in this analysis included Bismuth types I through III. Post-ERCP cholangitis may occur if contrast is injected into undrained segments. Antibiotics in the peri-procedure time may help to avoid this but most of these patients require bilateral stenting. Some physicians prefer an MRCP before attempt at ERCP to obtain a "road map." Hintze and colleagues [69] had 100% technical success in placement of a unilateral stent in 35 patients with Bismuth type III and IV tumors. Plastic or SEMS may be placed in the hilum. Many studies demonstrate the benefit in the placement of SEMS in palliation of distal CBD strictures. There are no large studies for the management of hilar strictures. A small, prospective randomized trial compared the use of bilateral SEMS and plastic stents for palliation of hilar cholangiocarcinoma [70]. Wallstents were placed in 9 patients and 11 patients received plastic stents. The Wallstent group had lower rates of cholangitis and fewer hospitalizations. The distal ends of the stent should be placed at the same level to reaccess the bile duct if needed in the future.

Photodynamic therapy

Photodynamic therapy (PDT) may be complementary to biliary stenting for palliation of locally advanced cholangiocarcinoma. A photosensitizer given to the patient accumulates in tumor tissue and is activated by light to cause tumor necrosis. A laser fiber with a cylindric light diffuser is placed across the stricture with fluoroscopic guidance. Ortner and colleagues [71] published the first randomized prospective study of PDT for nonresectable cholangiocarcinoma. Thirty-nine patients were enrolled in the study. One group received PDT and bilateral stenting and the other group received bilateral stenting alone. The study was terminated prematurely because of the encouraging results. The median survival of the PDT and stent group was 493 days as compared with 98 days for the stent group ($P < .0001$). Zoepf and colleagues [72] published similar encouraging results. Some centers encourage the use of PDT for nonresectable cholangiocarcinoma, given the low rate of adverse events.

Sphincter of Oddi dysfunction

Sphincter of Oddi dysfunction is a greatly debated topic among gastroenterologists. There are three types of SOD (Box 2) [73]. It is difficult to determine if there are three distinct entities or rather a condition at different stages or degree of severity. All three types consist of biliary-type pain. Most of the research has focused on the diagnosis and management of type I and type II SOD. Studies have shown that patients with type I SOD will benefit from an ERCP with sphincterotomy. Sphincter manometry is not necessary in this group [74]. Patients with type II SOD may benefit from a sphincterotomy, and these patients should have sphincter manometry.

Box 2. Geenen-Hogan classification of sphincter of Oddi dysfunction

Type I
Right upper quadrant (RUQ) pain and
Liver function tests elevated (AST and ALT 2× normal) and
Dilated CBD > 10 mm

Type II
RUQ pain and
Liver function tests elevated or
Dilated CBD > 10 mm

Type III
RUQ pain only

Geenan and colleagues [16] studied 47 patients with SOD type II. All patients had manometry and then the group was divided into those where
a sphincterotomy was performed and a sham group. The majority of patients that had documented elevated basal sphincter pressure (greater
than 40 mm Hg) and then had a sphincterotomy were clinically improved.
The benefit was seen in a 4-year follow-up. Toouli and colleagues [75] published similar findings. Patients with type III SOD have no significant benefit from sphincterotomy, and routine manometry is not recommended in
this group [74]. Larger studies are needed in this patient group. In earlier
studies of the management of SOD, there were reports of an increased
rate of post-ERCP pancreatitis [76]. It is now felt that the cause of the pancreatitis is not necessarily related to the manometry. Freeman and colleagues [77] recognized that there are certain patients, such as young,
female patients with small ducts, who have a higher incidence of post-
ERCP pancreatitis. Unfortunately, those characteristics are similar to those
patients with SOD.

Summary

Endoscopy now plays a major role in the diagnosis and therapy of biliary
disorders. Endoscopic retrograde cholangiopancreatography remains a risky
procedure. Risk is best reduced by strictly limiting its use, a strategy made
possible by newer accurate and safe imaging for diagnosis, such as MRI
and EUS.
Choledocholithiasis is ideally suited for endoscopic management. It is
doubtful that laparoscopic cholecystectomy would have enjoyed its appeal
without support of ERCP for bile duct problems. Strictures are treated endoscopically, with effectiveness equal to orthodox surgery but without the
substantial morbidity and mortality. Dominant strictures in sclerosing cholangitis are effectively diagnosed and treated endoscopically, while orthodox
surgery could be deleterious. Surgery, however, is the only hope for cure of
malignant biliary lesions. Unfortunately, many of these lesions are noncur-
able or found in patients unsuitable for surgery, and endoscopic methods
can usually provide effective palliation. Dysfunction of the sphincter of
Oddi remains controversial. Carefully studied and selected patients have
been shown to benefit from endoscopic sphincterotomy.

References

[1] Gupta K, Mallery S, Hunter D, et al. Endoscopic ultrasound and percutaneous access for
    endoscopic biliary and pancreatic drainage after initially failed ERCP. Rev Gastroenterol
    Disord 2007;7:22–37.
[2] Freeman ML. Adverse outcomes of endoscopic retrograde cholangiopancreatography:
    avoidance and management. Gastrointest Endosc Clin N Am 2003;13:775–98.

[3] Freeman ML, DiSario JA, Nelson DB, et al. Risk factors for post-ERCP pancreatitis: a prospective multicenter study. Gastrointest Endosc 2001;54:425–34.

[4] Masci E, Toti G, Mariani A, et al. Complications of diagnostic and therapeutic ERCP: a prospective multicenter study. Am J Gastroenterol 2001;96:417–23.

[5] Lieb JG II, Draganov PV. Early successes and late failures in the prevention of post endoscopic retrograde cholangiopancreatography pancreatitis. World J Gastroenterol 2007;13: 3567–74.

[6] Classen M, Demling L. Endoscopic sphincterotomy of the papilla of Vater and extraction of stones from the choledochal duct. Dtsch Med Wochenschr 1974;99:496–7.

[7] Kawai K, Akasaka Y, Murakami K, et al. Endoscopic sphincterotomy of the ampulla of Vater. Gastrointest Endosc 1974;20:148–51.

[8] Ko C, Lee S. Epidemiology and natural history of common bile duct stones and prediction of disease. Gastrointest Endosc 2002;56:S165–70.

[9] Sugiyama M, Atomi Y. Endoscopic ultrasonography for diagnosing choledocholithiasis: a prospective comparative study with ultrasonography and computed tomography. Gastrointest Endosc 1997;45(2):143–6.

[10] Kaltenthaler E, Vergel YB, Chilcott J, et al. A systematic review and economic evaluation of magnetic resonance cholangiopancreatography. Health Technol Assess 2004;8(10):iii, 1–89.

[11] Romagnuolo J, Bardou M, Rahme E, et al. Magnetic resonance cholangiopancreatography: a meta-analysis of test performance in suspected biliary disease. Ann Intern Med 2003; 139(7):547–57.

[12] Tse F, Liu L, Barkun AN, et al. EUS: a meta-analysis of test performance in suspected choledocholithiasis. Gastrointest Endosc 2008;67(2):235–44.

[13] Ang TL, Teo EK, Fock KM. Endosonography vs. endoscopic retrograde cholangiopancreatography-based strategies in the evaluation of suspected common bile duct stones in patients with normal transabdominal imaging. Aliment Pharmacol Ther 2007;26(8): 1163–70.

[14] NIH State of the Science statement on endoscopic retrograde cholangiopancreatography (ERCP) for diagnosis and therapy. NIH Consens State Sci Statements 2002; 19(1):1–26.

[15] Liu TH, Consorti ET, Kawashima A, et al. Patient evaluation and management with selective use of magnetic resonance cholangiography and endoscopic retrograde cholangiopancreatography before laparoscopic cholecystectomy. Ann Surg 2001;234:33–40.

[16] Geenan JE, Hogan WJ, Dodds WJ, et al. The efficacy of endoscopic sphincterotomy after cholecystectomy in patients with sphincter of Oddi dysfunction. N Engl J Med 1989;320: 82–7.

[17] Baron T, Harewood GC. Endoscopic balloon dilation of biliary sphincter compared to endoscopic biliary sphincterotomy for removal of common bile duct stones during ERCP: a metal-analysis of randomized, controlled trials. Am J Gastroenterol 2004;99:1455–60.

[18] DiSario JA, Freeman ML, Bjorkman DJ, et al. Endoscopic balloon dilation compared with sphincterotomy for extraction of bile duct stones. Gastroenterology 2004;127:1291–9.

[19] Tsujino T, Kawabe T, Komatsu H, et al. Endoscopic papillary balloon dilation for bile duct stones: immediate and long-term outcomes in 1000 patients. Clin Gastroenterol Hepatol 2007;5:130–7.

[20] Hintz R, Adler A, Veltzke W. Outcome of mechanical lithotripsy of bile duct stones in an unselected series of 704 patients. Hepatogastroenterology 1996;43:473–6.

[21] Garg PK, Randon RK, Ahuja V, et al. Predictors of unsuccessful mechanical lithotripsy and endoscopic clearance of large bile duct stones. Gastrointest Endosc 2004;59(6):601–5.

[22] Cipolletta L, Costamanga G, Bianco MA, et al. Endoscopic mechanical lithotripsy of difficult common bile duct stones. Br J Surg 1997;84(10):1407–9.

[23] Chen YK, Pleskow DK. SpyGlass single-operator peroral cholangiopancreatoscopy system for the diagnosis and therapy of bile-duct disorders: a clinical feasibility study. Gastrointest Endosc 2007;65(6):832–41.

[24] Bergman JJ, Rauws EA, Tijsses JG, et al. Biliary endoprosethesis in elderly patients with en-doscopically irretrievable common bile duct stones: report on 117 patients. Gastrointest En-dosc 1995;42(3):195–201.

[25] Boerma D, Rauws EA, Keulemans YC, et al. Wait and see policy or laparoscopic cholecys-tectomy after endoscopic sphincterotomy for bile duct stones: a randomized trial. Lancet 2002;360:761–5.

[26] MacFadyen BV Jr, Vecchio R, Ricardo AE, et al. Bile duct injury after laparoscopic chole-cystectomy. The United States experience. Surg Endosc 1998;12:315–21.

[27] Costamagna G, Shah SK, Tringali A, et al. Current management of postoperative compli-cations and benign biliary strictures. Gastrointest Endosc Clin N Am 2003;13:635–48.

[28] Kozarek RA. Endoscopic techniques in management of biliary tract injuries. Surg Clin North Am 1994;74:883–93.

[29] Heiss FW. Commentary: endoscopic techniques in management of biliary tract injuries. Surg Clin North Am 1994;74:895–6.

[30] Bergman J, Burgemeister L, Bruno M, et al. Long-term follow-up after biliary stent place-ment for postoperative bile duct stenosis. Gastrointest Endosc 2001;54:154–61.

[31] Costamagna G, Pandolfi M, Mutignani M, et al. Long-term results of endoscopic manage-ment of post-operative bile duct strictures with increasing numbers of stents. Gastrointest Endosc 2001;54:162–8.

[32] Warshaw AL, Schapiro RH, Ferrucci JT, et al. Persistent obstructive jaundice, cholangitis, and biliary cirrhosis due to common bile duct stenosis in chronic pancreatitis. Gastroenterol 1976;70:562–7.

[33] Judah JR, Draganov PV. Endoscopic therapy of benign biliary strictures. World J Gastro-enterol 2007;13:3531–9.

[34] Catalano MF, Lindor JD, George S, et al. Treatment of symptomatic distal common bile duct stenosis secondary to chronic pancreatititis: comparison of single vs. multiple simulta-neous stents. Gastrointest Endosc 2004;60:945–52.

[35] Shah JN. Endoscopic treatment of bile leaks: current standards and recent innovations. Gastrointest Endosc 2007;65:1069–72.

[36] Zyromski NJ, Lillemoe KD. Current management of biliary leaks. Adv Surg 2006;40:21–46.

[37] Sandha MB, Bourke MJ, Haber GB, et al. Endoscopic therapy for bile leak based on a new classification: results in 207 patients. Gastrointest Endosc 2004;60:567–74.

[38] Enns R, Eloubeidi MA, Mergener K, et al. Predictors of successful clinical and laboratory outcomes in patients with primary sclerosing cholangitis undergoing endoscopic retrograde cholangiopancreatography. Can J Gastroenterol 2003;17(4):243–8.

[39] May GR, Bender CE, LaRusso NF, et al. Non-operative dilation of dominant strictures in primary sclerosing cholangitis. Am J Roentgenol 1985;145:1061–4.

[40] Farges O, Malassagne B, Sebagh M, et al. Primary sclerosing cholangitis: liver transplanta-tion or biliary surgery. Surgery 1995;117:146–55.

[41] Baluyut AR, Sherman S, Lehman G, et al. Impact of endoscopic therapy on the survival of patients with primary sclerosing cholangitis. Gastrointest Endosc 2001;53:308–12.

[42] Van Milligen deWit AW, Van Bracht J, Rauws EA, et al. Endoscopic stent therapy for dominant extrahepatic bile duct strictures in primary sclerosing cholangitis. Gastrointest Endosc 1996;44(3):293–9.

[43] Ponsioen CY, Lam K, Van Milligen de Wit AW, et al. Four years experience with short term stenting in primary sclerosing cholangitis. Am J Gastroenterol 1999;94(9):2403–7.

[44] Pugliese V, Conio M, Nicolo G, et al. Endoscopic retrograde forceps biopsy and brush cytology of biliary strictures: a prospective study. Gastrointest Endosc 1995;42(6):520–6.

[45] Harewood GC, Baron TH, Stadheim LM, et al. Prospective, blinded assessment of factors influencing the accuracy of biliary cytology interpretation. Am J Gastroenterol 2004;99:1464–9.

[46] DeBellis M, Fogel EL, Sherman S, et al. Influence of stricture dilation and repeat brushing on the cancer detection rate of brush cytology in the evaluation of malignant biliary obstruction. Gastrointest Endosc 2003;58(2):176–82.

[47] Kipp BR, Stadheim LM, Halling SA, et al. A comparison of routine cytology and fluorescence in situ hybridization for the detection of malignant bile duct strictures. Am J Gastroenterol 2004;99:1675–81.

[48] Rosch T, Hofrichter K, Frimberger E, et al. ERCP or EUS for tissue diagnosis of biliary strictures? A prospective comparative study. Gastrointest Endosc 2004;60(3):390–6.

[49] Carr-Locke DL, Ball TJ, Connors PJ, et al. Mulitcenter randomized trial of Wallstent biliary endoprosthesis versus plastic stents. Gastrointest Endosc 1993;39:A310.

[50] Freeny PC. Radiologic diagnosis and staging of pancreatic ductal adenocarcinoma. Radiol Clin North Am 1989;27:121–8.

[51] Muller MR, Meyenberger C, Bertschinger P, et al. Pancreatic tumors: evaluation with endoscopic US, CT, and MR imaging. Radiology 1994;190:745–51.

[52] Soriano A, Castells A, Ayuso C, et al. Preoperative staging and tumor respectability assessment of pancreatic cancer: prospective study comparing endoscopic ultrasonography, helical computed tomography, magnetic resonance imaging, and angiography. Am J Gastroenterol 2004;99:492–501.

[53] Eloubeidi MA, Chen VK, Eltoum IA, et al. Endoscopic ultrasound-guided fine needle aspiration biopsy of patients with suspected pancreatic cancer: diagnostic accuracy and acute and 30-day complications. Am J Gastroenterol 2003;98:2663–8.

[54] Agarwal B, Abu-Hamda E, Molke KL, et al. Endoscopic ultrasound-guided fine needle aspiration and multidetector spring CT in the diagnosis of pancreatic cancer. Am J Gastroenterol 2004;99:844–50.

[55] Ballinger AB, McHugh M, Catnach SM, et al. Symptom relief and quality of life after stenting for malignant bile duct obstruction. Gut 1994;35:467–70.

[56] Abraham NS, Barkun JS, Barkun AN, et al. Palliation of malignant biliary obstruction: a prospective trail examining impact on quality of life. Gastrointest Endosc 2002;56:835–41.

[57] Saleh MM, Norregaard P, Jorgensen HL, et al. Preoperative endoscopic stent placement before pancreaticoduodenectomy: a meta-analysis of the effect on morbidity and mortality. Gastrointest Endosc 2002;56(4):529–34.

[58] Davids PH, Groen AK, Rauws EA, et al. Randomized trial of self-expanding metallic stents versus polyethylene stents for distal malignant biliary obstruction. Lancet 1992;340:1488–92.

[59] Knyrim K, Wagner HJ, Pausch J, et al. A prospective, randomized controlled trial of metal stents for malignant obstruction of the common bile duct. Endoscopy 1993;25:207–12.

[60] Kahaleh M, Tokar J, Conaway MR, et al. Efficacy and complications of covered Wallstents in malignant distal biliary obstruction. Gastrointest Endosc 2005;61:528–33.

[61] Shephard HA, Royale G, Ross AP, et al. Endoscopic biliary endoprosthesis in the palliation of malignant obstruction of the distal common bile duct: a randomized trial. Br J Surg 1988; 75:1166–8.

[62] Andersen JR, Sorensen SM, Kruse A, et al. Randomised trial of endoscopic endoprosthesis versus operative bypass in malignant obstructive jaundice. Gut 1989;30:1132–5.

[63] Smith AC, Dowsett JF, Russell RC, et al. Randomised trial of endoscopic stenting versus surgical bypass in malignant low bile duct obstruction. Lancet 1994;28:299–301.

[64] Raikar GV, Melin MM, Ress A, et al. Cost effective analysis of surgical palliation versus endoscopic stenting in the management of unresectable pancreatic cancer. Ann Surg Oncol 1996;3(5):470–5.

[65] Nakeeb A, Pitt HA, Sohn TA, et al. Cholangiocarcinoma: a spectrum of intrahepatic, perihilar, and distal tumors. Ann Surg 1996;224:463–73.

[66] Manfredi R, Barbaro B, Masselli G, et al. Magnetic resonance imaging of cholangiocarcinoma. Semin Liver Dis 2004;24:155–64.

[67] Khan SA, Davidson BR, Goldin R, et al. Guidelines for the diagnosis and treatment of cholangiocarcinoma: consensus document. Gut 2002;51(Suppl 6):V11–19.

[68] De Palma GD, Galloro G, Siciliano S, et al. Unilateral versus bilateral endoscopic hepatic duct drainage in patients with malignant hilar biliary obstruction: results of a prospective study, randomized, and controlled study. Gastrointest Endosc 2001;53:547–53.

[69] Hintze RE, Abou-Rebyeh H, Adler A, et al. Magnetic resonance cholangiopancreatography-guided unilateral endoscopic stent placement for Klatskin tumors. Gastrointest Endosc 2001;53:40–6.

[70] Wagner HJ, Knyrim K, Vakil N, et al. Plastic endoprostheses versus metal stents in the palliative treatment of malignant hilar biliary obstruction: a prospective and randomized trial. Endoscopy 1993;25:213–8.

[71] Ortner ME, Caca K, Berr F, et al. Successful photodynamic therapy for nonresectable cholangiocarcinoma: a randomized prospective study. Gastroenterology 2003;125:1355–63.

[72] Zoepf T, Jakobs R, Arnold JC, et al. Palliation of nonresectable bile duct cancer: improved survival after photodynamic therapy. Am J Gastroenterol 2005;100:2426–30.

[73] Hogan WJ, Geenan JE, Dodds WJ. Dysmotility disturbances of the biliary tract: classification, diagnosis and treatment. Semin Liver Dis 1987;7(4):302–10.

[74] Prajapati DN, Hogan WJ. Sphincter of Oddi dysfunction and other functional biliary disorders: evaluation and treatment. Gastroenterol Clin North Am 2003;32:601–18.

[75] Toouli J, Roberts-Thomson IC, Kellow J, et al. Manometry based randomized trial of endoscopic sphincterotomy for sphincter of Oddi dysfunction. Gut 2000;46:98–102.

[76] Sherman S, Ruffolo TA, Hawes RH, et al. Complications of endoscopic sphincterotomy. Gastroenterology 1991;101:1068–75.

[77] Freeman ML, Nelson DB, Sherman S, et al. Complications of endoscopic biliary sphincterotomy. N Engl J Med 1996;335(13):909–18.

ELSEVIER
SAUNDERS

SURGICAL
CLINICS OF
NORTH AMERICA

Surg Clin N Am 88 (2008) 1241–1252

Cholecystitis

David R. Elwood, MD

Surgical Associates of Marietta and Kennestone Hospital, 790 Church Street,
Suite 570, Marietta, GA 30060, USA

Overview

Cholecystitis in its varied forms is the most prevalent surgical entity afflicting populations of industrialized countries. The most common cause of cholecystitis and biliary colic is cholelithiasis. Autopsy findings show that 11% to 35% of American adults, or roughly 25 million people, have gallstones. Some 1% to 2% of people who have cholelithiasis develop symptoms or complications per year [1]. These complications include biliary colic, acute or chronic cholecystitis, choledocholithiasis, cholangitis, pancreatitis, and gallbladder carcinoma. It has been estimated that nearly 700,000 cholecystectomies are performed yearly in the United States. This article addresses the pathophysiology and clinical management of symptomatic cholelithiasis, acute calculous and acalculous cholecystitis, chronic cholecystitis, and complications of cholecystitis.

Symptomatic cholelithiasis: gallstones

Symptomatic cholelithiasis is defined as gallbladder pain in the presence of gallstones. Gallstones arise from the precipitation of cholesterol and calcium salts in supersaturated bile. They are classified by their content of cholesterol as either cholesterol stones or pigmented stones. Pigmented stones receive their color from their concentration of calcium bilirubinate. Black stones are small and tarry and are typically found associated with cirrhosis and hemolytic disorders, such as sickle cell disease and hereditary spherocytosis. Brown gallstones are more common in Asian populations and are associated with disorders of biliary motility and bacterial infection. In the United States, 70% to 80% of gallstones are of the cholesterol variety.

E-mail address: drelwood@gmail.com

0039-6109/08/$ - see front matter © 2008 Elsevier Inc. All rights reserved.
doi:10.1016/j.suc.2008.07.008   *surgical.theclinics.com*

Clinical manifestations and diagnosis

It is estimated that 20% of individuals who have gallstones have biliary colic. This term describes the constellation of symptoms experienced by a patient when the gallbladder contracts against an outlet obstruction, usually a gallstone lodged in the gallbladder neck or in the Hartman pouch. It is typically described as a sharp cramping pain localized to the right hypogastrium, often radiating to the right scapula or interscapular area. The symptoms commonly occur following large or fat-rich meals, and often at night when they awaken the patient from sleep. Associated symptoms include nausea, chills, malaise, bloating, belching, and occasionally diarrhea. Biliary colic is frequently indistinct or mild, limited to waves of nausea or gastric reflux symptoms. Uncomplicated biliary colic usually resolves spontaneously within 30 minutes to 6 hours, or with the administration of an analgesic. Nevertheless, once individuals begin to experience symptoms, the symptoms tend to become recurrent.

On physical examination, the patient may have localized right upper quadrant tenderness. Between episodes of biliary colic, however, the physical examination may be unimpressive and without tenderness. The workup for symptomatic cholelithiasis, particularly in the emergency room setting, oftentimes needs to exclude from the differential diagnosis angina, nephrolithiasis, pancreatitis, gastritis, and peptic ulcer disease. Laboratory studies, including leukocyte count, are generally normal. The transabdominal ultrasound of the right upper quadrant is the gold standard for diagnostic imaging. Although sensitive for identifying gallstones or sludge, ultrasound is limited by obesity, bowel gas, and operator skills. Gallbladder wall thickening or pericholecystic fluid suggests acute or chronic cholecystitis. Given that 20% of gallstones are radiopaque, some stones may occasionally be identified on CT scan or plain radiographs of the abdomen.

Treatment

Treatment of symptomatic cholelithiasis is electively scheduled routine laparoscopic cholecystectomy. An alternative approach described by some centers is the mini-cholecystectomy performed through a 5-cm midline incision [2]. Before surgery, the patient is advised to maintain a strictly low-fat diet and avoid heavy meals. Patients must also be counseled regarding the signs and symptoms that suggest progression to cholecystitis and the need for more urgent therapy.

Acute calculous cholecystitis

Pathophysiology

The primary cause of obstructive cholecystitis is gallstones. Of all individuals who have gallstones, 1% to 3% develop cholecystitis. Other causes of obstructive cholecystitis include primary tumors of the gallbladder or common duct, benign gallbladder polyps, parasites, metastatic tumors to the gallbladder or the periportal lymph nodes, and even foreign bodies, such as bullets [3–6]. Prolonged gallbladder outlet obstruction leads to acute cholecystitis. Obstruction at the neck of the gallbladder causes increased intraluminal pressure leading to venous congestion, compromised blood supply, and impaired lymphatic drainage. The mucosa becomes ischemic, releasing inflammatory mediators, such as prostaglandins I_2 and E_2. Localized mucosal trauma causes lysosome release of phospholipase, converting lecithin in the supersaturated bile to lysolecithin. Lecithin normally protects the mucosa against bile acids, but lysolecithin is a detergent and toxic to the mucosa. Wall thickening occurs with edema, vascular congestion, and intramural hemorrhage. Mucosal ulcers develop with focal areas of wall necrosis. Histologically, there is dense infiltration of neutrophilic leukocytes, microabscesses, and secondary vasculitis [7]. Eventually there may be secondary bacterial infection, accumulation of purulent fluid with the formation of an empyema, and perforation with widespread peritonitis with sepsis. Other complications of acute cholecystitis include hepatic abscess and intra-abdominal abscess.

Primary bacterial infection is not believed to play an initial role in cholecystitis, but secondary infection may complicate up to 50% of clinical courses. Some 40% to 50% of acute cholecystitis cases have been shown to have positive bile cultures. Bacteria that infect the bile include gram-negative bacilli (*Escherichia coli, Klebsiella* spp, *Enterobacter* spp), anaerobes (*Bacteroides, Clostridia* spp, *Fusobacterium* spp) and gram-positive cocci (enterococci) [8]. Overgrowth of gas-producing bacteria within the gallbladder can lead to emphysematous cholecystitis.

Clinical manifestations

The average patient presenting with acute cholecystitis ranges from 40 to 80 years old. Most men presenting with biliary colic present with acute cholecystitis. Because the incidence of stones in females is higher, however, overall there are more female patients who have acute cholecystitis. The female/male ratio is approximately 3:1.

Patients present with right upper quadrant or epigastric colic that either persists or escalates over 12 to 24 hours. Although it may be ameliorated by administration of analgesia, it does not typically resolve entirely. Commonly, patients have a history of more mild, sometimes escalating antecedent episodes of biliary colic. Other symptoms include chills, malaise, nausea, vomiting, and anorexia. The examiner must remember to question the patient about icteric orange-tea–colored urine or clay-colored stool, which would raise the suspicion of a common duct obstruction.

On physical examination, patients often have low- to moderate-grade fever, tachycardia, and marked right upper quadrant tenderness. Up to 25%

of patients have a palpable distended gallbladder. The classic Murphy sign, the abrupt inhibition of inspiration with palpation directly over the gallbladder fossa, is commonly seen. Abdominal wall guarding or rigidity must raise the suspicion of gangrenous cholecystitis or perforation.

Laboratory and radiologic diagnosis

Laboratory examination often demonstrates a mild to pronounced leukocytosis with left shift. The bilirubin, alkaline phosphatase, transaminases, and the amylase may be mildly elevated. A total bilirubin greater than 3 mg/dL should raise concerns for choledocholithiasis. Generally laboratory values are nonspecific, but they can be useful in ruling out alternative diagnoses, such as acute pancreatitis.

Plain films of the abdomen are of minimal value in diagnosing acute cholecystitis. In the global evaluation of the acute abdomen, however, plain films assist in ruling out intra-abdominal free air that can be seen with diverticulitis or a perforated peptic ulcer. Ultrasound of the right upper abdomen is sensitive and specific for the diagnosis of acute calculous cholecystitis. The identification of choleliths or sludge, wall thickening (>4 mm), or pericholecystic fluid all support the diagnosis of acute cholecystitis. The sonographic Murphy sign, which involves painful replication of the biliary colic and inhibition of inspiration by palpating the gallbladder in real time while visualizing it, is helpful in the diagnosis of cholecystitis. The measured common bile duct diameter is also important to consider. Although normal common bile duct caliber is often slightly increased in the elderly population, a diameter greater than 8 mm must raise concern over common duct obstruction. CT scan of the abdomen also demonstrates many of the radiologic features of cholecystitis, but is a much less sensitive and more time-consuming and expensive imaging modality.

The HIDA scan (99 m Tc-HIDA cholescintigraphy) is the most accurate test for cholecystitis, with a sensitivity of 97% and specificity of 87% [9]. The gallbladder is usually visualized within 30 minutes, and the absence of radiotracer uptake by 4 hours is considered positive for cystic duct occlusion. A prolonged fasting state diminishes the accuracy of the HIDA scan, and a false-positive rate of up to 40% has been seen after 5 days of non per os (NPO) status. Identification of radiotracer in the pericholecystic space indicates perforation. Generally, the HIDA scan is unnecessary in most cases of acute calculous cholecystitis given the availability of an ultrasound examination. Most practitioners reserve use of the HIDA scan for clinical situations in which there is diagnostic ambiguity. One example is the evaluation of incidental cholelithiasis and gallbladder wall thickening identified by ultrasound in a patient who does not have signs or symptoms of cholecystitis. A second example can occur during a sepsis evaluation in an obtunded or heavily sedated ICU patient who cannot provide an accurate history or physical examination. Third, patients who have hepatitis or cirrhosis commonly have abdominal complaints mimicking cholecystitis, and ultrasound findings of gallbladder wall edema, ascites, and gallbladder distension when fasting. In these patients, the HIDA scan can help to rule out cholecystitis, thereby avoiding consideration of cholecystectomy or unnecessary antibiotic treatment.

Treatment

Treatment of acute calculous cholecystitis commences with fluid resuscitation, making the patient NPO, providing analgesia, and initiating antibiotic therapy. The role of antibiotics in uncomplicated acute cholecystitis has not been fully determined when surgical treatment is completed in a timely fashion [8]. It is often difficult to clinically evaluate whether secondary bacterial infection has occurred, however, or whether the cholecystitis has evolved to gangrene and perforation. Broad-spectrum antibiotic coverage is therefore recommended. Commonly used regimens are ampicillin with gentamicin, ampicillin-sulbactam, piperacillin-tazobactam, a third- or fourth-generation cephalosporin, or a third-generation fluoroquinolone, such as moxifloxacin.

Laparoscopic cholecystectomy is currently the standard definitive management for acute calculous cholecystitis. It is well recognized to be more difficult in the acute setting, but with adequate experience it has been shown to be effective and safe [10]. Thickening of the gallbladder wall and friability can make the gallbladder difficult to grasp and limit the surgeon's ability to elevate the fundus or retract the infundibulum for exposure. Inflammation around the triangle of Calot can impair visualization of the ductal anatomy and the cystic artery. Conversion to an open cholecystectomy must be considered if there is any uncertainty about the anatomy before clipping or dividing ductal or arterial structures. Conversion to an open surgery must not be considered a failure and the possibility of conversion should be discussed preoperatively with the patient and included on the surgical permit.

Even during an open cholecystectomy, there may be such a dense inflammatory reaction at the base of the gallbladder as to preclude safe ligation of the cystic duct without endangering the portal structures. In these cases, one can consider performing a partial cholecystectomy, where a small portion of the gallbladder wall at the base is left behind. A permanent stitch can be carefully placed within the gallbladder to occlude the orifice of the cystic duct. The remnant mucosa is fulgurated and a surgical drain placed. If a postoperative bile leak occurs, an endoscopic retrograde cholangiopancreatography (ERCP) with common duct stent placement can be performed.

The timing of cholecystectomy for acute calculous cholecystitis has been a matter of much discussion in the literature. It is recognized that the presence of fever, marked leukocytosis, or diffuse abdominal tenderness portends possible necrosis, empyema, or rupture, and that emergent surgery within 12 to 24 hours is indicated. Patients who have diabetes often present later secondary to neuropathic impairment of pain sensation, and they have rapid disease progression and greater infectious complications [11]. These patients warrant early cholecystectomy. Similarly, urgent cholecystectomy for acute cholecystitis is indicated in the elderly and the immunocompromised, because they often present with vague, nonspecific symptoms and co-morbid medical conditions, and they have a higher incidence of complications [12].

Most patients who have uncomplicated acute cholecystitis can be treated supportively and scheduled for urgent cholecystectomy within 24 to 48 hours of presentation. Patients who undergo cholecystectomy within 48 hours of symptom onset have a 4% chance of conversion to an open proce-dure compared with a 23% chance of open cholecystectomy if surgery is de-layed [13]. It has been recognized that patients presenting with symptom duration greater that 72 hours have higher rates of complications and con-version to open cholecystectomy. The practice of treating patients with acute cholecystitis with antibiotics and then a planned interval cholecystec-tomy 4 to 8 weeks later with the hope of operating when the acute inflam-mation has abated is no longer supported. Of those patients treated with antibiotics with intention of doing an interval cholecystectomy, 20% to 30% will re-present and require urgent surgery during the interval period [14–16]. The conversion rate can still be as high as 30%, even with an inter-val cholecystectomy [17]. Delayed interval surgery does not reduce the mor-bidity or conversion rate, and it increases the overall hospital stay [18].

It is not infrequent that the surgeon is asked to evaluate a patient who has acute cholecystitis in the critical care setting with overwhelming medical co-morbidities that preclude safe surgical intervention. Often the cholecystitis is a major contributor to the patient's critical status. For the patient who is a poor surgical candidate, antibiotic and supportive care and percutaneous transhepatic cholecystostomy is adequate intervention. This procedure can be performed under local anesthesia with CT scan guidance or by ultrasound guidance at the bedside. For severe acute cholecystitis, percutaneous cholecys-tostomy is superior to gallbladder aspiration [19]. Eventually definitive treat-ment should be considered when possible; roughly half of patients reaccumulate gallstones within 5 years, even if all the gallstones are removed by cholecystostomy. If the patient's condition improves and he or she can tol-erate surgery later, interval cholecystectomy can be performed in 3 to 6 months.

Acute acalculous cholecystitis

Epidemiology

Acute inflammation of the gallbladder in the absence of cholelithiasis ac-counts for roughly 2% to 15% of acute cholecystitis cases and is the indica-tion for 1% to 2% of laparoscopic cholecystectomies. Risk factors include old age, critical illness, burns, trauma, major surgical operations, long-term total parenteral nutrition, diabetes, immunosuppression, and childbirth. Acute acalculous cholecystitis occurs in 0.2% of surgical intensive care admissions and has a mortality rate as high as 40% [20]. A higher proportion of patients who have acute acalculous cholecystitis are male. Children can be affected, especially after severe viral infections. Patients who have HIV and opportunistic infections, such as cytomegalovirus, cryptosporidium, *Mycobacterium tuberculosis*, *Mycobacterium avium intracellulare*, or mycotic infections, have been reported to develop acute acalculous cholecystitis. Complications, such as gangrene, empyema, and perforation, are more common with acalculous cholecystitis than with calculous cholecystitis. Deterioration of clinical status can be rapid.

Pathophysiology

The precise pathophysiology of acute acalculous cholecystitis remains poorly understood. Most known risk factors are associated with bile stasis within the gallbladder, leading to increased viscosity and the formation of sludge, which likely contributes to bacterial overgrowth. In elderly patients and patients on vasoconstrictor medications to support blood pressure, mucosal ischemia likely contributes to local inflammation and necrosis of the mucosal barrier. Histologically there are no specific differences between acute calculous and acalculous cholecystitis.

Clinical manifestations

Timely diagnosis of acute acalculous cholecystitis can be difficult and requires a high index of suspicion. Patients may present with biliary colic and fever, or they may have nonspecific or subtle complains, such as fatigue, indigestion, or nausea. Acalculous cholecystitis may be uncovered during an evaluation of fevers of unknown cause, especially in ICU patients for whom reliable physical examination is difficult. Laboratory findings are similar in acalculous and calculous cholecystitis. Ultrasound usually demonstrates gallbladder wall thickening and pericholecystic fluid, but no gallstones. It is difficult to interpret the findings of gallbladder wall edema or localized ascites in critically ill patients who have congestive heart failure, renal insufficiency, or hepatic disease, in which there is generalized anasarca. In these situations, the HIDA scan can be critical to determining the diagnosis. Often, however, the surgeon must rely on imperfect data and overall clinical impression.

Treatment

Treatment of acute acalculous cholecystitis is similar to that of calculous cholecystitis; supportive care, antibiotics, and emergent laparoscopic cholecystectomy. With acalculous cholecystitis, however, a greater proportion of patients are too ill to undergo anesthesia and surgery. In these situations, percutaneous transhepatic cholecystostomy is advised. Ninety percent of these patients demonstrate clinical improvement [21]. Once the patient has recovered, the cholecystostomy tube can be removed without sequelae, as long as there is confirmation that the gallbladder contains no stones. Interval cholecystectomy is not necessary.

Although mentioned earlier as a possible complication of calculous cholecystitis, emphysematous cholecystitis most often occurs in the absence of gallstones. Men are affected three times as often as women, and it typically occurs in patients who have diabetes mellitus and are between 50 and 80 years of age [7]. Small vessel occlusive disease involving the cystic artery is believed to be a major contributing factor. Nearly half of bile cultures from these patients contain *Clostridia welchii*. The gallbladder characteristically contains malodorous gas and purulent bile. CT scan, and occasionally abdominal plain films, demonstrates gas within the gallbladder and gallbladder wall pneumatosis. Emergency intervention is indicated. Emphysematous cholecystitis can lead to rapid clinical deterioration with mortality as high as 15% because of gangrene or perforation.

Chronic cholecystitis

Pathophysiology

Chronic inflammation of the gallbladder is the indication for nearly 3% of cholecystectomies in adults. Chronic cholecystitis has many forms and the pathophysiology is poorly understood. It is believed that in most instances an evolving inflammatory process occurs with repeated episodes of low-grade gallbladder obstruction, resulting in recurrent mucosal trauma [7]. There is little correlation between the number of choleliths or their overall volume and the degree of gallbladder wall inflammation. In fact, 12% to 13% of patients who have chronic cholecystitis have no demonstrable stones. Bacterial infection of the bile does not seem to play a role; less than one third of bile cultures contain *E coli* or enterococci. As each episode of acute inflammation resolves, neutrophilic infiltration is replaced with lymphocytes, plasma cells, macrophages, and eosinophils. Focal ulcerations and necrotic tissue are replaced by granulation tissue and collagen deposits. The gallbladder wall may become thickened or remain thin. The mucosa can remain intact, develop accentuated folds, or be flattened.

Particular mention should be made of several specific forms of chronic cholecystitis. Chronic obstruction by stones, tumor, fibrosis, or external compression of the cystic duct can lead to hydrops, wherein the gallbladder becomes markedly distended and the bile replaced with a clear or mucoid fluid. Gallbladder hydrops occurs in 3% of gallbladders removed in adults. When lymphocyte proliferation leads to the formation of prominent lymphoid follicles in the wall, the term "follicular cholecystitis" is applied. Xanthogranulomatous cholecystitis is found in 1.8% of removed gallbladders, wherein the gallbladder wall contains poorly demarcated firm yellow masses that are histologically characterized by focal infiltrates of foamy histiocytes, plasma cells, lymphocytes, and fibrosis. Last, when there is chronic penetration of bile through ulcers or fissures in the mucosa into the subepithelium of the gallbladder wall, chronic scarification and deposition of dystrophic calcifications give the gallbladder a firm rock-hard quality. The phenomenon, called porcelain gallbladder, is associated with an increased risk for gallbladder carcinoma.

Clinical manifestations

The symptoms of chronic cholecystitis vary from classic severe biliary colic to vague or nonspecific complaints. Patients may report only intermittent episodes of nausea, reflux symptoms, food intolerance, or bloating. Symptoms may be as subtle as low-grade fever, mild upper abdominal discomfort, or chronic fatigue. Not infrequently patients who have chronic cholecystitis have been treated for gastritis, ulcer disease, or irritable bowel syndrome without appreciable improvement in their complaints.

The evaluation for chronic cholecystitis usually occurs in the outpatient or urgent care setting, often initiated by the primary care physician or gastroenterologist. The physical examination is typically unremarkable except when there is massive distension of the gallbladder associated with hydrops or a hard mass in the right upper quadrant associated with porcelain gallbladder. Specific laboratory abnormalities are unusual and ultrasound may show cholelithiasis with or without wall thickening. Dystrophic calcification of the gallbladder is well demonstrated by CT scan. Many patients are taken to the operating room with a diagnosis of symptomatic cholelithiasis only to find histologic evidence for chronic cholecystitis on pathologic examination. In cases with inconclusive constellations of symptoms and lack of objective studies to implicate the gallbladder, a cholescintigraphy study with cholecystokinin challenge, or emptying study, can help to identify biliary dyskinesia. Most patients diagnosed with significant biliary dysmotility experience symptomatic relief with cholecystectomy. There are frequently histopathologic changes of chronic inflammation present in these specimens. It remains uncertain whether impaired gallbladder emptying leads to chronic inflammation or vice versa. When the diagnosis is not straightforward, it is recommended to consider endoscopic gastroduodenoscopy, colonoscopy, CT scan, and in some instances, cardiology evaluation before scheduling a patient for cholecystectomy to exclude other causes, such as peptic ulcer disease, angina, tumor, or pancreatitis.

Two complications of cholecystitis: Mirizzi syndrome and gallstone ileus

Two clinical entities result from long-term inflammation of the gallbladder and deserve mention in a discussion of cholecystitis: Mirizzi syndrome and gallstone ileus.

Mirizzi syndrome

Mirizzi syndrome is the partial obstruction of the common hepatic bile duct secondary to stone impaction and chronic inflammation in the adjacent gallbladder Hartman pouch. This inflammatory process can evolve into an erosive fistula to the anterior or lateral wall of the duct. The Csendes classification stratifies the degree of injury, from type I or simple external compression of the common hepatic duct, to type IV, or complete destruction of the entire wall of the duct [22]. Hepatic duct involvement by inflammation has been demonstrated to be present in 0.3% to 3% of patients undergoing cholecystectomy. It is only diagnosed preoperatively in 8% to 62.5% of cases. Mirizzi syndrome can lead to an increased risk for bile duct injury during cholecystectomy (up to 22.2%) and to an increased risk for conversion to open cholecystectomy. Preoperatively, ultrasound imaging may show a large immovable stone in the neck of a contracted gallbladder and proximal biliary dilatation. On CT scan there may be an irregular cavity near the neck of the gallbladder with stones outside of the lumen. ERCP, MRCP, or percutaneous transhepatic cholangiography can usually delineate the cause and level of a fistula.

Open cholecystectomy is the standard surgical approach to repair in Mirizzi syndrome. If no fistula is present, a subtotal cholecystectomy is adequate. With a small fistula (type II), a subtotal cholecystectomy can be performed and a T tube inserted into the fistula, closing the gallbladder remnant around the tube. For larger fistulae (types III and IV), the standard treatment is hepaticojejunostomy. In 6% to 27.8% of patients determined to have Mirizzi syndrome preoperatively, carcinoma of the gallbladder was the final diagnosis [23]. Frozen section histology should be performed intraoperatively in all cases of Mirizzi syndrome and preoperative preparations made for possible radical cholecystectomy.

Gallstone ileus

The second clinical entity, gallstone ileus, occurs after the gallbladder has spontaneously fistulized to the bowel. Gallstones may then pass directly into the gastrointestinal tract, and if large enough, cause a mechanical obstruction. In 68% of cases the fistula is a cholecystoduodenal fistula, in 5 % cholecystocolonic, and in 5% cholecystoduodenocolonic [24]. Typically the obstruction occurs at the narrow ileocecal junction. The term Bouveret syndrome is applied when the stone enters and obstructs the duodenum, creating a gastric outlet obstruction.

Gallstone ileus accounts for 1% of all small bowel obstructions. It is implicated in 25% of patients older than the age of 65 years when obstruction is not attributable to adhesive disease or hernias [25]. Most of the patients have no known history of cholecystitis. The diagnosis can be made preoperatively 73% of the time. Findings on plain abdominal films include dilated loops of small bowel consistent with obstruction, and in 40% of cases, intrabiliary gas. The latter finding is pathologic in any patient who has not had common duct instrumentation or a choledochoenterostomy. Unless the passed stone contains significant calcium, it is not appreciable on plain films or CT scan. In addition to intrabiliary gas, CT scan may demonstrate a small contracted gallbladder and a short bezoar at the obstruction transition point.

At laparotomy, the obstructing cholelith is identified by manual inspection of the bowel. It is extracted by way of a transverse enterotomy or by performing a small bowel resection if there is evidence for pressure necrosis of the bowel wall. Care must be taken in searching for additional stones proximally, because in 16% of cases there is more than one stone. Missing a second intraluminal cholelith risks a recurrent obstruction in the immediate postoperative period.

Considerable debate in the literature has focused on the appropriate approach to treatment of the cholecystenteric fistula. Several reports describe chronic cholecystitis or cholangitis if the fistula is left intact. Others have found that the fistula can close spontaneously. Typically there is a dense cicatrix involving the contracted and shriveled gallbladder and the involved bowel. There is appreciable risk for ductal injury, and the need to repair a defect in the duodenum or colon in a setting of acute or chronic inflammation. A single-staged procedure to treat the acute bowel obstruction and the fistula is feasible if the patient is stable and able to tolerate an extended operation. In one study, the associated mortality was 16.9%. Only 10% of patients who had the gallbladder left in place had continued biliary symptoms and the recurrence of gallstone ileus was less than 5%. If no large choleliths are palpable in the gallbladder fossa at the time of initial exploration for obstruction, it is safe to leave the fistula and decide future surgical intervention based on the patient's clinical course.

Summary

Rather than a single clinical entity, cholecystitis is a class of related disease states with different causes, degrees of severity, clinical courses, and management strategies. Appropriate care of the patient who has a diseased gallbladder requires a broad understanding of the acute, chronic, and acalculous cholecystitis syndromes, and awareness of their particular clinical nuances and potential complications.

References

[1] Glasgow RE, Cho M, Hutter MM, et al. The spectrum and cost of complicated gallstone disease in California. Arch Surg 2000;135:1021–5.
[2] O'Dwyer PJ, Murphy JJ, O'Higgins NJ. Cholecystectomy through a 5 cm incision. Br J Surg 1990;77:1189–90.
[3] Kuzu MA, Ozturk Y, Ozbek H, et al. Acalculous cholecystitis: ascariasis as an unusual cause. J Gastroenterol 1996;31(5):747–9.

[4] Langley RG, Bailey EM, Sober AJ. Acute cholecystitis from metastatic melanoma to the gall-bladder in a patient with a low-risk melanoma. Br J Dermatol 1997;136(2):279–82.

[5] Petersen JM, Knight TT. Gunshot cholecystitis. J Clin Gastroenterol 1995;21(4):320–2.

[6] Cappell MS, Marks M, Kirschenbaum H. Massive hemobilia and acalculous cholecystitis due to benign gallbladder polyp. Dig Dis Sci 1993;38(6):1156–61.

[7] Jessurun J, Albores-Saavedra J. Gallbladder and extrahepatic biliary ducts. In: Damjanov I, Linder J, editors. Anderson's pathology. 10th edition. St. Louis (MO): Mosby; 1996. p. 1959–90.

[8] Johannsen EC, Madoff LC. Infections of the liver and biliary system. In: Mandell GL, Bennett JE, Dolin R, editors. Principles of practice of infectious diseases. 6th edition. Philadelphia: Elsevier; 2005. p. 951–8.

[9] Ralls PW, Coletti PM, Halls JM, et al. Prospective evaluation of 99m TC-IDA cholescintigraphy in the diagnosis of acute cholecystitis. Radiology 1982;144:369–71.

[10] Kiviluoto T, Siren J, Luukkonen P, et al. Randomised trial of laparoscopic versus open cholecystectomy for acute and gangrenous cholecystitis. Lancet 1998;351(9099):321–5.

[11] Ikard RW. Gallstones, cholecystitis and diabetes. Surg Gynecol Obstet 1990;171(6):528–32.

[12] Tagle FM, Lavergne J, Barkin JS, et al. Laparoscopic cholecystectomy in the elderly. Surg Endosc 1997;11:636–8.

[13] Willsher PC, Sanabria JR, Gallinger S, et al. Early laparoscopic cholecystectomy for acute cholecystitis: a safe procedure. J Gastrointest Surg 1999;3:50–3.

[14] Lau H, Brooks DC. Transitions in laparoscopic cholecystectomy: the impact of ambulatory surgery. Surg Endosc 2002;16:323–6.

[15] Calland JF, Tanaka K, Foley E, et al. Outpatient laparoscopic cholecystectomy: patient outcomes after implementation of a clinical pathway. Ann Surg 2001;233:704–15.

[16] Papi C, Catarci M, D'Ambrosio L, et al. Timing of cholecystectomy for acute calculous cholecystitis: a meta-analysis. Am J Gastroenterol 2004;99(1):147–55.

[17] Lo CM, Liu CL, Fan ST, et al. Prospective randomized study of early versus delayed laparoscopic cholecystectomy for acute cholecystitis. Ann Surg 1998;227:461–7.

[18] Lai PB, Kwong KH, Leung KL, et al. Randomized trial of early versus delayed laparoscopic cholecystectomy for acute cholecystitis. Br J Surg 1998;85:764–7.

[19] Ito K, Fujita N, Noda Y, et al. Percutaneous cholecystostomy versus gallbladder aspiration for acute cholecystitis: a prospective randomized controlled trial. Am J Roentgenol 2004; 183(1):193–6.

[20] Kalliafas S, Ziegler DW, Flancbaum L, et al. Acute acalculous cholecystitis, risk factors, diagnosis and outcome. Am Surg 1998;64:471–5.

[21] Barie PS, Eachempati SR. Acute acalculous cholecystitis. Curr Gastroenterol Rep 2003;5(4): 302–9.

[22] Csendes A, Diaz JC, Burdiles P, et al. Mirizzi syndrome and cholecystobiliary fistula: a unifying classification. Br J Surg 1989;76:1139–43.

[23] Lai EC, Lau WY. Mirizzi syndrome: history, present and future development. Aust N Z J Surg 2006;76(4):251–7.

[24] Clavien PA, Richon J, Burgan S, et al. Gallstone ileus. Br J Surg 1990;77(7):737–42.

[25] Reisner RM, Cohen JR. Gallstone ileus: a review of 1001 reported cases. Am Surg 1994; 60(6):441–6.

SURGICAL
CLINICS OF
NORTH AMERICA

Surg Clin N Am 88 (2008) 1253–1272

Biliary Dyskinesia

Melina C. Vassiliou, MD, MEd,
William S. Laycock, MD, MSc*

*Department of General Surgery, Division of Minimally Invasive Surgery,
Dartmouth-Hitchcock Medical Center, One Medical Center Drive, Lebanon, NH 03756, USA*

The flow of bile through the biliary system is a complex process that depends on the hormonal environment, digestive phase, and functional response of the gallbladder and sphincter of Oddi to all of these factors. This article reviews functional causes of biliary pain, also referred to as biliary dyskinesia, of which there are three types. Gallbladder dyskinesia (GBD) is described as typical biliary pain in the absence of gallstones and is currently diagnosed by the demonstration of abnormal gallbladder emptying. There is some debate about the best method to establish the diagnosis and whether or not ejection fraction is an accurate predictor of outcome. GBD is effectively treated by laparoscopic cholecystectomy. Sphincter of Oddi dysfunction (SOD) can be either biliary or pancreatic and is further classified into types I to III based on diagnostic criteria. These criteria help to establish guidelines for evaluation, treatment, and prognosis of these disorders. In recent years, there has been a shift toward less invasive diagnostic methods to minimize endoscopic retrograde cholangiopancreatography (ERCP)–related complications. The current gold standard for diagnosis of SOD is sphincter of Oddi manometry (SOM), and the most popular treatment is endoscopic sphincterotomy.

Gallbladder dyskinesia

Epidemiology

GBD has been referred to as gallbladder spasm, cystic duct syndrome, and chronic acalculous cholecystitis [1]. It refers to the clinical entity of right upper quadrant pain or symptoms of biliary colic in the absence of

---

* Corresponding author.
E-mail address: william.s.laycock@hitchcock.org (W.S. Laycock).

0039-6109/08/$ - see front matter © 2008 Elsevier Inc. All rights reserved.
doi:10.1016/j.suc.2008.07.004   *surgical.theclinics.com*

gallstones or sludge. The true prevalence of this disorder is unknown. A large epidemiologic study estimated the prevalence of biliary pain without stones to be about 2.4% [2]. Another Italian study using ultrasound screening detected biliary pain without stones in 7.6% of men [3] and up to 20.7% of women [4]. The pathophysiology of functional gallbladder pain is not completely understood, but the most widely accepted theory is one of abnormal motility of the gallbladder in response to usual stimuli. The concept of biliary pain is also subject to interpretation by clinicians because many of the symptoms can overlap with other gastrointestinal disorders, such as peptic ulcer disease, irritable bowel, or other functional disorders [5].

Diagnostic criteria

The vague nature of functional gastrointestinal disorders prompted the development of the Rome Criteria. In 1994, a group of international investigators developed a classification system for functional gastrointestinal disorders in an attempt to provide a common foundation from which to do research and deliver patient care [6]. The criteria have most recently been updated for the second time in 2006 and are listed for GBD in Box 1 [7].

Box 1. Functional gallbladder and sphincter of Oddi dysfunction—Rome III criteria

Episodes of right upper quadrant or epigastric pain and all of the following:
Pain lasts 30 minutes or longer
Recurrent symptoms occurring at different intervals (not daily)
The pain builds up to a steady level
The pain is moderate to severe enough to interrupt the patient's daily activities or lead to an emergency department visit
The pain is not relieved by bowel movements, postural change, or antacids
Other structural disease that would explain the symptoms is excluded

Supportive criteria
Pain with one or more of the following: nausea and vomiting, radiation to the back or right subscapular area, awakening from sleep related to pain

Functional gallbladder disorder
Fulfills criteria above
Gallbladder present
Normal liver enzymes, conjugated bilirubin, and amylase/lipase

---

The Rome Committee also proposed three criteria after treatment to confirm GBD in long-term follow-up studies. These include absence of sludge, stones, or microlithiasis, abnormal ejection fraction (EF) (less than 40%) after a continuous infusion of cholecystokinin over 30 minutes, and a positive therapeutic response with absence of recurrent pain for longer than 12 months [8].

Physiology and pathophysiology

Functional biliary pain with an intact gallbladder is most often attributed to abnormal gallbladder motility or obstruction at the cystic duct [9]. The true pathophysiology of this disorder remains elusive and it may represent a constellation of biliary disorders that present similarly. Different hypotheses have been proposed to explain GBD, such as visceral hyperalgesia or functional disorders of surrounding structures, including the sphincter of Oddi. Gastric and other intestinal motility disorders have been associated with decreased gallbladder emptying [10] in addition to other conditions, such as pregnancy, diabetes, obesity, and cirrhosis. Medications, including atropine, morphine, octreotide, nifedipine, and progesterone, can also impair gallbladder emptying [11].

The muscular layer of the gallbladder is longitudinal in the body and around a circular axis about the neck. The gallbladder contracts in response to various stimuli, the most well known being cholecystokinin (CCK). Bile flows in and out of the cystic duct, depending on the digestive phase, and sometimes the contractions are not propulsive suggesting that there may be a "mixing" effect to prevent stasis [12]. Overall, bile is stored between meals and is emptied during the digestive phase. In the normal GB, the continued infusion of CCK causes emptying of most of the bile contained in the organ, about 20 to 30 mL.

Although stasis is a well-known player in the pathogenesis of gallstones, most patients clinically diagnosed with GBD do not have stones at the time of surgery. Small series have reported stones in 5% to 15% of patients [13–15] who have cholesterolosis observed in approximately one quarter of patients who have GBD [16]. Velanovich [17] sampled the bile of patients who had clinical GBD and a gallbladder ejection fraction (GBEF) of less than 35% and compared the presence of crystals in bile or in the gallbladder wall on pathology with patients undergoing surgery for known stones. They found no differences between the two groups, and both groups had similar evidence of chronic cholecystitis. The authors proposed that acalculous biliary disease is along the spectrum of calculous disease and suggested that eventually these patients would go on to develop stones. Some authors have also argued that the presence of cholesterolosis itself may impair gallbladder motility, and not the other way around. Neither of these theories has been proved.

Evaluation of patients who have suspected gallbladder dyskinesia

In patients who present with biliary pain, the more common causes, such as gallstone disease, should be ruled out. A transabdominal ultrasound, liver panel, and pancreatic enzymes should be obtained. In the absence of gallstones, upper endoscopy is recommended before proceeding with other tests [18]. Transabdominal ultrasound can detect stones larger than 3 to 5 mm in diameter [19].

Endoscopic ultrasound and biliary sampling

If these tests do not reveal a cause for the pain, additional, more specific testing can be performed. Analysis of a bile sample or endoscopic ultrasound (EUS) for microlithiasis are options. Dahan and colleagues [20] prospectively evaluated 45 patients who had normal transabdominal ultrasounds, but suspicious biliary pain, for microlithiasis using EUS and microscopic examination of duodenal bile. EUS was more sensitive (96%) than bile examination (67%), and they had similar specificities (86% and 91%, respectively). They also noted that none of the 16 patients who had both negative bile and EUS had stones. More recently, Thorboli and colleagues [21] used EUS alone to prospectively investigate 35 patients who had negative abdominal ultrasounds. Stones were detected in 52.4% and confirmed on postoperative pathology in 87% of patients. For microscopic examination, the bile sample must be obtained from direct cannulation during ERCP or after CCK stimulation during endoscopy making this a cumbersome and impractical investigation. Because EUS may not be readily available in many centers and ERCP is invasive, these tests are not routinely recommended. After initial blood work, transabdominal ultrasound, and upper endoscopy, if the symptoms warrant it, the next investigation in the algorithm is CCK-stimulated cholescintigraphy (CCK-CS).

Cholecystokinin

CCK is a polypeptide secreted by the duodenal mucosa in response to a meal, particularly one containing fat. Its numerous effects include contraction of the gallbladder, relaxation of the sphincter of Oddi, contraction of the pylorus, inhibition of gastric emptying, and relaxation of the lower esophageal sphincter. It also serves as a stimulus for increased secretion of hepatic bile and pancreatic enzymes [22]. CCK has been used in other clinical tests to assist in the diagnosis of acalculous biliary pain, but the least invasive and most reproducible examination remains cholescintigraphy.

Pain provocation with cholecystokinin

The CCK provocation test involves infusion of CCK and is considered positive if the patient reports reproduction of the right upper quadrant symptoms they initially consulted for. This test is fraught with bias and pain is a subjective outcome, despite attempts by some groups to use objective pain scores. In addition, the accuracy is compromised because CCK stimulates other organs that may contribute to the pain. Overall, the literature does not show this test to be useful in selecting patients who will benefit from cholecystectomy and it has essentially been abandoned [23].

Volume changes assessed by ultrasound after cholecystokinin infusion

This method has not been widely used in the evaluation of patients who have suspected abnormal gallbladder motility. It consists of measurement of gallbladder volume using real-time ultrasound in the fasting state and after CCK infusion. There may be a role for this in selected patients, but the results are operator dependent and the technique has not been subjected to randomized controlled studies [18].

Hepatobiliary iminodiacetic acid cholecystokinin cholescintigraphy

This procedure uses the radioactive biomarker technetium 99m–labeled iminodiacetic acid to calculate GBEF after the infusion of a CCK bolus [24]. Although this test has become the standard test to establish the diagnosis of GBD, there has been considerable variability in the literature regarding the optimal technique. The variability exists in whether sincalide (the only commercially available CCK analog available in the United States) or a fatty meal was used, how much was used, over how long it was infused, and what was defined as abnormal. The corollary of this is that there are inconsistencies in the literature regarding the value of this test in selecting patients who will respond to surgery. The current "definition" of what constitutes an abnormal EF is based on a small study of 40 asymptomatic volunteers who underwent CCK-CS (infusion of CCK over 45 minutes). The mean EF was 74.5% ± 12.2% and thus the pathologic EF was arbitrarily set at 40% (3 SD below the mean) [9]. In the original description by Krishnamurthy, the GBEF in the 6 asymptomatic patients who were studied ranged from 0 to 78% [24]. Furthermore, in one report, 35% of normal volunteers had an EF less than 35% [25]. For a thorough review of the various doses of CCK, the durations of infusion, and the different cutoff criteria for abnormal emptying, see Rastogi and colleagues [1]. In summary, the most reliable and physiologic method, proposed by Ziessman [22], involves an infusion of 0.02 μg/kg of sincalide in 30 mL infused over 30 minutes performed in patients who have been fasting for 3 to 4 hours.

Does gallbladder ejection fraction predict success?

Despite these differences in technique, there are myriad reports in the literature providing evidence for the usefulness of CCK-HIDA in confirming GBD and predicting successful therapy [9,13,15,26–32]. The two most convincing studies published to date were both published in 1991. The first by

Yap and colleagues [9] was mentioned earlier with regard to establishment of normal gallbladder emptying. The second part of their study consisted of a prospective evaluation of 21 patients who had GBEF less than 40% randomly assigned to open cholecystectomy or observation. Ninety-one percent of treated patients had resolution of their symptoms and more than 90% had histologic evidence of chronic cholecystitis. All of the patients in the observation group remained symptomatic and 2 eventually underwent cholecystectomy. The second study by Fink-Bennett and colleagues [28] was a retrospective review of 374 patients who underwent CCK-CS for recurrent biliary pain in the absence of stones. One hundred and eight of 115 (94%) patients who had abnormal EF who underwent cholecystectomy had pathologic findings postoperatively. Of those 108 patients, only 1 was not improved and 2 were lost to follow-up. Among the patients treated medically, 88% who had abnormal EFs remained symptomatic. The false-negative rate of CCK-CS in this study was 6% [28].

There are, nonetheless, several studies, including two reviews, that do not confirm these findings and call for more rigorous establishment of technique and the conduction of randomized trials [16,23,33–38]. In their 2003 review, DiBaise and Oleynikov [34] commented on 23 publications that met their inclusion criteria, and considered all the studies to be of poor methodologic quality. There were only 3 studies that were not retrospective case series, of which 2 were prospective and 1 was randomized. Overall, 19 of those studies found the GBEF to be a useful predictor of successful outcome in patients who had acalculous biliary pain. The authors concluded, however, that there is a paucity of quality evidence to provide definitive recommendations about the value of CCK-CS in the diagnosis and management of GBD.

A meta-analysis on this topic was also published in 2003. Only nine studies met the criteria, totaling 974 patients who had functional biliary pain, of whom 362 underwent cholecystectomy [35]. The method of CCK-CS varied from infusion rates of 30 to 45 minutes in three studies to 2 to 3 minutes in the remaining six studies. The EF cutoff was less than 50 in three studies, less than 40 in one, and less the 35 in the rest. Mean follow-up ranged between 12 and 34 months. The outcomes after cholecystectomy were good, regardless of the preoperative ejection fraction, and were 94% in the abnormal group and 85% in the normal group. The odds ratio for positive outcome was 1.37, which was not statistically significant ($P = 0.56$).

Treatment

The overall number of cholecystectomies has increased dramatically since the introduction and rapid adoption of laparoscopic techniques [39]. Specifically, from 1986 to 1995 the number of gallbladders being removed for biliary dyskinesia increased by 348% [40]. In some series, up to 30% of all cholecystectomies are performed for acalculous disease [39,41]. The effectiveness of cholecystectomy in improving or relieving symptoms is less predictable when compared with calculous disease [42]. Ponsky and colleagues [43] conducted a meta-analysis examining the effectiveness of surgery in patients who had biliary dyskinesia defined as biliary pain and EF of less than 40%. Symptom outcome was not addressed in patients who had normal gallbladder emptying. They included five studies involving 274 patients, 200 of whom underwent cholecystectomy. They suggest in their tables and conclusions that these procedures were all performed laparoscopically, but this is not clear from the source articles. In addition, they pooled reports of complete and partial relief into the successful category and concluded that 98% of patients improved with cholecystectomy compared with 32% of patients without. The authors determined that patients who had biliary dyskinesia were 2.79 times more likely to experience symptomatic relief with surgery than without.

Medical therapy

Medical therapy for this disorder has not been studied comprehensively and there are no current effective medical treatments. Medications, such as bile acid composition modifiers, promotility agents, and anti-inflammatories, have been used, but there is no evidence that they are effective or that any one is more effective than the other [44].

Conclusions

Symptom relief after laparoscopic cholecystectomy for gallstone disease is between 85% and 90%. The data are not as good for patients who have GBD and are of poor quality [44,45]. They suggest that about 65% to 70% of patients will be cured and 20% to 30% will improve with cholecystectomy. Approximately 60% to 80% of patients who have acalculous biliary pain have an abnormal EF on CCK-HIDA depending on the method used and the definition of abnormal [32]. The severity of dyskinesia does not seem to be a good predictor of outcome [34,46]. A prospective, randomized trial using uniform diagnostic criteria (such as those put forth by the Rome committee) and standardized CCK-CS methods (such as those recommended by Ziessman) is needed with patients randomized to laparoscopic cholecystectomy or observation and long-term follow-up.

Patients who meet Rome criteria for functional biliary pain should undergo CCK-CS with infusion of sincalide over 30 minutes after a 4- to 6-hour fast. Those who have a GBEF less than 35% to 40% should be offered laparoscopic cholecystectomy. Patients who have typical symptoms and GBEF greater than 40% present a challenge. They may benefit from further tests, such as EUS, looking for microlithiasis, or could be placed on a medication trial and observed for a period of time. The recommendation for cholecystectomy should be made on a case-by-case basis with an in-depth discussion about the limitations of our current understanding of this disease process.

Sphincter of Oddi dysfunction

SOD has been referred to as papillitis, papillary stenosis, papillary spasm, tachyoddia, biliary dyskinesia, and postcholecystectomy syndrome, to name a few. It is a term used to describe benign obstruction to the flow of bile or pancreatic secretions secondary to stenosis (structural) or primary motility (functional) disorders of the sphincter mechanism. Depending on the sphincter involved, patients present with persistent or recurrent biliary pain or idiopathic recurrent pancreatitis.

Epidemiology

Clinically, it is difficult to distinguish these different etiologies and they have therefore been grouped into one single entity. Although biliary SOD has been described in patients who have intact gallbladders, it is most often diagnosed in the postcholecystectomy patient [47,48]. The incidence of this disorder is difficult to glean from the literature because there are varying definitions and ways to establish the diagnosis. Biliary pain postcholecystectomy has been reported in up to 20% of patients [49], with symptoms suggesting SOD noted in 1.5% of patients, females outnumbering males [50]. In a group of patients who had postcholecystectomy pain, SOD was detected manometrically in 14% of patients and in the overall cohort of patients the frequency was 1% [51]. The incidence of pancreatic SOD among patients initially presumed to have idiopathic pancreatitis varies anywhere between 15% and 72% [52–54].

Anatomy of the choledocho-pancreatico-duodenal junction

The sphincter of Oddi was first described by Rugero Oddi in 1887; he was also the first to suggest that its malfunction could cause clinical symptoms [55]. The common bile duct and pancreatic duct become parallel as they approach the duodenum. The pancreatic duct enters the common duct most consistently 2 to 3 mm proximal to the papilla of Vater. In most cases (85%), a common channel is present; in 9% the ducts have separate duodenal openings; and 6% of the time the ducts open separately onto the papilla, but close to one another. The sphincter mechanism is actually composed of four sphincters (three biliary and one pancreatic) composed of longitudinal and circular fibers, which function independently of the duodenal musculature. Boyden [56] describes the anatomy of the sphincter in great detail . The three portions of the biliary sphincter include the superior portion (proximal to the duodenum), the intraduodenal portion, and the inferior portion located in the ampulla. The pancreatic sphincter is located in the intramural portion of the pancreatic duct.

Physiology of the sphincter of Oddi

The sphincter of Oddi may play several roles: active pumping of sphincter contents into the duodenum, phasic antegrade contractions that prevent reflux of duodenal contents and may have a housekeeping role to keep the conduits free of debris, and simultaneous or retrograde contractions that may promote filling of the gallbladder. Under normal circumstances, the pressure within the bile duct, through the various phasic contractions and relaxations of this sphincter complex, are kept within a narrow, low-pressure range thereby ensuring free flow of contents from the liver [57].

Sphincter of Oddi manometry

SOM has been performed for decades and is the gold standard for the diagnosis of SOD [58]. Direct pressure measurements during ERCP are made using pressure catheters (passed through the biopsy channel of the scope) inserted in a retrograde fashion through the sphincter into the bile duct. It is an invasive and specialized procedure that should be performed in high-volume centers [59]. Historically high rates of pancreatitis and other complications have been reported, particularly if the bile duct is of small caliber [60]. In one retrospective series of 100 patients, the rate of post-ERCP pancreatitis was 17% in patients undergoing manometry for SOD (compared to 5% in patients undergoing ERCP for other indications). The rates were higher in patients who underwent manometry followed by ERCP (9.3% manometry versus 26.1% manometry and ERCP), but were not affected by the performance of a sphincterotomy [61]. The authors proposed that this observation might prompt performance of the ERCP at an alternate time, but this has not been investigated and does not seem practical. The complication rates seem to be decreased with the technique of continuous aspiration from the pancreatic duct, which is performed using a triple lumen catheter.

Over the years, many different dynamic pressure measurements have been reported, but these have largely been replaced by simple basal pressure readings, which have been shown to have superior interrater and test-retest reliabilities [62,63]. Pressure measurements have included amplitude, duration, frequency, and propagation pattern of the phasic waves, paradoxical response to CCK, and increased frequency of retrograde waves. Normal basal sphincter pressure is approximately 15 mm Hg, but ranges from 3 to 35 mm Hg. Pressure greater than 40 mm Hg is defined as abnormal (3 SD above normal) [64]. Basal sphincter pressure greater than 40 mm Hg for either sphincter is the only accepted manometric criterion used to make the diagnosis of SOD.

Biliary sphincter of Oddi dysfunction

As for GBD, the Rome committee has also established a set of criteria to establish the diagnosis of both biliary and pancreatic SOD [18]. In its third revision, the Rome committee made some modifications to the most well-known classification system for biliary dyskinesia proposed by Hogan and Geenen [57], referred to as the Milwaukee classification. The modifications are intended to minimize the use of ERCP thereby limiting the inherent complications of this invasive procedure. The diagnostic criteria and the classification (shown in Table 1) are intended to guide workup and subsequent treatment of biliary SOD (BSOD) (Box 2).

Evaluation of patients who have suspected biliary sphincter of Oddi dysfunction

Most patients present with biliary pain in the epigastrium radiating to the right upper quadrant or back. The symptoms tend to occur approximately 5 years postcholecystectomy and resemble the pain before the surgery. The pain pattern can be related to fatty meals and can occur at intervals ranging from daily to many weeks [66]. The initial workup should include pancreatic and liver biochemistries and imaging studies to determine if there are structural causes for the patient's symptoms, such as stones or strictures of the bile ducts. These studies might include transabdominal or EUS, CT scan, and magnetic resonance cholangiopancreatography (MRCP). If the diagnosis of Type I dyskinesia is made based on these investigations, then there is no need for manometry to proceed with endoscopic sphincterotomy.

Table 1
Revised Milwaukee biliary group classification [65]

		Patients who have basal pressure >40 mm Hg on manometry (%)	Patients benefitting from sphincterotomy
Type I	Two or more occasions of documented increase in liver enzymes, bilirubin, or alkaline phosphatase AND bile duct >8 mm on ultrasound	70–100	90%–95%
Type II	Two or more occasions of documented increase in liver enzymes, bilirubin, or alkaline phosphatase OR bile duct >8 mm on ultrasound	40–86	P>40, 85% P<40, 35%
Type III	No laboratory or imaging abnormalities detected	20–55	P>40, 55%–65% P<40, <10%

Abbreviation P, pressure. All patients present with biliary-type pain.
Data from George J, Baillie J. Biliary and gallbladder dyskinesia. Curr Treat Options Gastroenterol 2007;10(4):322–7.

Box 2. Sphincter of Oddi disorders—Rome III criteria

Biliary SOD
Fulfills criteria above (see section on GBD)
Normal amylase/lipase

For patients who have suspected types II and III disease, other investigations have been proposed before proceeding with ERCP. Choledochoscintigraphy has been used with increasing promise for patients who do not have gallbladders. The gallbladder can serve as a reservoir for the flow of bile diverted away from the SO, thus preventing dilation of the sphincter, and most of these patients have normal rates of isotope emptying [67]. In cholecystectomized patients, quantitative cholescintigraphic data can be obtained, such as hilum-duodenum transit time, and this has been compared to manometric data with conflicting results [68–71]. Further data are needed before recommending widespread use of this noninvasive modality. Ultrasound of the bile ducts has also been reported; however, it is difficult to visualize the pancreatic duct and it is extremely operator dependent.

Patients who have suspected Type II SOD (episodic elevation of enzymes or increased duct caliber) should undergo ERCP, manometry, and sphincterotomy if indicated. Patients who have suspected Type III SOD should not undergo ERCP and manometry unless all other potential sources of pain have been ruled out. A trial of medical therapy is also recommended as first-line therapy for Type III SOD, with ERCP, manometry, and sphincterotomy being a last resort.

Treatment of biliary sphincter of Oddi dysfunction

Type I

The Milwaukee classification system is used to guide workup and treatment. Patients who have Type I BSOD have true papillary stenosis related to fibrosis, and are effectively treated by endoscopic sphincterotomy. There are no randomized trials specifically treating type I patients. There is a single randomized trial that does include Type I patients, but the outcome data for this subset are not presented separately [72]. Success rates for sphincterotomy are based on retrospective studies with small numbers of patients and limited follow-up. Based on these data, outcomes for these patients postsphincterotomy are good and range from 90% to 95% relief of symptoms. These patients do not require manometry to establish the diagnosis. Manometry is reported to be normal in 14% to 35% of patients who have type I disease who still obtain relief from sphincterotomy and may only confuse the picture [73,74]. Patients who have classic biliary or pancreatic pain, episodes of abnormal biochemistry, and radiographic evidence of duct dilatation, in whom other structural or pathologic causes have been ruled out should undergo ERCP and sphincterotomy without manometry.

Types II and III

The group of patients falling into these two classifications can be quite heterogeneous and it is unclear if they suffer from different pathologic conditions all named sphincter of Oddi dysfunction. The best data to date are derived from two randomized controlled trials that used appropriate classification criteria, manometry, and sphincterotomy [72,75]. These trials were also the only two that were analyzed in a Cochrane review examining the usefulness of sphincterotomy in patients who had BSOD [76]. Geenen and colleagues [75] randomized 47 patients believed to have Type II SOD into a treatment group and a sham group. All patients underwent manometry, and sphincterotomy was performed in the treatment group. Ten of 11 patients who had elevated basal pressures (>40 mm Hg) in the treatment group were improved compared to 3 of the 12 in the sham group. Subsequently, 7 patients who had elevated pressures in the sham group crossed over. With 4-year follow-up, they demonstrated improvement in symptoms in 17 of 18 patients who had elevated pressures who underwent sphincterotomy. Sphincterotomy was not found to be any more beneficial than sham in patients who had normal manometric findings [75].

The second study by Toouli and colleagues [72] included mostly type II patients, with small numbers of types I and III. In contrast to the Geenen study, these patients were randomized after manometry was performed into groups with the following characteristics: elevated basal pressure, phasic contraction abnormalities (termed "dyskinesia"), and normal manometry. The only group that benefited from sphincterotomy more than sham was the group with basal pressures greater than 40 mm Hg [72]. The Cochrane review combines these two studies and concludes that in the 49 patients who had elevated basal pressures, sphincterotomy was more effective than placebo with a highly significant Peto odds ratio of 9.08. The 77 patients who had normal basal pressures did not benefit from sphincterotomy, with a nonsignificant odds ratio of 1.28 [76].

There are many nonrandomized case series and cohort studies that challenge the usefulness of manometry in predicting successful outcomes in patients who have type II BSOD. Some of these series did not demonstrate a strong correlation between elevated basal pressures and response to sphincterotomy [77–79]. When considering the Cochrane review and the randomized studies described above, one must bear in mind that one of the authors of the review (Toouli) was also an author in both of the trials. Currently, the recommendations are to perform manometry and sphincterotomy in patients who have suspected type II BSOD, but further studies by different groups are needed.

Type III

The need to make a distinction between types II and III has been challenged in the literature [79]. A study by Botomon and colleagues [79] demonstrated a similar frequency of sphincter hypertension and response to sphincterotomy in these two groups suggesting that perhaps the current classification has limited clinical value. Type III patients (patients who have pain in the absence of objective findings) have sparked the most controversy in the literature. There are some who suggest that the pain cannot be reliably differentiated into biliary and pancreatic origins and that type III SOD should encompass both biliary and pancreatic subtypes [80]. Furthermore, given the suboptimal response rates of 40% to 50% in manometry-guided therapy, the consideration of other causes for the pain or a more generalized gastrointestinal motility disorder in these patients must also be considered [81].

Pancreatic sphincter of Oddi dysfunction

A similar but less popular classification system has been proposed for pancreatic SOD (Table 2). Most patients present with recurrent episodes of pancreatitis, and SOD is detected in 15% to 72% of these patients (Box 3) [52,53,82].

Evaluation of patients who have pancreatic sphincter of Oddi dysfunction

The initial evaluation includes a thorough history, physical, and liver and pancreatic biochemistries. All attempts should be made to exclude structural causes of pancreatitis, such as microlithiasis or pancreas divisum. Imaging studies should start with a transabdominal ultrasound or CT scan followed by EUS or ERCP. Finally, ERCP with possible manometry and sphincterotomy can be performed. Basal pressures are the best predictors of response

Table 2
Classification for pancreatic sphincter of Oddi dysfunction

Patients who had basal pressure >40 mm Hg on manometry (%)		
Type I	Elevated pancreatic enzymes (>1.5 × normal) with pain AND pancreatic duct >6 mm (head) and >5 mm (body) by ERCP. Delayed drainage of contrast by ERCP (>9 min)	92
Type II	One or two of the Type I criteria	58
Type III	None of the Type I criteria	35

All patients present with recurrent pancreatic or typical pancreatic pain.
Data from Sherman S, Troiano FP, Hawes RH, et al. Frequency of abnormal sphincter of Oddi manometry compared with the clinical suspicion of sphincter of Oddi dysfunction. Am J Gastroenterol 1991;86(5):586–90.

Box 3. Pancreatic sphincter of Oddi dysfunction

Fulfills criteria above (see section on GBD)
Elevated amylase/lipase

---

to sphincterotomy and both the biliary and pancreatic pressures must be measured because there are some patients who have a normal pressure in one sphincter and an abnormal pressure in the other.

Secretin

The injection of secretin with subsequent monitoring of pancreatic duct caliber by ultrasound or MRCP has been performed in small studies [83–85]. Secretin administration demonstrated an increase in pancreatic duct diameter on MRCP but did not predict manometry results in patients who had suspected SOD. One study demonstrated a sensitivity and specificity of 88% and 82% for the ultrasound secretin stimulation test compared with SOM [83]. These tests are highly specialized and operator dependent, but may serve as less invasive alternatives to manometry if they can be reliably shown to correlate with manometry and to predict outcomes of sphincterotomy.

Treatment

The best currently available treatment to prevent further episodes of pancreatitis remains complete division of the biliary and pancreatic sphincters and the septum [86–88]. This procedure can now be successfully performed endoscopically, but has traditionally been done surgically by means of a transduodenal sphincteroplasty. The placement of a pancreatic stent has been shown to reduce rates of post-ERCP pancreatitis from 26% to 7% in one series [89,90]. Botox has been tried and may be useful in predicting response to sphincterotomy, but the effects from the injection are temporary and therefore not appropriate as a definitive therapy [91].

Surgery

There are no data to suggest that surgical sphincterotomy is more effective than endoscopic division of the sphincters for SOD [92]. One large retrospective series of 446 patients who underwent surgical sphincteroplasty reported a morbidity of 38.4%. This cohort included 372 patients who had SOD, with improvement in 86.8% of patients. There may still be a role for surgical sphincteroplasty in the treatment of this entity, however. Two potential advantages of surgical over endoscopic therapy might include: difficulty dividing the septum endoscopically, which may result in incomplete pancreatic sphincterotomy, and the theoretical reduction in scarring and recurrent stenosis. Smaller surgical series have reported symptom improvement in about 50% to 60% of patients who have biliary and pancreatic symptoms, but the diagnostic criteria have been highly variable [87, 93–96]. Patients who have pancreatic symptoms may have worse outcomes possibly related to the presence of fibrosis and chronic pancreatitis that was not apparent preoperatively [94].

Pharmacologic

The most commonly prescribed medications to treat SOD have been those that cause relaxation of smooth muscle, such as calcium channel blockers and nitrates. In one series nifedipine and or nitrates were effective in about 50% of patients [97]. Vasoactive side effects are commonly observed, but a trial of medical therapy, particularly in type III patients, seems warranted.

Summary

Functional disorders of the sphincter of Oddi can result in biliary pain or recurrent pancreatitis. Classification systems have been developed to guide diagnosis, treatment, and discussion of these complex problems. They also provided a framework that can help to predict successful outcomes with endoscopic therapy. Patients who have abnormal enzymes and biliary or pancreatic duct dilation are believed to have papillary stenosis and they should undergo ERCP and sphincterotomy without the need for manometry. Based on the limited data available, success of sphincterotomy in type II patients can be predicted by elevated basal pressures, and these patients should have SOM. Type III SOD patients represent a clinical challenge because they may not benefit from sphincterotomy even if they have elevated basal pressures. There is shift away from SOM to medical and conservative management of these patients. Further studies examining alternative, less invasive diagnostic modalities are needed in addition to larger-scale randomized trials by independent groups.

References

[1] Rastogi A, Slivka A, Moser AJ, et al. Controversies concerning pathophysiology and management of acalculous biliary-type abdominal pain. [see comment]. Dig Dis Sci 2005;50(8):1391–401.
[2] Barbara L, Sama C, Morselli Labate AM, et al. A population study on the prevalence of gallstone disease: the Sirmione study. Hepatology 1987;7(5):913–7.
[3] The epidemiology of gallstone disease in Rome, Italy. Part I. Prevalence data in men. The Rome Group for Epidemiology and Prevention of Cholelithiasis (GREPCO). Hepatology 1988;8(4):904–6.

[4] Prevalence of gallstone disease in an Italian adult female population. Rome Group for the Epidemiology and Prevention of Cholelithiasis (GREPCO). Am J Epidemiol 1984;119(5): 796–805.

[5] Kellow JE, Miller LJ, Phillips SF, et al. Altered sensitivity of the gallbladder to cholecysto-kinin octapeptide in irritable bowel syndrome. Am J Physiol 1987;253(5 Pt 1):G650–5.

[6] Drossman DA. Rome III: the new criteria. Chin J Dig Dis 2006;7(4):181–5.

[7] Drossman DA. The functional gastrointestinal disorders and the Rome III process. Gastro-enterology 2006;130(5):1377–90.

[8] Drossman DA, Dumitrascu DL. Rome III: new standard for functional gastrointestinal dis-orders. J Gastrointestin Liver Dis 2006;15(3):237–41.

[9] Yap L, Wycherley AG, Morphett AD, et al. Acalculous biliary pain: cholecystectomy alle-viates symptoms in patients with abnormal cholescintigraphy. Gastroenterology 1991; 101(3):786–93.

[10] Moriarty KJ, Dawson AM. Functional abdominal pain: further evidence that whole gut is affected. Br Med J (Clin Res Ed) 1982;284(6330):1670–2.

[11] Marzio L. Factors affecting gallbladder motility: drugs. Dig Liver Dis 2003;35(Suppl 3): S17–9.

[12] Lanzini A, Jazrawi RP, Northfield TC. Simultaneous quantitative measurements of absolute gallbladder storage and emptying during fasting and eating in humans. Gastroenterology 1987;92(4):852–61.

[13] Misra DC Jr, Blossom GB, Fink-Bennett D, et al. Results of surgical therapy for biliary dys-kinesia. Arch Surg 1991;126(8):957–60.

[14] Ozden N, DiBaise JK. Gallbladder ejection fraction and symptom outcome in patients with acalculous biliary-like pain. Dig Dis Sci 2003;48(5):890–7.

[15] Poynter MT, Saba AK, Evans RA, et al. Chronic acalculous biliary disease: cholecystokinin cholescintigraphy is useful in formulating treatment strategy and predicting success after cholecystectomy. Am Surg 2002;68(4):382–4.

[16] Young SB, Arregui M, Singh K. HIDA scan ejection fraction does not predict sphincter of Oddi hypertension or clinical outcome in patients with suspected chronic acalculous chole-cystitis. Surg Endosc 2006;20(12):1872–8.

[17] Velanovich V. Biliary dyskinesia and biliary crystals: a prospective study. Am Surg 1997; 63(1):69–74.

[18] Behar J, Corazziari E, Guelrud M, et al. Functional gallbladder and sphincter of Oddi dis-orders. Gastroenterology 2006;130(5):1498–509.

[19] Zeman RK, Garra BS. Gallbladder imaging. The state of the art. Gastroenterol Clin North Am 1991;20(1):127–56.

[20] Dahan P, Andant C, Levy P, et al. Prospective evaluation of endoscopic ultrasonography and microscopic examination of duodenal bile in the diagnosis of cholecystolithiasis in 45 patients with normal conventional ultrasonography. Gut 1996;38(2):277–81.

[21] Thorboll J, Vilmann P, Jacobsen B, et al. Endoscopic ultrasonography in detection of cho-lelithiasis in patients with biliary pain and negative transabdominal ultrasonography. Scand J Gastroenterol 2004;39(3):267–9.

[22] Ziessman HA. Cholecystokinin cholescintigraphy: clinical indications and proper methodol-ogy. Radiol Clin North Am 2001;39(5):997–1006.

[23] Smythe A, Majeed AW, Fitzhenry M, et al. A requiem for the cholecystokinin provocation test? [see comment]. Gut 1998;43(4):571–4.

[24] Krishnamurthy GT, Bobba VR, Kingston E. Radionuclide ejection fraction: a technique for quantitative analysis of motor function of the human gallbladder. Gastroenterology 1981; 80(3):482–90.

[25] Ziessman HA, Fahey FH, Hixson DJ. Calculation of a gallbladder ejection fraction: advan-tage of continuous sincalide infusion over the three-minute infusion method. J Nucl Med 1992;33(4):537–41.

[26] Yost F, Margenthaler J, Presti M, et al. Cholecystectomy is an effective treatment for biliary dyskinesia. Am J Surg 1999;178(6):462–5.

[27] Chen PF, Nimeri A, Pham QH, et al. The clinical diagnosis of chronic acalculous cholecystitis. Surgery 2001;130(4):578–81.

[28] Fink-Bennett D, DeRidder P, Kolozsi WZ, et al. Cholecystokinin cholescintigraphy: detection of abnormal gallbladder motor function in patients with chronic acalculous gallbladder disease. J Nucl Med 1991;32(9):1695–9.

[29] Khosla R, Singh A, Miedema BW, et al. Cholecystectomy alleviates acalculous biliary pain in patients with a reduced gallbladder ejection fraction. South Med J 1997;90(11):1087–90.

[30] Sorenson MK, Fancher S, Lang NP, et al. Abnormal gallbladder nuclear ejection fraction predicts success of cholecystectomy in patients with biliary dyskinesia. Am J Surg 1993;166(6):672–4.

[31] Majeski J. Gallbladder ejection fraction: an accurate evaluation of symptomatic acalculous gallbladder disease. Int Surg 2003;88(2):95–9.

[32] Middleton GW, Williams JH. Diagnostic accuracy of 99Tcm-HIDA with cholecystokinin and gallbladder ejection fraction in acalculous gallbladder disease. Nucl Med Commun 2001;22(6):657–61.

[33] Goncalves RM, Harris JA, Rivera DE. Biliary dyskinesia: natural history and surgical results. Am Surg 1998;64(6):493–7.

[34] DiBaise JK, Oleynikov D. Does gallbladder ejection fraction predict outcome after cholecystectomy for suspected chronic acalculous gallbladder dysfunction? A systematic review. [see comment]. Am J Gastroenterol 2003;98(12):2605–11.

[35] Delgado-Aros S, Cremonini F, Bredenoord AJ, et al. Systematic review and meta-analysis: does gall-bladder ejection fraction on cholecystokinin cholescintigraphy predict outcome after cholecystectomy in suspected functional biliary pain? Aliment Pharmacol Ther 2003;18(2):167–74.

[36] Mishkind MT, Pruitt RF, Bambini DA, et al. Effectiveness of cholecystokinin-stimulated cholescintigraphy in the diagnosis and treatment of acalculous gallbladder disease. Am Surg 1997;63(9):769–74.

[37] Westlake PJ, Hershfield NB, Kelly JK, et al. Chronic right upper quadrant pain without gallstones: does HIDA scan predict outcome after cholecystectomy? Am J Gastroenterol 1990;85(8):986–90.

[38] Adams DB, Tarnasky PR, Hawes RH, et al. Outcome after laparoscopic cholecystectomy for chronic acalculous cholecystitis. Am Surg 1998;64(1):1–5.

[39] Legorreta AP, Silber JH, Costantino GN, et al. Increased cholecystectomy rate after the introduction of laparoscopic cholecystectomy. JAMA 1993;270(12):1429–32.

[40] Johanning JM, Gruenberg JC. The changing face of cholecystectomy. Am Surg 1998;64(7):643–7.

[41] Lam CM, Murray FE, Cuschieri A. Increased cholecystectomy rate after the introduction of laparoscopic cholecystectomy in Scotland. Gut 1996;38(2):282–4.

[42] Fenster LF, Lonborg R, Thirlby RC, et al. What symptoms does cholecystectomy cure? Insights from an outcomes measurement project and review of the literature. Am J Surg 1995;169(5):533–8.

[43] Ponsky TA, DeSagun R, Brody F. Surgical therapy for biliary dyskinesia: a meta-analysis and review of the literature. J Laparoendosc Adv Surg Tech A 2005;15(5):439–42.

[44] Hansel SL, Dibaise JK. Gallbladder dyskinesia. Curr Treat Options Gastroenterol 2008;11(2):78–84.

[45] Tabet J, Anvari M. Laparoscopic cholecystectomy for gallbladder dyskinesia: clinical outcome and patient satisfaction. Surg Laparosc Endosc Percutan Tech 1999;9(6):382–6.

[46] Patel NA, Lamb JJ, Hogle NJ, et al. Therapeutic efficacy of laparoscopic cholecystectomy in the treatment of biliary dyskinesia. Am J Surg 2004;187(2):209–12.

[47] Ruffolo TA, Sherman S, Lehman GA, et al. Gallbladder ejection fraction and its relationship to sphincter of Oddi dysfunction. Dig Dis Sci 1994;39(2):289–92.

[48] Choudhry U, Ruffolo T, Jamidar P, et al. Sphincter of Oddi dysfunction in patients with intact gallbladder: therapeutic response to endoscopic sphincterotomy. Gastrointest Endosc 1993;39(4):492–5.

[49] Black NA, Thompson E, Sanderson CF. Symptoms and health status before and six weeks after open cholecystectomy: a European cohort study. ECHSS Group. European Collaborative Health Services Study Group. Gut 1994;35(9):1301–5.

[50] Drossman DA, Li Z, Andruzzi E, et al. U.S. householder survey of functional gastrointestinal disorders. Prevalence, sociodemography, and health impact. Dig Dis Sci 1993;38(9): 1569–80.

[51] Bar-Meir S, Halpern Z, Bardan E, et al. Frequency of papillary dysfunction among cholecystectomized patients. Hepatology 1984;4(2):328–30.

[52] Sherman S, Troiano FP, Hawes RH, et al. Frequency of abnormal sphincter of Oddi manometry compared with the clinical suspicion of sphincter of Oddi dysfunction. Am J Gastroenterol 1991;86(5):586–90.

[53] Toouli J, Roberts-Thomson IC, Dent J, et al. Sphincter of Oddi motility disorders in patients with idiopathic recurrent pancreatitis. Br J Surg 1985;72(11):859–63.

[54] Geenen JE, Nash JA. The role of sphincter of Oddi manometry and biliary microscopy in evaluating idiopathic recurrent pancreatitis. Endoscopy 1998;30(9):A237–41.

[55] Toouli J. Biliary motility disorders. Baillieres Clin Gastroenterol 1997;11(4):725–40.

[56] Boyden EA. The anatomy of the choledochoduodenal junction in man. Surg Gynecol Obstet 1957;104(6):641–52.

[57] Hogan WJ, Geenen JE. Biliary dyskinesia. Endoscopy 1988;20(Suppl 1):179–83.

[58] Bar-Meir S, Geenen JE, Hogan WJ, et al. Biliary and pancreatic duct pressures measured by ERCP manometry in patients with suspected papillary stenosis. Dig Dis Sci 1979;24(3): 209–13.

[59] Cohen S, Bacon BR, Berlin JA, et al. National Institutes of Health State-of-the-Science Conference Statement: ERCP for diagnosis and therapy, January 14-16, 2002. [see comment]. Gastrointest Endosc 2002;56(6):803–9.

[60] Sherman S, Ruffolo TA, Hawes RH, et al. Complications of endoscopic sphincterotomy. A prospective series with emphasis on the increased risk associated with sphincter of Oddi dysfunction and nondilated bile ducts. Gastroenterology 1991;101(4):1068–75.

[61] Maldonado ME, Brady PG, Mamel JJ, et al. Incidence of pancreatitis in patients undergoing sphincter of Oddi manometry (SOM). Am J Gastroenterol 1999;94(2):387–90.

[62] Smithline A, Hawes R, Lehman G. Sphincter of Oddi manometry: interobserver variability. Gastrointest Endosc 1993;39(4):486–91.

[63] Thune A, Scicchitano J, Roberts-Thomson I, et al. Reproducibility of endoscopic sphincter of Oddi manometry. Dig Dis Sci 1991;36(10):1401–5.

[64] Guelrud M, Mendoza S, Rossiter G, et al. Sphincter of Oddi manometry in healthy volunteers. Dig Dis Sci 1990;35(1):38–46.

[65] George J, Baillie J. Biliary and gallbladder dyskinesia. Curr Treat Options Gastroenterol 2007;10(4):322–7.

[66] Toouli J. What is sphincter of Oddi dysfunction? Gut 1989;30(6):753–61.

[67] Funch-Jensen P, Drewes AM, Madacsy L. Evaluation of the biliary tract in patients with functional biliary symptoms. World J Gastroenterol 2006;12(18):2839–45.

[68] Madacsy L, Middelfart HV, Matzen P, et al. Quantitative hepatobiliary scintigraphy and endoscopic sphincter of Oddi manometry in patients with suspected sphincter of Oddi dysfunction: assessment of flow-pressure relationship in the biliary tract. Eur J Gastroenterol Hepatol 2000;12(7):777–86.

[69] Piccinni G, Angrisano A, Testini M, et al. Diagnosing and treating sphincter of Oddi dysfunction: a critical literature review and reevaluation. J Clin Gastroenterol 2004;38(4): 350–9.

[70] Vijayakumar V, Briscoe EG, Pehlivanov ND. Postcholecystectomy sphincter of oddi dyskinesia–a diagnostic dilemma—role of noninvasive nuclear and invasive manometric and endoscopic aspects. Surg Laparosc Endosc Percutan Tech 2007;17(1):10–3.

[71] Craig AG, Peter D, Saccone GT, et al. Scintigraphy versus manometry in patients with suspected biliary sphincter of Oddi dysfunction. Gut 2003;52(3):352–7.

[72] Toouli J, Roberts-Thomson IC, Kellow J, et al. Manometry based randomised trial of endoscopic sphincterotomy for sphincter of Oddi dysfunction. Gut 2000;46(1):98–102.

[73] Rolny P, Geenen JE, Hogan WJ. Post-cholecystectomy patients with "objective signs" of partial bile outflow obstruction: clinical characteristics, sphincter of Oddi manometry findings, and results of therapy. Gastrointest Endosc 1993;39(6):778–81.

[74] Cicala M, Habib FI, Vavassori P, et al. Outcome of endoscopic sphincterotomy in post cholecystectomy patients with sphincter of Oddi dysfunction as predicted by manometry and quantitative choledochoscintigraphy. Gut 2002;50(5):665–8.

[75] Geenen JE, Hogan WJ, Dodds WJ, et al. The efficacy of endoscopic sphincterotomy after cholecystectomy in patients with sphincter-of-Oddi dysfunction. N Engl J Med 1989;320(2):82–7.

[76] Craig AG, Toouli J. Sphincterotomy for biliary sphincter of Oddi dysfunction. Cochrane Database Syst Rev 2001;(3):001509.

[77] Viceconte G, Micheletti A. Endoscopic manometry of the sphincter of Oddi: its usefulness for the diagnosis and treatment of benign papillary stenosis. Scand J Gastroenterol 1995;30(8):797–803.

[78] Wehrmann T, Wiemer K, Lembcke B, et al. Do patients with sphincter of Oddi dysfunction benefit from endoscopic sphincterotomy? A 5-year prospective trial. Eur J Gastroenterol Hepatol 1996;8(3):251–6.

[79] Botoman VA, Kozarek RA, Novell LA, et al. Long-term outcome after endoscopic sphincterotomy in patients with biliary colic and suspected sphincter of Oddi dysfunction. Gastrointest Endosc 1994;40(2 Pt 1):165–70.

[80] Eversman D, Fogel EL, Rusche M, et al. Frequency of abnormal pancreatic and biliary sphincter manometry compared with clinical suspicion of sphincter of Oddi dysfunction. Gastrointest Endosc 1999;50(5):637–41.

[81] Petersen BT. Sphincter of Oddi dysfunction, part 2: Evidence-based review of the presentations, with "objective" pancreatic findings (types I and II) and of presumptive type III. Gastrointest Endosc 2004;59(6):670–87.

[82] Venu RP, Geenen JE, Hogan W, et al. Idiopathic recurrent pancreatitis. An approach to diagnosis and treatment. Dig Dis Sci 1989;34(1):56–60.

[83] Di Francesco V, Brunori MP, Rigo L, et al. Comparison of ultrasound-secretin test and sphincter of Oddi manometry in patients with recurrent acute pancreatitis. Dig Dis Sci 1999;44(2):336–40.

[84] Bolondi L, Gaiani S, Gullo L, et al. Secretin administration induces a dilatation of main pancreatic duct. Dig Dis Sci 1984;29(9):802–8.

[85] Aisen AM, Sherman S, Jennings SG, et al. Comparison of secretin-stimulated magnetic resonance pancreatography and manometry results in patients with suspected sphincter of Oddi dysfunction. Acad Radiol 2008;15(5):601–9.

[86] Tarnasky PR, Palesch YY, Cunningham JT, et al. Pancreatic stenting prevents pancreatitis after biliary sphincterotomy in patients with sphincter of Oddi dysfunction. Gastroenterology 1998;115(6):1518–24.

[87] Toouli J, Di Francesco V, Saccone G, et al. Division of the sphincter of Oddi for treatment of dysfunction associated with recurrent pancreatitis. Br J Surg 1996;83(9):1205–10.

[88] Elton E, Howell DA, Parsons WG, et al. Endoscopic pancreatic sphincterotomy: indications, outcome, and a safe stentless technique. Gastrointest Endosc 1998;47(3):240–9.

[89] Fogel EL, Eversman D, Jamidar P, et al. Sphincter of Oddi dysfunction: pancreaticobiliary sphincterotomy with pancreatic stent placement has a lower rate of pancreatitis than biliary sphincterotomy alone. Endoscopy 2002;34(4):280–5.

1272 VASSILIOU & LAYCOCK

[90] Tarnasky PR, Hawes RH. Endoscopic diagnosis and therapy of unexplained (idiopathic) acute pancreatitis. Gastrointest Endosc Clin N Am 1998;8(1):13–37.
[91] Wehrmann T, Schmitt TH, Arndt A, et al. Endoscopic injection of botulinum toxin in patients with recurrent acute pancreatitis due to pancreatic sphincter of Oddi dysfunction. Aliment Pharmacol Ther 2000;14(11):1469–77.
[92] Prajapati DN, Hogan WJ. Sphincter of Oddi dysfunction and other functional biliary disorders: evaluation and treatment. Gastroenterol Clin North Am 2003;32(2):601–18.
[93] Nardi GL, Michelassi F, Zannini P. Transduodenal sphincteroplasty. 5–25 year follow-up of 89 patients. Ann Surg 1983;198(4):453–61.
[94] Nussbaum MS, Warner BW, Sax HC, et al. Transduodenal sphincteroplasty and transampullary septotomy for primary sphincter of Oddi dysfunction. Am J Surg 1989;157(1):38–43.
[95] Anderson TM, Pitt HA, Longmire WP Jr. Experience with sphincteroplasty and sphincterotomy in pancreatobiliary surgery. Ann Surg 1985;201(4):399–406.
[96] Moody FG, Berenson MM, McCloskey D. Transampullary septectomy for post-cholecystectomy pain. Ann Surg 1977;186(4):415–23.
[97] Dobronte Z, Simon L, Patai A. [Management of Oddi sphincter dyskinesis. Results of drug therapy and sphincterotomy]. Orv Hetil 1995;136(40):2165–7 [Hungarian].

ELSEVIER
SAUNDERS

SURGICAL
CLINICS OF
NORTH AMERICA

Surg Clin N Am 88 (2008) 1273–1294

Open Cholecystectomy

David McAneny, MD, FACS

Section of Surgical Oncology and Endocrinology, Boston University School of Medicine, FGH Building, Suite 5008, 820 Harrison Avenue, Boston Medical Center, Boston, MA 02118, USA

There is but one way to perform a cholecystectomy: safely separate the gallbladder from its perfusion, the bile duct, and the liver. How one accomplishes this is at the surgeon's discretion, as it has been for over a century.

History

John Stough Bobbs (1809 to 1870), a Civil War surgeon from Pennsylvania, is credited with the first operation on a human gallbladder (Fig. 1). He performed a cholecystostomy in 1867, at the corner of Meridian and Washington Streets in Indianapolis [1]. Carl Johann August Langenbuch [2] (1846 to 1901) performed the first cholecystectomy on July 15, 1882, in his capacity as the chief at the Lazaruskrankenhaus, in what would much later be the French sector of West Berlin (Fig. 2). Langenbuch had practiced the operation on animals and cadavers before applying it in the clinical realm. Furthermore, he discussed this departure from the standard of care with the patient and allowed the 42 year-old man to consider the recommendation for several days before proceeding. As a result, some also have regarded Langenbuch as having pioneered the notion of informed consent [3]. The patient had an uncomplicated recovery, and Langenbuch ultimately presented a series of 24 patients who had undergone cholecystectomies to the Eighteenth Congress of the German Surgical Society in 1889, when he argued that their outcomes surpassed the results of other contemporary operations for cholelithiasis. Langenbuch reasoned that cholecystectomy removed both the offending gallstones and the organ that produced them. He published his first volume of "Chirurgie der Leber und Gallenblase" (Surgery of the Liver and Gallbladder) in 1894. He was a master biliary surgeon, who also described techniques for choledocholithotomy, choledochoduodenostomy, and cholangioenterostomy [4]. Langenbuch died at the age of 55 years, likely

E-mail address: david.mcaneny@bmc.org

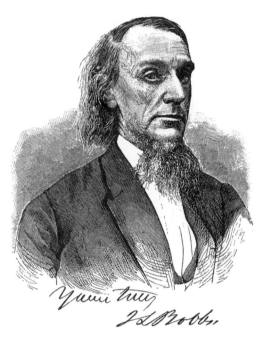

Fig. 1. John Stough Bobbs (1809 to 1870) reported the first gallbladder operation, a cholecystostomy, in 1867. (*Courtesy of* Nancy L. Eckerman, MLS, Special Collections Librarian, Ruth Lilly Medical Library, Indiana University School of Medicine.)

from acute appendicitis and resultant peritonitis, ironically just 3 months after a presidential address to the Freie Vereinigung der Chirurgen Berlins about the surgical management of generalized peritonitis.

During the decades immediately after Langenbuch's momentous operation, surgeons debated the merits and hazards of cholecystectomy versus cholecystostomy, as the latter originally was associated with less mortality and morbidity. Interestingly, Langenbuch himself had adapted the suffix "ektomie" to refer to the removal of an organ, so it was appropriate that he led the nascent camp of gallbladder resectionists.

The ability to preoperatively examine the gallbladder and biliary tract is critical to the selection of appropriate candidates for cholecystectomy. The biliary tract originally was imaged radiographically in 1918, when Reich [5] injected bismuth paste and petrolatum into a biliary fistula. Cole [6], a surgical resident working in Evarts Graham's laboratory, obtained the first positive image of a human gallbladder in 1924. A nurse was injected with 5.5 g of calcium tetrabromphenolphthalein, and a dense gallbladder shadow developed at 24 hours. The absence of radiographic lucencies led to the identification of a right ureteral obstruction as the source of her symptoms. Mirizzi [7] reported the first series of intraoperative cholangiograms in 1932.

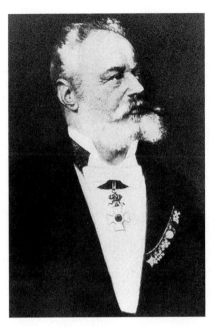

Fig. 2. Carl Johann August Langenbuch (1846 to 1901) performed the first cholecystectomy in 1882.

Cholecystectomies were performed by sundry groups of surgeons (including general practitioners) with widely variable levels of training and apprenticeship during the early 20th century. The operations eventually became the exclusive province of surgeons, and uniform guidelines for surgical training were established. One survey revealed a lower mortality rate for cholecystectomies performed by fellows of the American College of Surgeons or board-certified surgeons than for those performed by nonfellows or nonboard-certified surgeons [8]. Another study demonstrated that board-certified surgeons had fewer abdominal complications after complex biliary operations than did nonboard-certified surgeons [9]. An historical vignette of those times involved the saga of a British politician, who later became the prime minister. Anthony Eden developed bile duct complications after a cholecystectomy on April 12, 1953, and he underwent an open drainage of a subhepatic bile collection 17 days later. He was transferred to the care of Dr. Richard Cattell (and later Dr. John Braasch) for biliary reconstruction at the Lahey Clinic, in the United States, about 2 months after the cholecystectomy [10]. Some British officials, concerned and likely embarrassed that their youngest-ever foreign secretary had not undergone the operative revision in their homeland, reportedly explained that American surgeons were better suited to handle this problem, as the complication was common in the "colonies" but rather rare in Great Britain. (Editor's note: In personal communication with Dr. Braasch, it was pointed out that Sir Anthony was transported and treated postoperatively aboard the Royal yacht, Britannia, making a protocol visit to Boston.) Interestingly, Anthony Eden's protracted illness from recurrent biliary sepsis likely influenced the conduct of British foreign affairs and indeed world events, including the Suez Canal crisis in late 1956. As standards for surgeons evolved, and surgical training became more uniform, the incidence of complications significantly decreased.

The origin of laparoscopic surgery for the gallbladder was the nexus of several factors, including technological advances, public demand for less invasive treatments, and perhaps even the specter of lithotripsy and gallstone dissolution therapy encroaching upon the surgical domain. Nonetheless, laparoscopic cholecystectomy initially was greeted with some skepticism and derision. In an effort to assert the superiority of the traditional open cholecystectomy, many surgeons compared the lengths of their standard right upper quadrant incisions with the aggregate lengths of laparoscopic trocar incisions. Some surgeons continue to champion minicholecystectomy, which is performed through a small incision. This operation preserves the abdominal wall musculature, avoids the insufflation of a pneumoperitoneum, and does not require cumbersome equipment or specially fitted operating rooms. Furthermore, some have demonstrated that this technique is a safer and less expensive alternative to laparoscopic cholecystectomy [11].

Indications

Most cholecystectomies are performed for symptomatic gallstone disease or for complications of the stones (eg, acute cholecystitis, acute pancreatitis, obstructive jaundice), and over 90% of those operations are performed laparoscopically. Most open cholecystectomies are performed when surgeons convert from laparoscopic cholecystectomies, and the most common cause of conversion is the presence of profound inflammation that precludes identification of the anatomy within the triangle of Calot (Fig. 3) [12]. The triangle of Calot is, by definition, bordered by the cystic duct, cystic artery, and the common hepatic duct; the hepatocystic triangle is defined by the cystic duct, common hepatic duct, and the liver. Throughout this article, references to the triangle of Calot imply a full mobilization of the gallbladder neck to precisely define the divisible structures within the hepatocystic triangle. Strasberg refers to this as the "critical view" in laparoscopic surgery, but it is just as critical during an open operation, and one should not divide structures if this exposure cannot be established (Fig. 4) [13]. A multivariate analysis demonstrated that predictors of conversion to an open operation were:

Age greater than 60 years
Male sex
Weight greater than 65 kg

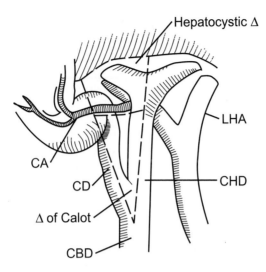

Fig. 3. Triangle of Calot and hepatocystic triangle. The triangle of Calot is bordered by the cystic duct (CD), the common hepatic duct (CHD), and the cystic artery (CA). The hepatocystic triangle is defined by the cystic duct, the common hepatic duct, and the liver. CBD, common bile duct; LHA, left hepatic artery.

The presence of acute cholecystitis, a history of prior upper abdominal surgery. A history of prior upper abdominal surgery.
Higher glycosylated hemoglobin level (among diabetic patients)
A less experienced surgeon [12]

If one cannot operate on a patient within 2 to 3 days of the onset of acute cholecystitis, it may be best to nonoperatively manage the initial episode and

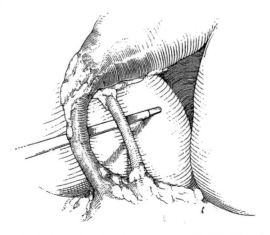

Fig. 4. Strasberg's critical view. (*From* Strasberg SM, Hertl M, Soper NJ. An analysis of the problem of biliary injury during laparoscopic cholecystectomy. J Am Coll Surg 1995;180:113; with permission.)

perform an interval cholecystectomy about 6 weeks later, to permit resolution of the intense inflammatory reaction. The decision to convert to an open cholecystectomy is ultimately a function of the surgeon's expertise, the pathology of the gallbladder and adjacent viscera, intraoperative challenges, and the patient's condition.

Hemorrhage is the second most common cause of conversion to an open operation. Although unexpected hemorrhage often can be managed laparoscopically, a conversion to an open operation is indicated if bleeding cannot be controlled expeditiously and without compromise to the structures of the porta hepatis or other adjacent viscera.

When one is preoperatively aware of the presence of a suspicious gallbladder mass, it is best to perform an open operation, anticipating the possibility of a portal lymph node dissection, as well as an en bloc resection of the gallbladder, a portion of the liver, and perhaps a segment of the bile duct. About 1% of gallbladders removed laparoscopically are found to contain carcinomas. This is a compelling argument to have the pathologist examine the specimen during the operation when there are any concerns about the gallbladder. If a carcinoma is recognized immediately, the operation can be converted to an open, radical technique, presuming the proper expertise is available. If this operation is not within the surgeon's realm of practice and the local capabilities, the patient may be referred to an expert for re-exploration. A multivariate analysis revealed that gallbladder carcinoma resectability and stage are independent predictors of survival, but a prior exploration (eg, open or laparoscopic cholecystectomy) does not adversely affect long-term outcome [14]. If a radical operation is performed after a laparoscopic cholecystectomy, the resection also should include the original trocar wounds to eradicate potential sites of tumor implants. Whether an open operation should succeed a laparoscopic cholecystectomy, when a malignancy is discovered upon final pathology, is a function of the depth of primary tumor invasion. One may avoid a radical resection if the tumor is confined to the mucosa and submucosa (T1a), but invasion of the gallbladder muscularis (T1b or deeper) warrants a radical resection [15]. A harbinger of malignancy may be a porcelain gallbladder [16]; so one should have a low threshold of converting to an open cholecystectomy in this situation. However, recent series have suggested that this concern may have been overstated and that a calcified gallbladder wall does not portend malignancy [17]. These conflicting reports might reflect whether gallbladder mural calcification is detected by radiography or microscopy.

Patients who have severe cardiopulmonary disease are occasionally unable to tolerate the physiologic effects of the pneumoperitoneum, even at reduced pressure [18]. It is reasonable to attempt a laparoscopic cholecystectomy in these patients, with plans to evacuate the pneumoperitoneum and perform an open operation, if necessary. Another option is minicholecystectomy.

Cirrhosis can make a cholecystectomy a daunting endeavor, depending upon the severity of liver disease and associated portal hypertension. In fact, operative mortality was as high as 7% to 26% for cholecystectomy in the setting of cirrhosis just a couple decades ago [19], and in one series of cirrhotic patients, all five who underwent bile duct operations died of massive hemorrhage and sepsis [20]. More recently, and with proper patient selection, laparoscopic cholecystectomy was performed safely and without mortality among cirrhotic patients, albeit with a greater incidence of complications and longer hospital stays than among patients without cirrhosis [12,21]. Notably, one randomized series comparing laparoscopic with open cholecystectomy demonstrated a lower complication rate, less blood loss, and shorter hospitalization for the former technique [19]. Preoperatively, the surgeon should maximize the patient's liver function, including a reduction of ascites and correction of coagulopathy. Intraoperative findings such as a stiff liver, portal varices, abdominal wall varices, and fused, vascular portal tissues may warrant a conversion to an open operation. If significant bleeding develops upon dissecting the gallbladder from the liver, an option is to leave the posterior wall of the gallbladder in situ and to coagulate its mucosa. Intraoperative chemical adjuncts, including octreotide or vasopressin infusion, may also decrease the amount of hemorrhage. More ominous signs of hepatic decompensation, such as a coagulopathy, ascites, or malnutrition, should provoke consideration of whether it may be safer to leave the gallbladder in situ or to perform an operation such as a cholecystolithotomy or a subtotal cholecystectomy.

It is occasionally necessary to remove the gallbladder during pregnancy, and the decision to operate weighs the relative risks (to both mother and fetus) of the gallstone disease versus the hazards of cholecystectomy. Less than 1% of women manifest gallstone disease during pregnancy, but this can result in fetal loss, preterm labor, preterm delivery, and other problems. For example, gallstone pancreatitis has been associated with a 70% incidence of recurrent symptoms or complications of gallstones during the same pregnancy, and a 10% to 20% chance of fetal loss [22]. On the other hand, any operation during pregnancy risks fetal teratogenicity, spontaneous abortion, preterm labor or delivery, uterine trauma, and an increased chance of the mother developing an incisional hernia, thromboembolic complications, or pulmonary compromise. Recent experiences indicate that laparoscopic cholecystectomy can be performed with reasonable safety during pregnancy, perhaps ideally during the second trimester to minimize teratogenicity [22]. Interestingly, a Markov decision analytic model has calculated that laparoscopic cholecystectomy is superior to nonoperative management of biliary tract disease during the first and second trimesters of pregnancy, relative to maternal health and fetal outcome [23]. The analysis demonstrated an average gain of 4 quality pregnancy weeks during the first trimester, and a gain of 2 quality pregnancy weeks for women in the second trimester. The size of the uterus during the third trimester increases the likelihood of direct injury to both the uterus and other viscera because of the lack of space to manipulate instruments. Consequently, an open cholecystectomy is generally necessary during the late stages of pregnancy, if the operation cannot be delayed until after delivery of the baby.

Open cholecystectomies are performed during various major abdominal operations, including pancreatoduodenectomy, liver resection, liver choledochal cyst excision, transduodenal sphincterotomy, bile duct resection, liver transplantation, and laparotomies for trauma, among others. Furthermore, there is merit to removing the gallbladder when stones or a mass are discovered during an operation on adjacent viscera. For example, one series demonstrated that concomitant cholecystectomy for asymptomatic gallstone disease does not increase the complication rate of colorectal surgery, whereas the long-term likelihood of the patient requiring a later cholecystectomy is significant [24]. Similarly, it may be reasonable to remove a denervated gallbladder that contains stones, such as when a vagotomy is performed for a peptic diathesis or during an esophagogastrectomy. Another indication for an open operation is the need to perform a common bile duct exploration when the bile duct is not amenable to either endoscopic stone extraction or laparoscopic exploration. The gallbladder may not bear evidence of severe inflammation when it is removed during another operation. Nevertheless, the surgeon should not mistakenly regard this as a minor component of the larger effort. For example, the gallbladder may be distended significantly in patients who have obstructive jaundice, so that the cholecystic veins are considerably more prominent than usual.

Two conditions, gallstone ileus and Mirizzi's syndrome, merit special mention, as they involve intense inflammatory reaction within the triangle of Calot and require open biliary operations. Gallstone ileus classically presents in elderly, infirm patients when a large stone spontaneously erodes through the gallbladder wall and creates a cholecystoenteric fistula, typically into the duodenum. The impaction of a stone in the gut lumen results in bowel obstruction. An enterolithotomy alone is sufficient for most patients in the acute setting, as profound inflammation invests the gallbladder and renders it dangerous to dissect. Furthermore, most patients will clinically tolerate the biliary fistula and only a minority will require an interval cholecystectomy. A concomitant (one-stage) cholecystectomy, closure of the fistula, and enterolithotomy are reserved for select patients who are fit and have a pressing indication to correct the biliary condition [25]. Mirizzi's syndrome develops when a gallstone becomes lodged in the cystic duct or gallbladder neck. The resultant inflammation extrinsically compresses the hepatic duct, causing obstructive jaundice and perhaps a cholecystobiliary fistula, and this fibrosis obliterates the triangle of Calot. The extent of bile duct involvement in Mirizzi's syndrome has been classified by Czendes and dictates the operative conduct. An open operation is necessary to: safely evacuate gallstones, remove a portion of the gallbladder, identify a fistula, and attend to the bile duct. Intraoperative cholangiography is valuable, and a T-tube often suffices to decompress the hepatic duct until the inflammation subsides. Another option to control a cholecystobiliary fistula is to create an anastomosis between the gallbladder remnant and the bowel. A significant disruption of the bile duct requires a Roux-en-Y hepaticojejunostomy [26].

Other causes of conversion from laparoscopic to open cholecystectomy include the presence of confounding adhesions, mechanical problems with laparoscopic equipment, aberrant anatomy, bile duct laceration or transection, bowel or vascular injury, gallbladder disruption with stone spillage, and discovering other abdominal pathology [27]. The reported rates of conversion from laparoscopic to open cholecystectomy have ranged from 1% to 30%, but are usually much less than 10% [28,29]. Conversion never should be regarded as a failure or complication, because the ultimate mission is the safe removal of the gallbladder.

Technique

Whether laparoscopic or open, the removal of a gallbladder is a serious operation that demands attention to detail and an expectation of encountering anomalous anatomy. The surgeon ignores the admonition that "there is no such thing as a routine gallbladder operation" at his or her own (and the patient's) peril.

The patient may be anesthetized already when the decision is made to perform an open cholecystectomy, typically during a laparoscopic cholecystectomy. As a result, most open cholecystectomies are performed under general anesthesia, but less common choices include regional (eg, epidural or spinal) techniques, and rarely local anesthesia. Pleural injection of local agents has been employed for perioperative analgesia, although this is not an ordinary element of current practice [30]. Prophylactic antibiotics are administered, and measures such as sequential compression boots or subcutaneous heparin reduce the likelihood of deep vein thrombosis.

The patient lies supine for the cholecystectomy, but it may be beneficial to place a folded blanket beneath the right back. The operating room table should be oriented so that cholangiography can be performed. This may involve reversing the bed so that the patient's head is located at the end that ordinarily is reserved for the feet. This affords space for the fluoroscopic C-arm, so that it is not hindered by the base of the bed. If static radiography is favored over a dynamic study, the surgeon should assure that a radiographic cassette can be placed beneath the patient's back to permit imaging of the biliary tract. The surgeon ordinarily stands on the patient's right side, opposite the assistant, although sinistrally dominant surgeons may prefer otherwise.

Most open cholecystectomies are performed through a right subcostal (Kocher) incision that is placed about two fingerbreadths inferior to the right costal margin. (The Kocher eponym also pertains to the transverse cervical incision common among thyroid and parathyroid operations.) Even when the surgeon intends to perform a laparoscopic cholecystectomy, trocar incisions should be planned so that as many as possible can be incorporated into a Kocher incision in the event of a conversion. Following the incision of the anterior fascia, the right rectus abdominis and lateral muscles (external oblique, internal oblique, and transversus abdominis) are divided, while maintaining hemostasis with electrocautery. Prominent abdominal wall vessels, such as the anastomosis between the deep epigastric and internal mammary vessels, are ligated, especially when portal hypertension is present. The ligamentum teres may be secured and divided, followed by an incision of a portion of the falciform ligament. A mobilized ligamentum teres, however, may serve as a valuable vascularized pedicle, to wrap about an anastomosis or along a staple line during operations such as pancreas resections, in which case it is preferable to divide the ligamentum at the level of the umbilicus [31]. A midline incision may be preferable when other operations are to be performed or if the patient has a narrow costal angle. The right paramedian (Mayo) incision for cholecystectomy has been relegated to an historical curiosity, although the author occasionally uses this exposure for pancreatoduodenectomy when it fits the patient's shape best.

To the extent possible, and based upon the patient's size and the presence of adhesions, the abdominal viscera should be inspected and palpated in a search for concomitant pathology. This effort may have had a greater yield prior to the widespread application of cross-section imaging, although it is still a valuable exercise, particularly for surgeons in training. A wound protector may be deployed to protect the soft tissues of the abdominal wall, especially when suppurative biliary disease is anticipated. Erector set-styled retractor systems are durable and have permitted a generation of medical students and junior residents to actually see the operation without developing fatigue, perspiration, or a disdain for the operating room.

The surgeon palpates and inspects the liver, and air is admitted into the subphrenic space to inferiorly displace the liver and to better expose its inferior surface. The colon, small bowel, and stomach are retracted atraumatically with laparotomy pads to expose the gallbladder, porta hepatis, and duodenum. When possible, hemostats are attached to the extracorporeal tags of the laparotomy pads to avoid inadvertently leaving foreign bodies in the abdomen. Adhesions are incised to expose the full length of the gallbladder, and the organ is palpated carefully for stones and masses. Severe inflammation may mimic a tumor, so hard, contracted gallbladders eventually should be opened (by the pathologist, or by the surgeon off the table) to evaluate for mucosal lesions. The surgeon may assess the porta hepatis by inserting a thumb into the foramen of Winslow and using the index and middle fingers to palpate for stones or tumor. Severe inflammation or cirrhosis with portal hypertension, however, may obliterate the foramen. The identification of a pulse along the lateral (right) aspect of the porta hepatis implies the presence of a replaced right hepatic artery, a variant that branches from the superior mesenteric artery and occurs in about 20% to 25% of the population.

It can be difficult to manipulate the gallbladder when it is distended markedly, as it may be when a stone is impacted in its neck or with obstructive jaundice. The surgeon can decompress the organ by inserting a metal trocar or large bore intravenous catheter into the fundus and aspirating bile by means of attached suction tubing. The absence of pigment in the aspirate suggests longstanding cystic duct obstruction. One should minimize the leakage of bile into the peritoneal cavity by applying a hemostat to the fundus upon withdrawal of the trocar. A longer hemostat is placed on the infundibulum to manipulate the organ. The gallbladder may be mobilized from its fundus towards the porta hepatis (retrograde technique), or by proceeding from the porta hepatis towards the fundus (anterograde technique). Young surgeons often favor the latter method, likely because of their laparoscopic experience [29].

The retrograde technique is standard for many experienced surgeons, and it is especially beneficial when severe inflammation is present (Fig. 5). The surgeon incises the visceral peritoneum of the gallbladder fundus about 1 cm from its attachment to the liver, and this incision is carried along the gallbladder, parallel to the liver. The assistant can use a tonsil-tipped

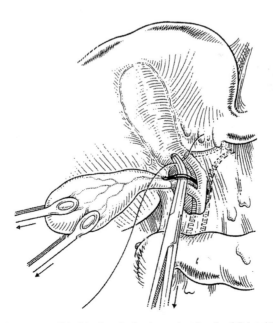

Fig. 5. Mobilization of the gallbladder from its fundus to the triangle of Calot. (*From* – Gertsch P. The technique of cholecystectomy. In: Blumgart LH, Fong Y, editors. Surgery of the liver and biliary tract, 3rd edition. Philadelphia: WB Saunders: 2000. p. 706; with permission.)

suction device to maintain a dry operative field and to develop a plane along the gallbladder fossa, while the surgeon secures and divides the attachments that typically include diminutive cholecystic veins. These veins usually are controlled with electrocoagulation, although ligation of prominent veins may be necessary in the presence of portal hypertension or gallbladder distension. Lacerations of the liver are managed with direct pressure and topical hemostatic agents. In this manner, the gallbladder is mobilized fully from the liver before dissecting within the triangle of Calot and along the porta hepatis. Thus, "no bridges are burned" before the critical structures are identified indisputably, and this should reduce the likelihood of a bile duct injury. It is occasionally beneficial, when significant inflammation is present, to insert a digit into the gallbladder lumen to guide its dissection and mobilization.

If the anterograde approach is employed, the gallbladder neck should be mobilized sufficiently from the liver to expose the triangle of Calot (Fig. 6), the notion that Strasberg has popularized as the critical view for laparoscopic cholecystectomy [13]. The cystic artery resides in this area, although one also may encounter structures such as the proper hepatic artery or its right branch, in a "caterpillar hump" configuration. About one third to one half of patients have classic textbook anatomy in the porta hepatis, so one should expect to find peculiar anomalies. Notably, postmortem dissections of 71 patients who had undergone open cholecystectomies revealed that the right hepatic artery (normal or replaced) had been ligated in 7% of cases [32]. None of these patients had evidence of liver atrophy or cirrhosis, supporting the contributions of portal venous blood flow and collateral arterial perfusion. The hepatic artery, however, cannot necessarily be ligated with impunity in the setting of sepsis, shock, obstructive jaundice, reduced

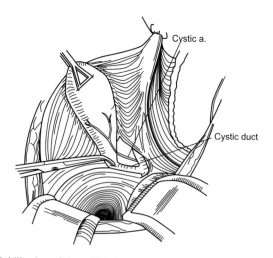

Fig. 6. Mobilization of the gallbladder from the triangle of Calot to the fundus.

portal circulation, or liver transplantation. The cystic duct and the cystic artery are divided once their courses are established. Prior to dividing the cystic duct, the surgeon should deliver any stones from the cystic duct into the gallbladder lumen by gentle manipulation. Anterior displacement of the gallbladder neck facilitates the amputation of the organ from the liver. The gallbladder bed ordinarily is not sutured closed, as was formerly practiced and may still be illustrated in older texts.

One must retract the gallbladder carefully without too much tension and dissect within the triangle so that the porta hepatis is not harmed. Tenting of the bile duct at the cystic duct junction can lead to a partial disruption of the duct's lateral wall. A blunt Kitner (peanut) device may expose the cystic artery and cystic duct, but it is best to dissect towards the portal structures. Stripping away from the porta hepatis can avulse tissue, harming the vasculature of the bile duct. In addition, devices that impart thermal energy (eg, monopolar or even bipolar electrocautery, radiofrequency, or high-frequency ultrasound) should be avoided immediately adjacent to the bile duct. The perfusion of the common bile duct courses along its medial and lateral aspects, in the 3:00 and 9:00 positions (Fig. 7). The lateral (9:00) duct wall vessel is at particular risk of harm during a cholecystectomy, caused by either a thermal injury or a direct injury from an imprudently applied hemostat. Sudden and brisk bleeding from the porta hepatis can be rather frightening, but the surgeon should try to maintain calm and order, arresting the hemorrhage with direct pressure and perhaps a Pringle maneuver. The value of adequate exposure and hemostasis cannot be overstated.

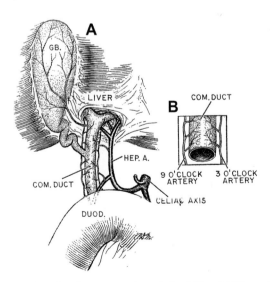

Fig. 7. The perfusion of the bile duct courses through the 3:00 and 9:00 vessels, with contributions from the hepatic, gastroduodenal, and cystic arteries. (*From* Bolton JS, Braasch JW, Rossi RL. Management of benign biliary stricture. Surg Clin North Am 1980;60:23; with permission.)

Venous bleeding may develop from small braches or even the main portal vein. Nonetheless, one should recall that, although the portal system has rapid blood flow, its pressure is relatively low. Consequently, hemorrhage often will arrest spontaneously with direct pressure, time, patience, and topical hemostatic agents. One must resist the temptation to blindly employ hemostats, sutures, or thermal energy along the porta hepatis in a frantic effort to control bleeding, as these measures may disrupt the lateral bile duct vessel and result in a later ischemic stricture. A review of operative notes of patients who develop remote postcholecystectomy strictures often suggests (if one reads between the lines) frenzied attempts to control significant bleeding, rather than an actual transection or partial disruption of the bile duct.

Surgeons should avoid using nonabsorbable suture material on the cystic duct stump, for a choledochotomy suture line, or for a biliary–enteric anastomosis. Silk sutures are notoriously lithogenic and may incite a chronic inflammatory reaction, even when used as external ligatures on the cystic duct stump. Synthetic material such as polyglactin 910 (Vicryl, Ethicon, Somerville, New Jersey), polydioxanone (PDS, Ethicon), or poliglecaprone 25 (Monocryl, Ethicon) is absorbable and effective for biliary tract operations. If the cystic duct stump is thickened markedly, it may be best to close it with an absorbable suture rather than a ligature, although mechanical staplers also can provide secure closure of the cystic duct when there is terrific mural thickening. Metallic (eg, titanium) clips are inert and commonly used during laparoscopic operations, but they are also practical in traditional open operations. Of course, it is imperative that the surgeon absolutely defines the anatomy before any structures are secured and divided.

Intense inflammation or portal hypertension can confound the dissection between the gallbladder and the liver. If a safe plane cannot be established between the viscera, a valuable maneuver is to leave a portion of the deep wall of the gallbladder attached to the liver. The full thickness of the organ's wall is incised circumferentially at the fundus and at the neck so that the remainder of the specimen is removed, along with the gallstones. The mucosa of the remnant is cauterized to hopefully prevent the development of a mucocele.

The surgeon infrequently may encounter inflammation so severe that the anatomy within the triangle of Calot cannot be defined, and the gallbladder cannot be removed safely without threat to the adjacent viscera, including the portal structures, the duodenum, and the hepatic flexure. In those situations, it may be prudent to perform a partial (subtotal) cholecystectomy. The surgeon amputates as much of the gallbladder as possible and removes stones from the remaining lumen. The gallbladder neck is sutured or stapled closed, leaving a stump of the infundibulum attached to the encased cystic duct. A catheter also may be placed into the gallbladder remnant, as described for an open cholecystostomy.

Another contingency option in the setting of severe inflammation, when the cystic duct cannot be exposed and dissected safely, is to simply drain the gallbladder with a cholecystostomy tube. The fundus is incised, and impacted gallstones are removed, to the extent possible, although intense scar tissue may thwart these efforts when the stones are densely impacted in the gallbladder neck. One should resist the temptation to blindly probe the cystic duct, as this could result in a false passage and injury to the porta hepatis. A large tube, such as a 28 French silicone Malecot catheter (Cook Medical, Bloomington, Indiana), is placed into the gallbladder lumen by means of the fundus wall, and it is secured with absorbable sutures. (The author generally avoids the Pessar catheter, as it is stiffer and more resistant to later removal.) The Malecot catheter also passes through omentum, which is anchored to the site of egress on the gallbladder fundus. A closed-suction drain is placed in the subhepatic space to capture any leakage about the catheter. It is gratifying when bile issues from the catheter within a few days, implying patency of the cystic duct. An eventual cholecystogram confirms passage of contrast through the cystic duct, assesses the presence of residual stones within the gallbladder or bile duct, and assures that no contrast extravasates from the gallbladder. The catheter may be occluded to permit retention of bile in the biliary tract, and the closed-suction drain is removed if no bile subsequently issues from it. The catheter is left in situ for 2 to 3 months to establish a mature tract; if stones remain in the gallbladder, they may be removed with interventional radiology techniques. The catheter ultimately can be removed without danger, especially if the cystic duct is patent. In these circumstances, the gallbladder is usually quite contracted and tantamount to a partial cholecystectomy. It may be safest to leave the gallbladder in situ, especially if it has been rendered stone-free and the patient is asymptomatic and elderly.

Drains were placed routinely during open cholecystectomy as recently as the 1980s, when their value was assessed critically. A randomized comparison of closed-suction drains (Baxter, Deerfield, Illinois) (eg, Jackson-Pratt) versus passive (eg, Penrose) drains (Bard, Covington, Georgia) determined that the former were associated with a lower wound infection rate [33]. A recent Cochrane review analyzed 28 randomized trials of drain usage (drain versus no drain) during uncomplicated open cholecystectomy [34]. Among the 3659 patients studied, drains did not affect the incidence of mortality, bile peritonitis, abdominal fluid collections, or abdominal abscesses. Patients without drains, however, had fewer wound infections and fewer chest infections, regardless of the types of drains used. Therefore, drains should not be placed following uncomplicated open cholecystectomy for symptomatic cholelithiasis. Exceptions to this recommendation may include situations such as a concomitant common bile duct exploration or the presence of acute cholecystitis, when inflamed tissues might preclude recognition and ligation of ducts of Luschka in the gallbladder fossa. It is advisable to use a closed-suction system when a drain is necessary, and the drain typically is removed within a few days if no bilious fluid emerges. If bile is present in the drainage, further investigation is indicated, such as a nuclear cholescintigraphy scan (eg, hepatobiliary iminodiacetic acid [HIDA] scan), ultrasonography, or cross-sectional imaging (computed tomography scanning), to assure that no undrained bile is accumulating in the abdomen.

The biliary tract may be assessed during open cholecystectomy with palpation, intraoperative cholangiography, and intraoperative ultrasonography. Cholangiograms generally are performed by securing a catheter within the cystic duct. The catheter may be advanced through a partial cholecystodochotomy or placed within the central stump of a divided cystic duct. Regardless, the surgeon first should palpate the biliary tract and gently milk any cystic duct stones into the gallbladder lumen if possible. Alternative methods of cannulating the biliary tract include either the insertion of a small (eg, 25 gauge) butterfly catheter through the anterior wall of the common bile duct (ie, when the cystic duct is not recognizable or of sufficient length or caliber), or the direct injection of contrast into the gallbladder (cholecystocholangiogram), particularly if the ductal anatomy is uncertain. Although the valves of Heister can hinder the introduction of the cholangiogram catheter, they usually can be negotiated safely with patience. Two syringes are connected to a stopcock that is attached to the catheter hub, one syringe with injectable saline solution, and the other with contrast (iodinated contrast or a noniodinated compound). Air must be eliminated from the system so that bubbles do not create a spuriously positive examination. The author uses half-strength contrast, because a denser agent may obscure bile duct stones. An antihistamine or corticosteroid may be administered if the patient has a history of a contrast reaction. To minimize sphincter of Oddi spasm, the saline and contrast should approximate body temperature, and one also may administer 1 mg of intravenous glucagon shortly before the injection of contrast. Contrast should be injected slowly to avoid cholangio-venous reflux or the provocation of pancreatitis. The patient is tilted slightly rightward to offset the biliary images from the spine, and one should accordingly adjust the angle of the C-arm or the portable radiography unit. Radiation protection measures are important for the operating room team, including lead shields. Dynamic cholangiography with a mobile C-arm image intensifier fluoroscopy system is ideal for thorough and efficient imaging. If fluoroscopy is not readily available, static cholangiography may be performed, but it is time-consuming. The surgeon injects a small amount (eg, 2 to 3 cc) of contrast with the first projection to minimize contrast filling the duodenum and preventing visualization of the distal bile duct, where small stones are most likely to reside. Further radiographic images are projected after an additional 15 to 20 cc of contrast are injected slowly. The cholangiogram hopefully will illustrate:

Opacification of the right and left hepatic ducts, the hepatic duct and common bile duct, the cystic duct junction, and the duodenum
The presence of bile duct lucencies (ie, stones)

Extravasation of contrast
The presence of altered anatomy or other pathology

One may need to tilt the patient (eg, into the Trendelenberg position), inject additional contrast, or adjust the catheter's location to accomplish these goals. Tilting also may discriminate between choledocholithiasis and air bubbles, as the latter will float to a nondependent position.

Intraoperative cholangiography has been used to define biliary tract anatomy, to assess the presence of unsuspected bile duct stones, and to identify bile duct injuries. However, surgeons have debated whether this technique should be applied selectively or routinely. A recent meta-analysis of cholangiography for laparoscopic cholecystectomy hopefully resolves this dispute [35]. The series revealed a 4% incidence of unsuspected stones retained in the bile duct, but the data suggest that only 15% of these would have manifested clinically. Furthermore, bile duct transections and minor injuries were rare, and their incidence did not differ between patients who had either routine or selective cholangiography. One also must recognize that cholangiograms convey some risk, in that false-positive studies may unnecessarily lead to the exploration of normal-sized bile ducts or to subsequent endoscopic retrograde cholangio-pancreatography (ERCP) with its inherent hazards. Considering the possibility of false-positive studies and the fact that only 0.6% of patients have occult but clinically significant bile duct stones, the study calculated the impact of detecting meaningful bile duct stones in a single patient. The authors determined that 167 patients would be subjected to unnecessary intraoperative cholangiograms, and eight unnecessary bile duct explorations or ERCPs would be conducted to find that patient. Another report estimated the financial cost of identifying one patient with a clinically significant occult bile duct stone to be nearly $500,000 [36]. Therefore, it is likely best to selectively perform intraoperative cholangiograms during cholecystectomy. Selective cholangiography is predicated upon:

Risk factors for choledocholithiasis (eg, a history of obstructive jaundice or of gallstone pancreatitis, elevated liver chemistries, an enlarged common bile duct or cystic duct, the presence of multiple small gallstones, and abnormal preoperative imaging)
Challenging anatomy
A short cystic duct
The possibility of a duct injury [37]

A numerical scoring system also has been devised to grade the likelihood of the patient harboring common bile duct stones and the resultant yield of cholangiography [38]. Of course, one should not hesitate to obtain a cholangiogram if the anatomy is in doubt.

Over 80% of litigated bile duct injuries from laparoscopic cholecystectomies are not recognized intraoperatively, and these are associated with a significant chance of death [28]. Some have argued that routine cholangiography may result in avoidance of injury or in the identification of a problem amenable to an immediate repair. On the other hand, not all surgeons or situations are suited for a durable repair such as a Roux-en-Y hepaticojejunostomy. In addition, one analysis suggested that 821 routine cholangiograms would have to be performed to permit detection of just one minor bile duct injury [35]. It is clear that routine cholangiography should not be a substitute for routine thorough dissection of the triangle of Calot.

When the cholecystectomy has been completed, the two musculoaponeurotic layers are closed separately, unless they are fused by scar tissue from a previous operation. The author favors a continuous heavy absorbable suture (eg, #1 PDS* II polydioxanone). The skin is closed primarily, unless the case is contaminated or dirty, when a delayed primary or secondary closure may be preferable.

The technique for minicholecystectomy is fairly comparable to the standard open operation described previously, but it employs a more focused exposure. The surgeon performs a 4 to 7 cm transverse incision about two to three fingerbreadths inferior to the xyphoid process, minimizing the division of the abdominal wall musculature. Small retractors and gauze sponges replace hands in the operative field, and a headlamp is valuable. Lighted retractors and suction devices are other useful instruments. Electrocoagulation is applied with an extended-tip device, and clips secure the cystic artery and cystic duct [11].

Complications

The frequency of complications following open cholecystectomies traditionally has ranged from 6% to 21%, although these data do not necessarily reflect contemporary practice [27]. Common problems such as wound infections, cardiopulmonary or thromboembolic complications, and urinary tract infections historically have developed with an incidence of 2% to 6% each [9]. In addition, about 3% to 5% of patients have required readmission to the hospital. Abdominal complications such as bleeding, peritonitis, bile leak, retained bile duct stones, bowel obstruction, ileus, hepatic dysfunction, abscess, pancreatitis, gastrointestinal bleeding, and the need to reoperate are relatively rare, occurring in less than 1% of patients. As with other operations, abdominal abscesses and perihepatic bile collections generally can be managed with percutaneous drainage. A complication of the Kocher incision is the development of chronic postoperative pain or paresthesias inferior to the scar, typically from the division of the ninth intercostal nerve. Neuralgia may respond to an injection of the nerve with a local anesthetic, or with an anti-inflammatory or neurolytic agent. Deaths followed cholecystectomy in over 6% of patients during the 1930s, primarily because of the underlying biliary tract disease, cirrhosis, surgical errors, and anesthesia complications. The mortality rate declined to less than 2% by

1950, and it was about 0.5%, mostly due to cardiovascular disease, during the 1980s. Mortality and morbidity are typically functions of advanced patient age and emergency operations (eg, acute cholecystitis), as might be expected.

The likelihood of complications, particularly wound problems and cardiopulmonary compromise, is much less after laparoscopic cholecystectomy than it has traditionally been for its open counterpart. In addition, hospital stays are shorter [12]. It is admittedly difficult to compare current discharge practices and duration of disability with older data for open cholecystectomy, especially considering contemporary anesthesia and analgesia techniques and external pressures to return patients to home and work. Perhaps a more fair comparison regards minicholecystectomy, which offers an intriguing alternative to the conventional open operation and results in as many as 88% of patients being discharged within 12 hours of surgery [11]. In one prospective, randomized trial that compared minicholecystectomy with laparoscopic cholecystectomy, the former was associated with a slightly longer length of hospital stay and a later return to work. Patients who underwent minicholecystectomies, however, had fewer intraoperative complications and shorter operating times, and their care was less costly. Overall complication rates were comparable between the two techniques [39]. Another randomized prospective trial also demonstrated that while minicholecystectomy required less operating time than the laparoscopic operation, the two operations were otherwise similar, including the complication rates, lengths of hospital stay, and return to work [40].

It is important to acknowledge that laparoscopic biliary surgery has increased the chances of certain complications that previously were not associated with gallbladder operations, such as bowel perforation and major vascular trauma. In addition, the incidence of bile duct injury has increased significantly, and remains about twofold greater after a laparoscopic cholecystectomy (1 injury per 200-5,000 cases) than after an open cholecystectomy [28,35]. This is particularly striking, because the more treacherous operations are often those that require an open approach. Furthermore, the nearly 20-year learning curve and formal training in laparoscopy have not dampened the higher risk of bile duct injuries. Some have attributed this phenomenon to the limited depth perception and altered spatial orientation that are inherent to laparoscopy. It is noteworthy that litigation is much more likely after laparoscopic bile duct trauma, and verdicts favor the plaintiffs in over half the cases.

The likelihood of permanent harm to patients is reduced dramatically when bile duct injuries are recognized during the cholecystectomy, whether laparoscopic or open. If the duct suffers a fairly simple laceration, such as a limited choledochotomy for the introduction of a cholangiogram catheter, it is reasonable to perform a primary repair, especially if the injury is on the anterior wall of the bile duct. A T-tube may not be necessary for a minor injury, particularly if the duct has a small caliber, although a closed-suction drain should be placed. A lateral injury, however, might disrupt the vasculature of the duct, in which case a more formal repair may be required. In general, a major injury of the bile duct (eg, a transection or a disruption of a significant portion of the duct wall) should be repaired with a reconstruction, typically a hepaticojejunostomy with a Roux-en-Y configuration [41]. A distal duct injury occasionally could be amenable to a choledocho-duodenostomy, if this can be accomplished in a tension-free manner, but this situation is uncommon. It is critical that the surrounding tissues be divided flush with the bile duct to avoid disrupting its perfusion, and one should not circumferentially dissect a long segment of the duct. If the porta hepatis is severely inflamed, it may be prudent to simply drain the bile duct and accept a controlled fistula; a biliary reconstruction can be performed at a later date when the tissues are no longer acutely inflamed. Similarly, if the surgeon is not accustomed to complex biliary operations, it is best to consult a more experienced colleague for the bile duct repair. If a local expert is not available, the bile duct should be drained rather than further manipulated, and the patient should be immediately transferred to a surgeon with expertise in biliary reconstruction [41].

Open cholecystectomy in the future

Although laparoscopic cholecystectomy has resulted in an increase in bile duct injuries, some have proposed an eventual swing of the pendulum so that open cholecystectomy might become associated with a greater chance of duct complications. This would be the result of a combination of factors, including selection bias and surgeon training. For example, the most profoundly inflamed gallbladders (those with the greatest risk of duct injury) are those that will be converted to open operations. In the near future, these operations will be performed by surgeons who have limited experience in complex biliary (and other open) operations, as the seasoned biliary surgeons leave practice. This scenario has yet to come to fruition, however, and bile duct injuries are still twice as likely to develop after laparoscopic than open cholecystectomy [28].

In the United States, the graduating chief surgical resident now performs an average of 12 open cholecystectomies, and less than two common bile duct explorations, in contrast to about 90 laparoscopic cholecystectomies [29]. Although there is nothing to suggest that this trend of diminishing exposure to open biliary surgery will reverse, the need for open cholecystectomy remains. Therefore, residents and young surgeons must flock to the operating room whenever these challenging cases arise, and they must be well-versed in the contingency measures described previously. One hopes that computer modules will offer realistic simulations of operative experiences to bridge the gap between clinical volume and training needs.

It certainly will be difficult, however, for software programs to generate:

The exact nature of acute inflammation
The fusion of tissue planes
The dense inflammatory rinds
The fragility of vasculature in the porta hepatis
What constitutes a safe amount of traction and countertraction
So many other experiences that the surgeon encounters and intuitively
appreciates

This type of virtual reality may not be available as soon as once hoped [42]. As with any operation, strong knowledge of anatomy, the possession of well-honed technical skills, and sound clinical judgment and problem-solving will guide the surgeon. Furthermore, the surgeon should not hesitate to call upon colleagues who have greater experience in complex biliary operations when difficult cases present.

References

[1] Davis CA, Landercasper J, Gundersen LH, et al. Effective use of percutaneous cholecystostomy in high-risk surgical patients. Arch Surg 1999;134:727–32.
[2] Langenbuch C. Ein Fall von Exstirpation der Gallenblase wegen chronischer Cholelithiasis: Heilung. Berliner Klin Wochenschr 1882;19:725–7.
[3] Harding Rains AJ. A thought for Carl Langenbuch (1846–1901): a centenary. Ann R Coll Surg Engl 1982;64:268–9.
[4] Halpert B. Fiftieth anniversary of the removal of the gallbladder. Arch Surg 1932;25:178–82.
[5] Reich A. Accidental injection of bile ducts with petrolatum and bismuth paste. J Am Med Assoc 1918;71:1555.
[6] Cole WH. The development of cholecystography: the first fifty years. Am J Surg 1978;136:541–60.
[7] Mirizzi PL. La cholangiografia durante las operaciones de las vias biliares. Bol Soc Cir Buenos Aires 1932;16:1133–61.
[8] Gallbladder survey committee. Ohio Chapter, American College of Surgeons. 28,621 cholecystectomies in Ohio. Am J Surg 1970;119:714–7.
[9] Scher KS, Scott-Conner CEH. Complications of biliary surgery. Am Surg 1987;53:16–21.
[10] Braasch JW. Anthony Eden's (Lord Avon) biliary tract saga. Ann Surg 2003;238:772–5.
[11] Seale AK, Ledet WP. Minicholecystectomy. Arch Surg 1999;134:308–10.
[12] Ibrahim S, Hean TK, Ho LS, et al. Risk factors for conversion to open surgery in patients undergoing laparoscopic cholecystectomy. World J Surg 2006;30:1698–704.
[13] Strasberg SM, Hertl M, Soper NJ. An analysis of the problem of biliary injury during laparoscopic cholecystectomy. J Am Coll Surg 1995;180:101–25.
[14] Fong Y, Jarnagin W, Blumgart LH. Gallbladder cancer: comparison of patients presenting initially for definitive operation with those presenting after prior noncurative intervention. Ann Surg 2000;232:557–69.
[15] Steinert R, Nestler G, Sagynaliev E, et al. Laparoscopic cholecystectomy and gallbladder cancer. J Surg Oncol 2006;93:682–9.
[16] Polk HC Jr. Carcinoma and the calcified gall bladder. Gastroenterology. 1966;50:582–5.
[17] Towfigh S, McFadden DW, Cortina GR, et al. Porcelain gallbladder is not associated with gallbladder carcinoma. Am Surg 2001;67:7–10.

[18] Gebhardt H, Bautz A, Ross M, et al. Pathophysiological and clinical aspects of the CO_2 pneumoperitoneum (CO_2-PP). Surg Endosc 1997;11:864–7.

[19] Ji W, Ling-Tang L, Wang Z-M, et al. A randomized controlled trial of laparoscopic versus open cholecystectomy in patients with cirrhotic portal hypertension. World J Gastroenterol 2005;11:2513–7.

[20] Schwartz SI. Biliary tract surgery and cirrhosis: a critical combination. Surgery 1981;90: 577–83.

[21] Cucinotta E, Lazzara S, Melita G. Laparoscopic cholecystectomy in cirrhotic patients. Surg Endosc 2003;17:1958–60.

[22] Glasgow RE, Visser BC, Harris HW, et al. Changing management of gallstone disease during pregnancy. Surg Endosc 1998;12:241–6.

[23] Jelin EB, Smink DS, Vernon AH, et al. Management of biliary tract disease during pregnancy: a decision analysis. Surg Endosc 2008;22:54–60.

[24] Juhasz ES, Wolff BG, Meagher AP, et al. Incidental cholecystectomy during colorectal surgery. Ann Surg 1994;219:467–74.

[25] Ayantunde AA, Agrawal A. Gallstone ileus: diagnosis and management. World J Surg 2007; 31:1292–7.

[26] Johnson LW, Sehon JK, Lee WC, et al. Mirizzi's syndrome: experience from a multi-institutional review. Am Surg 2001;67:11–4.

[27] The Southern Surgeons Club. A prospective analysis of 1518 laparoscopic cholecystectomies. N Engl J Med. 1991;324:1073–8.

[28] McLean TR. Risk management observations from litigation involving laparoscopic cholecystectomy. Arch Surg 2006;141:643–8.

[29] Visser BC, Parks RW, Garden OJ. Open cholecystectomy in the laparoscopic era. Am J Surg 2008;195:108–14.

[30] El-Naggar MA, Schaberg FJ, Phillips MR. Intrapleural regional analgesia for pain management in cholecystectomy. Arch Surg 1989;124:568–70.

[31] Ianniti DA, Coburn NG, Somberg J, et al. Use of the round ligament of the liver to decrease pancreatic fistulas: a novel technique. J Am Coll Surg 2006;203:857–64.

[32] Halasz NA. Cholecystectomy and hepatic artery injuries. Arch Surg 1991;126:137–8.

[33] Sarr MG, Parikh KJ, Minken SL, et al. Closed-suction versus Penrose drainage after cholecystectomy. A prospective, randomized evaluation. Am J Surg 1987;153:394–8.

[34] Gurusamy KS, Samraj K. Routine abdominal drainage for uncomplicated open cholecystectomy. Cochrane Database Syst Rev 2007;(2) CD006003. 10.1002/14651858.CD006003.pub2.

[35] Metcalfe MS, Ong T, Bruening MH, et al. Is laparoscopic intraoperative cholangiogram a matter of routine? Am J Surg 2004;187:475–81.

[36] Snow LL, Weinstein LS, Hannon JK, et al. Evaluation of operative cholangiography in 2043 patients undergoing laparoscopic cholecystectomy. Surg Endosc 2001;15:14–20.

[37] MacFadyen BV. Intraoperative cholangiography: past, present, and future. Surg Endosc 2006;20:S436–40.

[38] Sarli L, Iusco DR, Roncoroni L. Preoperative endoscopic sphincterotomy and laparoscopic cholecystectomy for the management of cholecystocholedocholithiasis: 10-year experience. World J Surg 2003;2:180–6.

[39] Ros A, Gustafsson L, Krook H, et al. Laparoscopic cholecystectomy versus minilaparotomy cholecystectomy: a prospective, randomized, single-blind study. Ann Surg 2001;234:741–9.

[40] Majeed AW, Troy G, Nicholl JP. Randomised, prospective, single-blind comparison of laparoscopic versus small-incision cholecystectomy. Lancet 1996;347:989–94.

[41] Sicklick JS, Camp MS, Lillemoe KD, et al. Surgical management of bile duct injuries sustained during laparoscopic cholecystectomy. Ann Surg 2005;241:786–95.

[42] Dunham R, Sackier JM. Is there a dilemma in adequately training surgeons in both open and laparoscopic biliary surgery? Surg Clin North Am 1994;74:913–21.

ELSEVIER
SAUNDERS

SURGICAL
CLINICS OF
NORTH AMERICA

Surg Clin N Am 88 (2008) 1295–1313

Laparoscopic Cholecystectomy

Demetrius E.M. Litwin, MD[a,b,*],
Mitchell A. Cahan, MD[a,b]

[a]Department of Surgery, University Campus, 55 Lake Avenue North, The University
of Massachusetts Medical School, Worcester, MA 01655, USA
[b]Department of Surgery, University Campus, 55 Lake Avenue North, University
of Massachusetts Memorial Medical Center, Worcester, MA 01655, USA

Laparoscopic cholecystectomy (LC) was first reported in Germany (1985) and France (1987) more than 2 decades ago [1–4]. Although not immediately universally adopted, LC has revolutionized general surgery. Management of biliary tract disease has evolved from the extensive procedure Karl Langenbuch [5] first performed in 1882 with its significant convalescence to a relatively safe and tolerable outpatient procedure today, offering early return to full activity [6]. In the early 1990s, there was widespread initial skepticism regarding the benefits of LC [7,8] but the number of LCs increased dramatically during these early years [9] driven by patient demand and the perception that the surgery had lower risk, shorter recovery, and less postoperative pain. By 1992, a National Institutes of Health Consensus Statement [10] endorsed LC as a legitimate tool in the surgeon's armamentarium for the treatment of symptomatic cholelithiasis, and by 1995, 10 years after the introduction of LC, the number of cholecystectomies performed (both open and laparoscopic) had increased by 25% to 30% [9,11], of which close to 80% were done laparoscopically. Laparoscopy has become the new gold standard for the treatment of symptomatic cholelithiasis and an increasing number of procedures are done for acute cholecystitis (AC) [12–16]. Despite the tremendous impact of LC on the management of biliary pathology, however, surgeons continue to face challenges in the application of LC in daily practice.

LC today can be a straightforward operation, but may also be an operative approach fraught with underlying complexities. Anatomic variations and the severity of underlying biliary disease make LC challenging in

* Corresponding author. Department of Surgery, University Campus, 55 Lake Avenue North, Worcester, MA 01655.
E-mail address: litwind@ummhc.org (D.E.M. Litwin).

0039-6109/08/$ - see front matter © 2008 Published by Elsevier Inc.
doi:10.1016/j.suc.2008.07.005   *surgical.theclinics.com*

many clinical situations. Many surgeons remain relatively inexperienced in laparoscopic surgery with regard to the technical nuances that allow for successful and safe completion of a difficult cholecystectomy. Visual misperception and altered depth perception can contribute to errors in judgment. Finally, most recently trained surgeons are far more familiar with LC than open cholecystectomy (OC); this suggests that the prospect of conversion to OC for many novice surgeons when encountering a difficult dissection presents significant potential problems because of a lack of experience with the open operation. As a result, LC tube placement could always be considered with drainage of the Morison pouch in difficult scenarios as opposed to conversion to OC. Indeed, percutaneous cholecystostomy (PC) should be considered ab initio in those patients who have profound gallbladder (GB) wall thickening and acute illness greater than 72 hours' duration. PC allows for resolution of the acute symptoms and the opportunity for interval cholecystectomy 6 to 8 weeks later. The importance of PC cannot be underestimated because common bile duct (CBD) injury occurs more frequently when the cholecystectomy was considered to be complex [17].

Indications

The indications for LC have remained relatively constant and include symptomatic gallstones manifesting as biliary colic, AC, chronic cholecystitis, gallstone pancreatitis, and biliary dyskinesia, and the complications of acute and chronic GB disease.

Contraindications

Patients who cannot tolerate general anesthesia or major surgery should not undergo LC. Other options, including PC, should be considered in these patients [18–20]. Conditions such as pregnancy, cirrhosis, and coagulopathy are no longer contraindications to the laparoscopic approach but require special care and preparation of the patient by the surgeon and a careful evaluation of risk versus benefit.

Technical considerations

Several concepts and strategies have been promoted to ensure safe LC. These include the establishment of the "critical view of safety" [21], the concept that we have used of broadly creating the open "window" of dissection, the strategy of medial and lateral rotation of the infundibulum to expose the triangle of Calot (the "flag technique") [22], and the use of the "top-down" (retrograde dissection) technique.

All of these strategies have been developed to ensure precise dissection within the triangle of Calot so that the cystic duct and the cystic artery are safely isolated from all other structures. The critical view mandates that only two structures remain attached to the GB: the cystic duct and the cystic artery. We meticulously dissect the cystic duct and cystic artery, and then separate the lower part of the GB from the liver bed to create the broad open window (Fig. 1) that is necessary to ensure that there is no confusion with the anatomy. The surgeon must have full confidence that the anatomy is understood.

Another aspect of technical success in LC that has been described involves the establishment of sufficient mobility of the GB away from the hepatic fossa by freeing the peritoneal reflections medially and laterally so that the infundibulum may be gently reflected as a flag back and forth to be able to view the triangle anteriorly and posteriorly.

At times the degree of inflammation makes it compulsory to alter the approach; in this instance one may use the top-down technique [23,24] to liberate the GB from the hepatic fossa starting with the fundus as used in OC, but this can prove difficult laparoscopically. Instead, we favor the transection approach we reported in 1999 [16], which uses division of the GB beyond the triangle of Calot and then retrograde dissection of the GB remnant (Fig. 2).

Common bile duct injury

In the early years of LC, the incidence of CBD injury was increased in LC when compared with open surgery. Although the CBD had always been at risk during GB surgery, referral centers began to see large numbers of complicated CBD injuries that coincided with the advent of LC [25]. The reasons for the increased injuries were multifactorial but learning curve phenomena and relative inexperience with laparoscopic techniques no doubt played an important role. Today surgeons who are trained in laparoscopy are more familiar with the anatomic view laparoscopically and have accommodated to

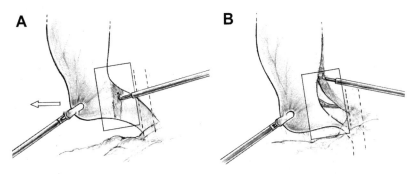

Fig. 1. Window of dissection. (*A*) Appropriate traction to patient's right exactly as depicted. Dissection begins in the triangle of Calot taking small bands and strands of tissue. (*B*) The open window. All tissue is divided except for the cystic duct and cystic artery, and the lower part of the GB is completely separated from the liver, allowing for confirmation that no duct or vessel re-enters the liver.

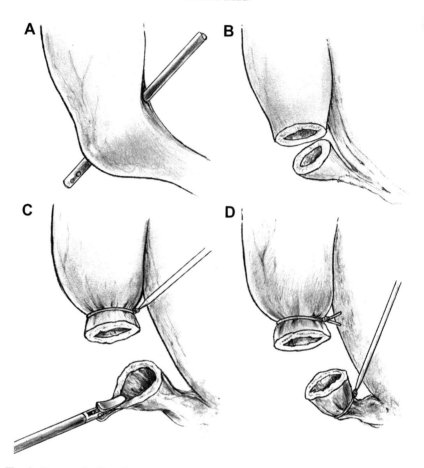

Fig. 2. Retrograde dissection technique. (*A*) Lower portion of GB separated from liver. (*B*) Transection of the GB above cystic duct junction; Endoloop upper GB cuff to avoid stone spill. (*C*) Caudad retraction of remnant with retrograde dissection (top-down) along GB wall toward the cystic artery and cystic duct. (*D*) Dissect to the cystic duct, GB junction. An Endoloop is then placed around the remnant cuff.

the lack of depth perception that is inherent in this technique. Their hand skills are better and the principles of laparoscopic surgery demand that there is little tolerance for obscurative bleeding, because most of the cues in laparoscopy are visual. One would hope that training and adherence to emerging principles of laparoscopic surgery would reduce the number of injuries to be consistent with, or better than, historical norms. A recent large population-based study of 1.6 million Medicare beneficiaries undergoing LC from 1992 to 1999 indicates undeniably that surgeons are much more likely to sustain CBD injury if they are operating on one of their first 20 cases [17]. These data are consistent with the Southern Surgeons Club study that demonstrated a higher risk for injury in the first 30 cases of a surgeon's experience [26,27]. Similarly, in a large institutional series recently published, it was noted that six bile duct injuries occurred in a cohort of 5200 LCs collected over 14 years, but that all six occurred in the first half of their LC experience [28]. Also, a large single-surgeon series (5500 patients who did not have CBD injury, Joseph Petelin, MD, personal communication, April 30, 2008) and a single institutional [29] series with no bile duct injuries, lend credence to the belief that laparoscopy does not inherently place the CBD at greater risk, but rather experience and critical dissection principles are the most important considerations.

Cholangiography

There remains ongoing controversy regarding the role of routine versus selective intraoperative cholangiography (IOC) [30–34]. It is argued that routine cholangiography prevents common bile duct injury, but this is controversial. Large population-based studies have indicated lower rates of CBD injury in those patients who had IOC, and also lower rates of CBD injury for those surgeons who practice a high rate of cholangiography, but these data are not conclusive [35,36]. These studies reviewed patients undergoing LC during the early period of adoption of this technique, and whether a cholangiogram was performed may have been related to the surgeon's ability to actually reliably perform IOC, so that IOC may have been a measure of overall laparoscopic competence. Also, in the study by Flum and colleagues [36], routine users were defined as such if they reached a threshold rate of performing IOC of 75%. Because cannulation rates in experienced hands approach 100%, it seems that almost all surgeons in the study practiced selective IOC. They simply exercised different judgment calls as to when, and how frequently. Proponents of selective IOC make this point, that IOC is an adjunct that should be used any time there is any uncertainty regarding the anatomy, but maintain that meticulous dissection is the key to prevention of CBD injury. Furthermore, IOC cannot prevent all injury. For example, when performing IOC, a CBD misidentified as the cystic duct would sustain a small cut, be cannulated, and be clipped to hold a cholangiocatheter in position to shoot the cholangiogram. CBD injury would have occurred, but with proper interpretation of the cholangiogram, there would be early recognition of the injury and repair could be performed.

Regarding stones in the CBD, routine IOC definitely demonstrates more choledocholithiasis. A selective IOC policy using strict criteria to delineate the presence of CBD stones misses only a small number of patients, however. Early in the LC era, Barkun and colleagues [37] reported a low postoperative prevalence of CBD stones when using aggressive preoperative criteria for imaging the bile duct by either endoscopic retrograde cholangiopancreatography (ERCP) or IOC. With 13 to 34 months of follow-up after surgery, the prevalence of retained CBD stones was 1.3%. Similarly, in a recent single-surgeon study, Nugent and colleagues [38] found a prevalence of retained CBD stones of 0.43% when IOC was performed using strict criteria for cholangiography. Both of these studies demonstrate that many unnecessary IOCs are required for every stone that is found, causing a significant increase in OR time and OR resources that would significantly add to health care costs.

There are additional dilemmas related to the routine versus selective IOC debate for which there are no easy answers. If surgeons are not trained to be facile in routine cholangiography, then they may not be experienced enough to obtain a cholangiogram laparoscopically when it really counts, nor may they be able to properly interpret the findings. Furthermore, without performing routine cholangiography, stone detection rates may be too low to allow surgeons to become expert in laparoscopic common bile duct exploration techniques.

We currently practice a liberal application of selective cholangiography. The criteria for cholangiography are as follows:

Elevated bilirubin, alkaline phosphatase, or transaminases (AST, ALT)
Small stones
Large cystic duct (especially if short)
History of jaundice, pale stools, or dark urine
History of gallstone pancreatitis
Dilated CBD or presence of stone
Unclear anatomy
Aberrant anatomy

Acute cholecystitis

LC has become the gold standard for most GB pathologies, but some conditions require more skill and a higher level of experience to safely perform the operation, whether the case is approached laparoscopically or open. Besides AC, several other clinical situations such as cholecystoduodenal fistula, Mirizzi syndrome, and the fibrotic or sclerotic GB, pose particular challenges.

The degree of operative difficulty increases substantially over time in AC and surgeons have typically used 72 hours as an arbitrary cutoff in degree of difficulty of the dissection [16,39,40]. Generally, in the first 48 to 72 hours of symptoms the tissue planes are edematous but structures are identifiable and the tissue planes separate without much difficulty. After 72 hours, the tissues become more friable and separate less well, the important structures are less likely to be seen well, and there is often more obscurative bleeding. For this reason it is important to consider operating early in AC if the patient does not respond to conservative measures and antibiotic therapy after 24 hours of observation. Often patients present late after many days of symptoms, however, or the GB appears extremely edematous and thick walled on ultrasound (US). Generally, all of these patients should be considered for LC unless they are extremely ill or significant comorbidities exist, in which case PC tube placement should occur [19,20]. If the patient goes to the operating room, an attempt at exposure of the Calot triangle and a trial dissection should be undertaken. If it is determined that safe LC cannot be performed, two potential options exist: (1) conversion to open surgery, or (2) LC tube placement. An open operation might not offer much additional benefit to a very experienced laparoscopic surgeon, and many recently trained surgeons today do not have a great deal of experience performing OC, so that conversion may not be that beneficial to the surgeon or the patient. Cholecystostomy tube placement should be part of the armamentarium of every surgeon. If the patient improves after cholecystostomy, a period of 6 to 8 weeks should pass before interval cholecystectomy occurs. These operations are performed laparoscopically and we have found them to be straightforward. We prefer to leave the cholecystostomy tube in place until interval cholecystectomy. The tube is removed at the time of surgery. In some instances, especially in the poor surgical candidate, the GB can remain in place and no further attempt is made for cholecystectomy after cholecystostomy tube removal [41,42].

Fibrotic/sclerotic gallbladder

Rarely chronic disease causes the gall bladder to be small, fibrotic, and contracted. The GB can be a small nubbin of tissue that is difficult to identify. Occasionally, this is the status of the GB with associated cholecystenteric fistula or Mirizzi syndrome, which makes cholecystectomy challenging. Often the contracted GB proves to be a surprising finding in the operating room, because the US was misinterpreted as showing a GB filled with stones. Invariably the duodenum was drawn up into the GB fossa and the gas-filled duodenum was mistaken by the ultrasonographer for the GB. Often there are dense adhesions between GB and duodenum or bile duct with or without the presence of a fistula. Because the GB may be difficult to identify, adhesions can be dense and surgical planes difficult to establish. This scenario can put the CBD and right hepatic artery at risk during the dissection as one tries to get one's bearings. The pronounced fibrosis tends to contract the space in the window so that there is not much room to dissect and the vital structures are closer to the GB fossa than one might expect. Slow meticulous dissection and adherence to the LC dissection principles are the keys to safe cholecystectomy.

Mirizzi syndrome

In AC, Mirizzi syndrome can occur when a large stone is impacted in the infundibulum or neck of the GB compressing the CBD and causing jaundice. Preoperative diagnostic imaging is important and a persistent or increasing bilirubin mandates visualization of the biliary tree by magnetic resonance cholangiopancreatography or ERCP. In these cases, when the patient is early in the course of AC and when no fistula is present, LC may be attempted. The GB can usually be bluntly dissected off the CBD. Often a more chronic process is present, however, with or without a fistula from GB to CBD. In these cases, the GB is often contracted and fibrotic, and a stone may be impacted in the fistula. Although an initial trial of dissection may be performed by an experienced laparoscopic biliary surgeon, one must be prepared for conversion and for biliary reconstruction. Endoscopic stone fragmentation at ERCP, with papillotomy, stone fragment extraction, and stenting, is a viable alternative to operative surgery to treat the acute situation in Mirizzi syndrome. Subsequent cholecystectomy may be performed if indicated.

Cholecystoduodenal fistula

Another challenging situation occurs when a patient is found to have a fistula between the GB and the alimentary tract, including the duodenum, small intestine, or colon. Gallstone ileus may also occur as a result of the fistula [43]. Although the removal of the stone and exploration of the remainder of the gastrointestinal tract for other stones represents a mandatory part of the procedure in the acute setting, the fistula may be addressed at the time of the initial procedure or postponed to a second operation after inflammation has subsided. Controversy exists regarding the management of the GB. Importantly, if there are no ongoing GB symptoms or if the GB is decompressed, then the approach may be individualized and cholecystectomy delayed. On the other hand, if symptoms persist, including pain, fever, or a clinical picture of recurring gallstone ileus, then cholecystectomy should be performed. Cholecystenteric fistula does not represent a contraindication to laparoscopic surgery, although it does require careful visualization of the anatomy of the GB. In these cases, the GB can be extremely shrunken and fibrotic. The principles of safe cholecystectomy must be followed. Although the GB is usually fibrotic and the intestine densely adherent, the intestine around the fistula tends to be supple and relatively easy to work with. The fistula should be sharply divided with a small ellipse of the intestine. Transverse interrupted closure in one or two layers with Vicryl or silk should be performed. Laparoscopic suturing skills are essential.

Pregnancy

The physiologic effects of pneumoperitoneum on the fetus are well documented and include hypertension, tachycardia, and hypercapnia with acidosis. Additionally, there is decreased uterine blood flow secondary to CO_2 pneumoperitoneum [44–46]. It is unclear whether these physiologic changes will have a detrimental outcome, but one certainly needs to regard pregnancy as a special situation that requires good surgical judgment, foresight, and planning. Although complications of biliary tract disease can have a high incidence of fetal loss, many patients who have biliary tract disease present with a single short-lived episode of typical biliary colic that can be managed with dietary modification with no subsequent attacks for a long period of time. On the other hand, if patients have multiple or prolonged attacks, or complications of biliary tract disease, then a cholecystectomy should be considered. Surgery in the second trimester of pregnancy is the safest period. In the third trimester, the risks for spontaneous labor are greater and the size of the uterus may pose technical problems. Patient undergoing surgery should be placed in a left lateral recumbent position to shift the weight of the gravid uterus off the vena cava. Insufflation pressure should be lowered to 10 to 12 mm Hg provided that visualization and operating space are not impaired. Maternal $Paco_2$ monitoring must be performed by measuring either arterial blood gases or end-tidal CO_2, but arterial $Paco_2$ may be more accurate [46]. It may be wise to maintain maternal end-tidal CO_2 somewhat below normal with mild hyperventilation because experimentation in the pregnant ewe model demonstrates that fetal $Paco_2$ runs higher than maternal $Paco_2$ with CO_2 pneumoperitoneum. Our experimentation with fetoscopy has demonstrated that fetal hypercarbic acidosis can be reduced by maternal hyperventilation [47]. Furthermore, maternal hypercapnia may be responsible for decreased uterine blood flow [48].

A multidisciplinary approach is imperative in the pregnant patient and a decision to operate can only be made in conjunction with the patient's obstetrician who has a better knowledge of the status of the pregnancy and the current health of mother and fetus. In situations in which maternal or fetal health is considered at risk, percutaneous cholecystostomy performed with ultrasound control is a viable option.

Conduct of surgery

Safe LC requires meticulous preoperative planning. Appropriate investigations include an US performed within 6 months of surgical evaluation. If the patient has experienced recent, severe symptoms other than a few episodes of classic short-lived biliary colic, one should obtain a repeat US before surgery. Key information US provides the surgeon includes GB size, the number and size of the stones, GB wall thickness, presence of mass or polyps, CBD size and presence of stones, inflammation or fluid around the GB, and the status of the pancreatic head. A small contracted GB or thickened wall of the GB alerts one to possible complexities during surgery and allows for appropriate expectations and planning.

Diagnostic laparoscopy

The operator places the laparoscope at the umbilicus. Mandatory inspection of the viscera beneath the trocar rules out injury, no matter how simple insertion has been, whether by Veress needle or cut-down technique. An important caveat involves alternative port placement at the pararectus muscle in the right upper quadrant (RUQ) if scarring precludes use of the umbilical site. The laparoscope is placed at that site and visualization and subsequent LC occurs from that eccentric visualizing site. Next, the surgeon inspects the liver to rule out any abnormality, evaluates the status of the GB, the presence of any adhesions, or any other pathology in the RUQ. Subsequent placement of ports is as depicted (Fig. 3A).

Triangulation with central visualization is key for successful LC. In general, the operator places the high epigastric port at the level of the liver edge so that it is at the level of the xiphisternum or between xiphoid and costal margin on the patient's right. The midclavicular (MCL) port is usually placed high up, lateral to the GB, and should be placed on a trajectory as if one were trying to impale the GB. The most lateral port should be at the anterior axillary line and is used for the fundus grasper. It is important to grasp the most floppy portion of the dome of the fundus with an atraumatic grasper and not to grasp too much tissue, because that makes it difficult to pull the GB up over the liver edge, a maneuver that allows for better traction on the GB. The fundus then needs to be pulled over the edge of liver and retracted toward the MCL, or even more laterally toward the right shoulder. More medial retraction closes the triangle of Calot, whereas traction toward the right shoulder tends to open this triangle up.

Exposure of the Calot triangle

Once retraction of the GB fundus has been established, the GB must be retracted in an appropriate fashion to splay open Calot's triangle (Fig. 4A–C). The GB body just proximal to the infundibulum must be retracted laterally, at a right angle to the CBD (see Fig. 4A). This retraction is imperative to open up a suitable window and allows for progressive distraction of the GB and cystic duct from the CBD. The dissection begins as an exact analog of the traditional open operation as commonly practiced. The anterior and posterior peritoneum overlying Calot's triangle is incised, usually with the L-hook, and the space is teased open from lateral to medial by gently pulling the peritoneum and fatty tissue away from the GB. This process invariably leaves small bands of tissue that can safely be divided by the L-hook. A blunt dissecting tool spreading the tissues apart, usually used parallel to the cystic duct/artery, can hasten this dissection and reveal small tethering bands or lymphatics that can be divided by the L-hook. None of these divided structures should be large enough to be considered to be a major duct or vessel (cystic duct, cystic artery, CBD, right hepatic artery). Mass division or clipping of any large clump of tissue or duct structure should not occur. Eventually, using this technique, the entire window must be opened. Opening this window allows for the critical view. Occasionally, the cystic artery is divided early. This procedure allows for more distraction of the GB laterally and opens the window even wider, lengthening the cystic duct and

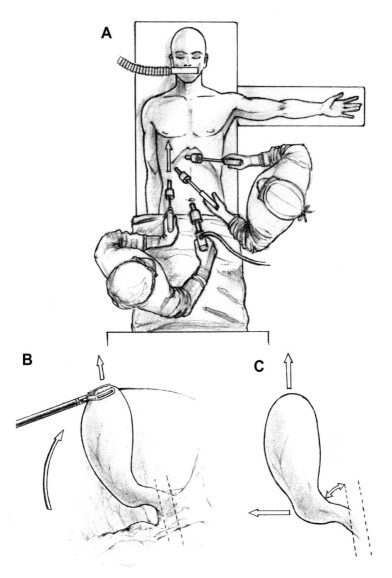

Fig. 3. Port placement and retraction strategies. (*A*) Conventional setup. Two-handed surgeon. Assistant retracts GB straight back to shoulder. (*B*) Internal view of retraction. (*C*) Retraction force vectors. Fundus pushed straight back, but infundibulum pulled straight laterally to open the triangle of Calot, open window, and increase distraction away from CBD.

enlarging the safety zone for dissection. The window is open when all tissue except for the cystic artery and cystic duct has been divided in the triangle of Calot, and the dissection has been performed so that there is separation of the GB well onto the liver bed, precluding the possibility that any ductal structure could reenter the liver unbeknownst to the surgeon.

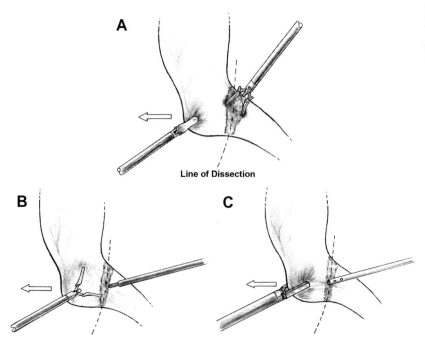

Fig. 4. Retraction strategies. (*A*) Standard retraction by grasping the Hartmann pouch and retracting laterally; separation of tissue to isolate structures in Calot's triangle. (*B*) Atraumatic manner with which to retract GB (fan technique) especially useful in AC. (*C*) In AC the big 10-mm claw grasper is used by way of the midclavicular port to grasp the thickened GB, or if a stone is impacted.

The direction of the retraction of the infundibulum of the GB is a critical maneuver (see Fig. 4A–C) and can be accomplished in several different ways. The GB can simply be grasped and retracted laterally. A common error is to grasp the GB in the wrong place, or to grasp too much tissue. Grasping too much tissue can actually crimp the tissues together, closing the window and making the tissues more difficult to tease apart. Occasionally using the grasping instrument as a fan retractor by holding the jaws open to deflect the GB laterally along the appropriate trajectory is a useful technique because it tends to broaden the window, make the structures more visible, and make dissection easier.

Cholangiography technique

Cholangiography (Fig. 5A–D) is an important technique with which all surgeons must be facile. The cholangiocatheter should enter the abdomen as depicted, between the two lateral ports and somewhat caudad to them. The small nick in the cystic duct should be at the GB/cystic duct junction (or as high as possible) to give one an adequate length of duct to work

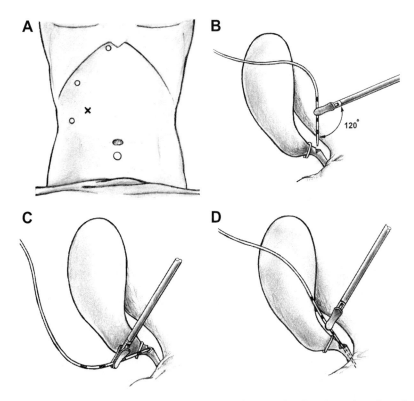

Fig. 5. Cholangiogram catheter insertion (*A*) Optimal cholangiocatheter insertion site. (*B*) Catheter should be grasped at a 120-degree angle to shaft of instrument. (*C*) Rotation of hand in the counterclockwise direction and advancement of tip to the orifice of the cut. (*D*) Clockwise rotation and simultaneous advancement of the tip achieves cannulation and the catheter is clipped in position.

with. The GB should be clipped just above the GB/cystic duct junction to allow for this. The cholangiocath should be gripped by the operating surgeon's right hand (high epigastric port) at about a 110- to 120-degree angle. The surgeon must then rotate his or her hand counterclockwise to allow the tip of the catheter to be placed into the small hole created in the cystic duct. Clockwise rotation and advancement of the catheter should occur simultaneously allowing for easy cannulation. The catheter is held in position with a clip.

Extent of dissection

The extent of dissection before division of the cystic artery and cystic duct is the most important feature of LC (see Fig. 1A, B). In every case a funnel must be seen and exposed (ie, the normal tapering of GB from body to infundibulum to cystic duct). There is no other normally occurring funnel in the biliary system. The window, in which the triangle of Calot is found, must be opened well onto the liver bed using the techniques described earlier to ensure that the tubular structures do not head back into the liver; for example, the right hepatic artery or CBD would be seen in the open window heading back into the liver if misidentified during dissection. Finally, the cystic duct must be dissected or visualized to the extent that when the lowest clip is placed on it a clearly tubular structure is seen below it; this prevents the inadvertent clipping of a tented CBD. One must be dogmatic about these dissection principles to minimize the risk for CBD injury. When training residents we insist that they (1) open the window, (2) identify the funnel, and (3) visualize a clear-cut tubular structure below the lowest clip. We never divide the cystic duct before these steps are performed.

Removal of the gallbladder

Once the cystic duct is clipped and transected, removal of the GB from the liver bed is facilitated by to-and-fro retraction (Fig. 6A, B). This process allows sequential dissection first of the peritoneum, the next layer of tissue on the medial aspect of the GB, and then the lateral aspect. Back and forth, each layer should be taken along a wide swath.

Acute cholecystitis

In AC grasping the GB can be difficult because it is thick and nonpliable and multiple attempts can macerate the fundus with subsequent bile leakage and stone spillage. When the GB cannot be grasped after one or two attempts because of wall thickness or lack of wall pliability, the following technique should be used (Fig. 7A–C). The top of the GB should be incised, usually with the L-hook, although any cutting device can be used. Suction must be available to immediately suction infected bile or pus, and then the suction tip should be placed in to the GB to remove infected bile or

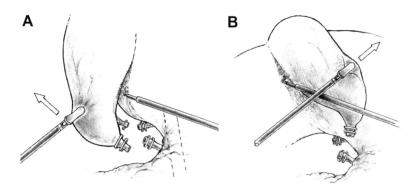

Fig. 6. To–and-fro retraction for dissection off liver bed. (*A*) Traction vector to divide medial attachments. (*B*) Traction vector for lateral attachments.

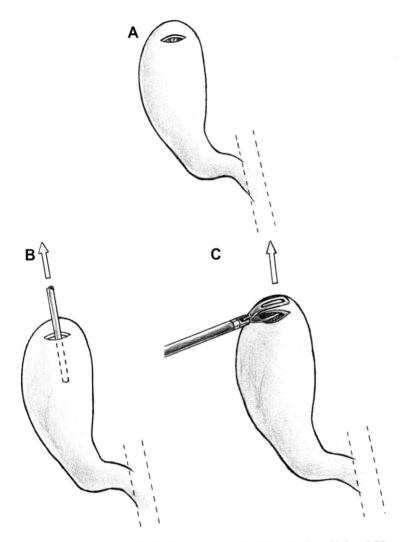

Fig. 7. Retraction strategy for AC. (*A*) Opening of the GB. (*B*) Aspiration of infected GB contents. (*C*) Grasping cut margin to elevate the GB.

pus because the GB is now open. One may irrigate the GB with the suction/irrigator to wash out infected fluid, but this could theoretically force stones into and down the cystic duct into the CBD. Once the top of the GB is opened, the cut margin can be easily grasped and the GB retracted in standard fashion with good purchase.

One of the most challenging aspects of performing LC in AC is providing adequate exposure, because of difficulty grasping and therefore retracting the GB. To accomplish this the 5-mm MCL port may need to be switched to a 10- to 12-mm port to allow a more robust tool. We favor the 10-mm claw instrument (see Fig. 4C), which can effectively grab almost any GB. The instrument should be applied and held without repeated applications because this will eventually tear the GB. Once placed, the heavier grasper allows for appropriate distraction of the GB laterally. Conversely, not grasping the GB at all and applying standard instrumentation using the fan technique (see Fig. 4B) can provide excellent exposure in the acute setting. Additionally, the mode of dissection is often altered in AC. Although the technique of iso-lating small bands and strands that are then divided by the L-hook is not aban-doned, there is a much heavier reliance on blunt dissection. The edematous and thickened tissues are apt to separate with blunt dissection. This separation can be assisted with traditional laparoscopic blunt dissecting tools or with the blunt-tipped 5-mm suction/irrigator, which functions as an outstanding blunt dissection tool, occasionally assisted by continuous irrigation, which keeps the field clean (especially if it is oozing) and provides a modicum of low-pressure hydrodissection. The Maryland dissector is too pointed and can deviate from established planes and puncture structures. Often using the blunt dissection technique the entire window can be opened in this way.

In the presence of acute inflammation, conventional dissection is some-times not possible in the triangle of Calot. In those instances, retrograde dis-section can be helpful and safer. At the same time, it is imperative that the GB traction remains intact to keep the liver elevated and the region of the triangle of Calot exposed. This process can be accomplished as depicted in Fig. 2A–D. In AC, a dissection plane can usually be easily established between GB and liver. After the peritoneum is opened, the edematous plane between liver and GB can be bluntly dissected and the GB encircled somewhat below its midportion and above the infundibulum. This location is safe and above any significant structures one would find in the window. After the GB is encircled it is transected (the harmonic scissors are useful for this). Generally, the upper segment is closed with an Endoloop to prevent stone spillage, and any stones spilled must be retrieved. The lower segment is cleared of stones and by visualizing the interior one can usually surmise the location of the cystic duct orifice. The remnant can then be grasped and retracted in a caudad direction to allow dissection along the wall of the GB to the GB/cystic duct junction. This retrograde dissection is probably safer than our usual approach. Often the tissue peels away easily and one is left with a ductular structure that can be safely clipped. Conversely, if dissection can only be safely taken to the GB/cystic duct junction, an Endoloop can be placed at that site to occlude the cystic duct at its orifice. The small GB remnant will necrose or redundant tissue can be resected. Endoloop closure is not as secure as a clip across the cystic duct, so the site must be drained.

Cholecystostomy tube

A cholecystostomy tube allows a surgeon to exit from a difficult situation with the potential for less morbidity, thereby allowing the acute inflammation to subside, and allowing the surgeon an opportunity to return in 6 to 8 weeks for a more elective cholecystectomy. For the experienced laparoscopic surgeon, or for the inexperienced open cholecystectomist, conversion is unlikely to render the difficult situation safer. Cholecystostomy tube insertion should therefore always remain an option. The fundus of the GB should be opened as in Fig. 7A. Typically this should be large enough for the suction irrigator. The inside of the GB can be washed out. I do not make an attempt to remove stones. Generally, a large Malecot stretched over a 5-mm instrument can be placed through the MCL port and placed into the hole in the fundus. Occasionally the hole in the fundus needs to be enlarged or stretched by spreading an instrument in the orifice. Once the Malecot is in the GB, one should be able to irrigate freely through it to prove that it is inside a luminal structure and to prove that it is not kinked; otherwise it might not drain well. Occasionally the opening in the fundus needs a stitch to narrow it around the catheter. A drain should always be placed in Morison's pouch and removed when it is free of biliary drainage.

Gallbladder retrieval

Routine extraction is through the umbilical port. If the GB is friable, or has a hole, it must be placed in a bag to avoid bile leakage or stone spillage.

Summary

LC has supplanted OC for most GB pathology. Experience has allowed the development of now well-established technical nuances, and training has raised the level of performance so that safe LC is possible. If safe cholecystectomy cannot be performed because of acute inflammation, LC tube placement should occur. A systematic approach in every case to open the window beyond the triangle of Calot, well up onto the liver bed, is essential for the safe completion of the operation.

Acknowledgments

The authors thank Richard Beane for creation of the figures in the manuscript.

References

[1] Reynolds W Jr. The first laparoscopic cholecystectomy. JSLS 2001;5(1):89–94.
[2] Mouret P. Celioscopic surgery. Evolution or revolution. Chirurgie 1990;116(10):829–32.
[3] Cuschieri A, Dubois F, Mouiel J, et al. The European experience with laparoscopic cholecystectomy. Am J Surg 1991;161(3):385–7.

[4] Delaitre B, Testas P, Dubois F. Complications of cholecystectomy by laparoscopic approach. Apropos of 6512 cases. Chirurgie 1992;118(1–2):92–9.

[5] Morgenstern L. Carl Langenbuch and the first cholecystectomy. Surg Endosc 1992;6:113–4.

[6] Zucker KA, Bailey RW, Gadacz TR, et al. Laparoscopic guided cholecystectomy. Am J Surg 1991;161(1):36–42.

[7] Tompkins RK. Laparoscopic cholecystectomy. Threat or opportunity? Arch Surg 1990; 125(10):1245.

[8] Keith RG. Laparoscopic cholecystectomy: let us control the virus. Can J Surg 1990;33(6): 435–6.

[9] Cohen MM, Young W, Theriault ME, et al. Has laparoscopic cholecystectomy changed patterns of practice and patient outcome in Ontario? CMAJ 1996;154(4):491–500.

[10] Gallstones and laparoscopic cholecystectomy. NIH Consens Statement 1992;10(3):1–28.

[11] Steiner CA, Bass EB, Talamini MA, et al. Surgical rates and operative mortality for open and laparoscopic cholecystectomy in Maryland. N Engl J Med 1994;330(6):403–8.

[12] Mosimann F. Laparoscopic cholecystectomy has become the new gold standard for the management of symptomatic gallbladder stones. Hepatogastroenterology 2006;53(69):1.

[13] Kitano S, Matsumoto T, Aramaki M. Laparoscopic cholecystectomy for acute cholecystitis. J Hepatobiliary Pancreat Surg 2002;9(5):534–7.

[14] Cuschieri A. Laparoscopic cholecystectomy. J R Coll Surg Edinb 1999;44(3):187–92.

[15] Sain AH. Laparoscopic cholecystectomy is the current "gold standard" for the treatment of gallstone disease. Ann Surg 1996;224(5):689–90.

[16] Wilsher PC, Sanabria JR, Gallinger S, et al. Early laparoscopic cholecystectomy for acute cholecystitis: a safe procedure. J Gastrointest Surg 1999;3(1):50–3.

[17] Flum DR, Cheadle A, Prela C, et al. Bile duct injury during cholecystectomy and survival in medicare beneficiaries. JAMA 2003;290(16):2168–73.

[18] Byrne MF, Suhocki P, Mitchell RM, et al. Percutaneous cholecystostomy in patients with acute cholecystitis: experience of 45 patients at a US referral center. J Am Coll Surg 2003; 197(2):206–11.

[19] Berber E, Engle KL, String A, et al. Selective use of tube cholecystostomy with interval laparoscopic cholecystectomy in acute cholecystitis. Arch Surg 2000;135(3):341–6.

[20] Patterson EJ, McLoughlin RF, Mathieson JR, et al. An alternative approach to acute cholecystitis. Percutaenous cholecystostomy and interval laparoscopic cholecystectomy. Surg Endosc 1996;10(12):1185–8.

[21] Strasberg SM, Hertl M, Soper NJ. An analysis of the problem of biliary injury during laparoscopic cholecystectomy. J Am Coll Surg 1995;180(1):101–25.

[22] Fabiani P, Iovine L, Katkhouda J, et al. Dissection du triangle de Calot par voie coelioscopique. Presse Med 1993;22(11):535–7.

[23] Sheth KR, Pappas TN. Operative management of cholecystitis and cholelithiasis. In: Yeo CJ, editor. Shackelford's surgery of the alimentary tract. 6th edition. Philadelphia: WB Saunders; 2007. p. 1471–81.

[24] Martin IG, Dexter SP, Marton J, et al. Fundus-first laparoscopic cholecystectomy. Surg Endosc 1995;9:203–6.

[25] Adams DB, Borowicz MR, Wootton FT 3rd, et al. Bile duct complications after laparoscopic cholecystectomy. Surg Endosc 1993;7(2):79–83.

[26] Moore MJ, Bennett CL. The learning curve for laparoscopic cholecystectomy. The Southern Surgeons Club. Am J Surg 1995;170(1):55–9.

[27] A prospective analysis of 1518 laparoscopic cholecystectomies. The Southern Surgeons Club. N Engl J Med 1991;324(16):1073–8.

[28] Lien HH, Huang CC, Liu JS. System approach to prevent common bile duct injury and enhance performance of laparoscopic cholecystectomy. Surg Laparosc Endosc Percutan Tech 2007;17(3):164–70.

[29] Misra M, Schiff J, Rendon G, et al. Laparoscopic cholecystectomy after the learning curve: what should we expect? Surg Endosc 2005;19(9):1266–71.

[30] Ludwig K, Bernhardt J, Steffen H, et al. Contribution of intraoperative cholangiography to incidence and outcome of common bile duct injuries during laparoscopic cholecystectomy. Surg Endosc 2002;16(7):1098–104.
[31] Carroll BJ, Friedman RL, Liberman MA, et al. Routine cholangiography reduces sequelae of common bile duct injuries. Sug Endosc 1996;10(12):1194–7.
[32] Robinson BL, Donohue JH, Gunes S, et al. Selective operative cholangiography. Appropriate management for laparoscopic cholecystectomy. Arch Surg 1995;130(6):625–30.
[33] Varadarajulu S, Eloubeide MA, Wilcox CM, et al. Do all patients with abnormal intraoperative cholangiogram merit endoscopic retrograde cholangiopancreatography? Surg Endosc 2006;20(5):801–5.
[34] Clair DG, Carr-Locke DL, Becker JM, et al. Routine cholangiography is not warranted during laparoscopic cholecystectomy. Arch Surg 1993;128(5):551–4.
[35] Fletcher ER, Hobbs MS, Tan P, et al. Complications of cholecystectomy: risks of the laparoscopic approach and protective effects of operative cholangiography. A population based study. Ann Surg 1999;229:449–57.
[36] Flum DR, Dellinger EP, Cheadle A, et al. Intraoperative cholangiography and risk of common bile duct injury during cholecystectomy. JAMA 2003;289(13):1639–44.
[37] Barkun JS, Fried GM, Barkun AN, et al. Cholecystectomy without operative cholangiography. Ann Surg 1993;218(3):371–9.
[38] Nugent N, Doyle M, Mealy K. Low incidence of retained common bile duct stones using a selective policy of biliary imaging. Surgeon 2005;3(5):352–6.
[39] Lo C, Liu C, Fan S, et al. Prospective randomized study of early versus delayed laparoscopic cholecystectomy for acute cholecystitis. Ann Surg 1998;227(4):461–7.
[40] Pessaux P, Tuech JJ, Rouge C, et al. Laparoscopic cholecystectomy in acute cholecystitis: a prospective study in patients with acute vs. chronic cholecystitis. Surg Endosc 2000; 14(4):358–61.
[41] McLoughlin RF, Patterson EJ, Mathieson JR, et al. Radiologically guided percutaneous cholecystostomy for acute cholecystitis: long-term outcome in 50 patients. Can Assoc Radiol J 1994;45(6):455–9.
[42] Patel M, Midema BW, James MA, et al. Percutaneous cholecystostomy is an effective treatment for high risk patients with acute cholecystitis. Am Surg 2000;66(1):33–7.
[43] VanLandingham SB, Broders CW. Gallstone ileus. Surg Clin North Am 1982;62(2):241–7.
[44] Hunter JG, Swanstrom L, Thornburg K. Carbon dioxide pneumoperitoneum induces fetal acidosis in a pregnant ewe model. Surg Endosc 1995;9(3):272–7.
[45] Curet MJ, Vogt DA, Schob O, et al. Effects of CO_2 pneumoperitoneum in pregnant ewes. J Surg Res 1996;63(1):339–44.
[46] Cruz AM, Southerland LC, Duke T, et al. Intraabdominal carbon dioxide insufflation in the pregnant ewe: uterine blood flow, intraamniotic pressure, cardiopulmonary effects. Anesthesiology 1996;85(6):1395–402.
[47] Saiki Y, Litwin DE, Bigras JL, et al. Reducing the deleterious effects of intrauterine CO_2 during fetoscopic surgery. J Surg Res 1997;69(1):51–4.
[48] Walker AM, Oakes GK, Ehrenkranz R, et al. Effect of hypercapnia on uterine and umbilical circulation in conscious pregnant sheep. J Appl Physiol 1976;41:727–33.

SURGICAL
CLINICS OF
NORTH AMERICA

Surg Clin N Am 88 (2008) 1315–1328

Common Bile Duct Exploration for Choledocholithiasis

Jennifer E. Verbesey, MD,
Desmond H. Birkett, MB, BS, FACS*

*Department of General Surgery, Lahey Clinic Medical Center,
Tufts University School of Medicine, 41 Mall Road, Burlington, MA 01805, USA*

Common bile duct stones represent a significant danger to patients, because they can lead to biliary colic, obstructive jaundice, cholangitis, or pancreatitis. Common bile duct stones either migrate from the gallbladder or form primarily within the bile ducts themselves. Primary stones are more common in South Asia and are usually sequelae of biliary infection and stasis. In the United States and other Western countries, common bile duct stones are predominantly secondary stones, having formed in the gallbladder. In patients who have gallstones, and in whom a cholecystectomy is considered, common bile duct stones can be found preoperatively, intraoperatively, or postoperatively. Ten percent to 15% of patients undergoing a cholecystectomy will be found to have choledocholithiasis at some point during their treatment [1–6]. Of these patients, it is estimated that approximately one third may pass the obstructing common duct stone within 2 months with no intervention [7]. The remainder will require an endoscopic or surgical intervention to relieve the obstruction. Because, at this time, it is impossible to predict into which group a patient will fall, it generally is accepted that in all situations where common bile duct stones are either suspected or confirmed, extraction should be performed.

Preoperative diagnosis and treatment

Choledocholithiasis is suspected preoperatively in those patients who have elevated liver function studies, jaundice, pancreatitis, radiologic signs

---

* Corresponding author.
E-mail address: desmond.h.birkett@lahey.org (D.H. Birkett).

0039-6109/08/$ - see front matter © 2008 Elsevier Inc. All rights reserved.
doi:10.1016/j.suc.2008.08.002   *surgical.theclinics.com*

of dilated intra- or extrahepatic ducts, or evidence of common bile duct stones by ultrasound. The most direct method of dealing with choledocholithiasis preoperatively is by endoscopic retrograde cholangiopancreatography (ERCP). ERCP first was reported in 1974 and has gained widespread usage. Decompression of the ductal system can be achieved by means of endoscopic removal of stones with or without sphincterotomy. This procedure has a reported success rate of 70% to 90% [8]. A normal examination, however, will be encountered in 40% to 60% of cases where common bile duct stones are suspected. Therefore, sphincterotomy should be reserved for those patients in whom there is good evidence that a stone is present in the common bile duct. Certainly, ERCP has its share of complications that need to be considered in the decision-making process. Published rates for morbidity from ERCP are approximately 5% to 19%, and mortality has been reported at 0% to 2.3% [8]. The use of magnetic resonance cholangiopancreatography (MRCP) to help select the patients who would benefit most from ERCP is discussed later in this article.

ERCP is an excellent therapeutic option in those centers where the equipment and experienced, qualified endoscopists are readily available, but it does add an extra procedure for the patient, which reduces the effectiveness and efficiency of a laparoscopic approach. Because the published morbidity rates for ERCP and laparoscopic common bile duct exploration are roughly equivalent, ERCP plus or minus sphincterotomy is a good starting point in patients in whom stones are known to be present or strongly suspected, and a laparoscopic cholecystectomy is planned. A recently published Cochrane meta-analysis concluded that, in past years, when open cholecystectomies were common, open common bile duct exploration was superior to ERCP. In the laparoscopic era, however, laparoscopic exploration and ERCP have very similar success and morbidity rates associated with common bile duct clearance [9].

Intraoperative diagnosis and treatment

If the patient has a history of elevated liver function tests or biliary pancreatitis preoperatively, it is important to perform an intraoperative cholangiogram to rule out persistent common bile duct stones. If stones are found during the course of a laparoscopic cholecystectomy, there are three ways of proceeding: laparoscopic common bile duct exploration (LCBDE), conversion to an open common bile exploration (CBDE), or completion of the cholecystectomy with postoperative ERCP. The inherent risk of the last option is that if ERCP is unsuccessful at retrieving the impacted stone, the patient will need to return to the operating room for yet another procedure. If the patient is undergoing an open cholecystectomy, then it is most logical to continue with an open common bile duct exploration.

Postoperative diagnosis and treatment

Occasionally, the patient will have no signs of common bile duct obstruction and a normal cholangiogram intraoperatively (or one is not performed), yet develop signs of choledocholithiasis postoperatively. Most frequently this is because of a stone being pushed down from either the gallbladder or cystic duct into the common bile duct in the course of performing a laparoscopic cholecystectomy. Because the surgery is already complete, the most sensible option for the patient is to undergo ERCP plus or minus sphincterotomy to deal with the problem.

Preoperative imaging

Radiologic assessment of the bile ducts has improved in the past decade. Transabdominal ultrasound often is used as a screening test for common bile duct stones; however, it is not extremely sensitive (sensitivity 0.3, specificity 1.00) [10–12]. In combination with clinical symptoms and laboratory abnormalities, ultrasound examination can help select the patients who need further imaging. With high specificity, if an ultrasound is negative and liver function tests are normal, there is a very small likelihood of common duct stones [12]. CT scans are commonplace, particularly in the emergency room workup of patients, and have been quoted as having sensitivity between 65% and 93%, and a specificity of 84% to 100% (Fig. 1) [13–15]. Better options include MRCP, with a sensitivity and specificity of greater than 90% [13,16–18] (Fig. 2), or endoscopic ultrasound (EUS), also with a sensitivity and specificity of greater than 90% (Fig. 3). All of these studies are purely diagnostic, whereas ERCP has the advantage of being both diagnostic and possibly therapeutic at the same time. Given the complication risk of ERCP, however, these other preoperative screening tools can be very helpful to select out those patients who would benefit most from ERCP.

Indications for common bile duct exploration

Common bile duct exploration is done based on the results of an intraoperative cholangiogram (IOC) or sonogram. Some surgeons advocate for IOC in every patient, because they would argue that, in addition to demonstrating the presence of common bile duct stones, it provides a map of the anatomy and decreases the incidence of bile duct misadventures. On the other hand, many feel that with a good preoperative history, appropriate laboratory tests, and preoperative imaging, extra biliary manipulation is unnecessary. For this group, indications for intraoperative cholangiogram include the history or presence of any of the following:

History of elevated liver function tests
History or presence of jaundice

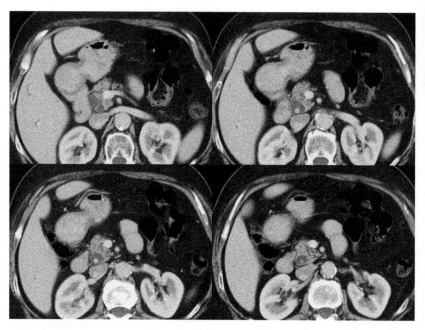

Fig. 1. CT scan demonstrating dilated cystic and common bile duct. Gallstone is seen in common bile duct.

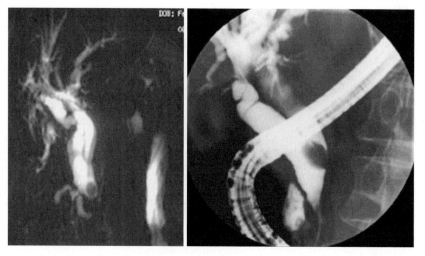

Fig. 2. Magnetic resonance cholangiopancreatography image documenting presence of stone in distal common bile duct. An endoscopic retrograde cholangiopancreatography later verified that finding, and the patient underwent a successful sphincterotomy.

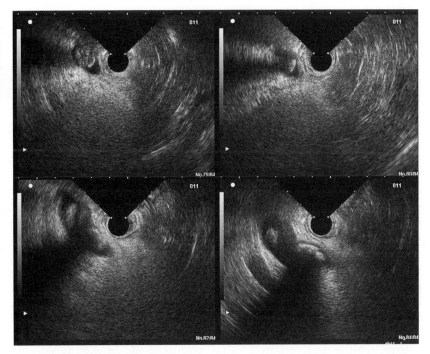

Fig. 3. Endoscopic ultrasound demonstrating common bile duct stone. Ultrasound probe is located in the duodenum, and multiple stones can be seen in the duct, causing shadowing distally.

Biliary pancreatitis
Radiographic evidence of a dilated ductal system
Radiographic visualization of common bile duct stones

Contraindications for laparoscopic or open exploration include an inexperienced surgical team not comfortable with the procedure or lack of necessary equipment.

Open common bile duct exploration

The first open common bile duct exploration was described in 1889 by New York surgeon Robert Abbé. He opened the duct of a 36-year-old woman with severe jaundice, removed a stone, sewed the duct closed with fine silk, and returned her to perfect health. Other sources give credit for the first exploration to Londoner J.K. Thornton, Swiss surgeon Ludwig Courvoisier, or Herman Kümmell of Hamburg, Germany [19].

Although very rare today given the success of stone removal by means of endoscopic or laparoscopic techniques, there are still several indications for proceeding with an open bile duct exploration. The most obvious example is those patients who are undergoing another open abdominal procedure or an open cholecystectomy because of concomitant problems or past surgeries, making a laparoscopic approach very difficult. In addition, some patients will undergo an open exploration because of conversion of a laparoscopic procedure to an open one. A relative indication for open exploration is large or multiple stones or the need to perform a transduodenal sphincteroplasty. Finally, open common bile duct exploration still is considered the gold standard for the removal of common bile duct stones. If the surgical team does not have the experience or feels uncomfortable with the laparoscopic approach, or qualified endoscopists are not available, an open technique should be employed.

The common bile duct is exposed in the free border of the lesser omentum, above the duodenum. If this is difficult because of dense adhesions or inflammation, a small needle can be used to aspirate bile from the structure thought to be the bile duct to confirm the anatomy. In addition, a transcystic intraoperative cholangiogram can be very helpful in verifying the anatomy. Two stay sutures using 4-0 chromic stitches are placed on either side of the planned bile duct incision. An anterior, vertical choledochotomy is made. Great care should be taken to not injure the posterior wall of the duct when making the initial incision. Some surgeons alternatively will place the stay sutures after making the incision.

The first tactic to remove the stones is flushing of the duct. A small red rubber catheter attached to a saline syringe is placed distally into the duct. The distal duct is irrigated, and small stones often will float back toward the choledochotomy and out. If the saline injection is not returning out the incision, the catheter is too far in and past the sphincter. At this point, some surgeons will flush the proximal duct, but more frequently this is avoided because of the fear of pushing small stones further up into small hepatic radicals, where they can become very difficult to dislodge.

A Fogarty balloon catheter, with the balloon deflated, is passed distally through the choledochotomy and advanced distally into the duodenum. The balloon is inflated, and the catheter is withdrawn until resistance is felt at the sphincter of Oddi (Fig. 4). At that point, the balloon is deflated, tension on the catheter released, and the catheter withdrawn a small amount and then reinflated; this is repeated until the catheter is just above the sphincter. The catheter is then gently completely withdrawn, hopefully bringing out any remaining stones with it through the choledochotomy (Fig. 5). The catheter then is passed proximally to retrieve any proximal stones also (Fig. 6) [20].

After attempting to clear the duct with irrigation and balloon catheters, direct vision using a flexible fiber choledochoscope needs to be performed. If a stone is seen using the choledochoscope, then a retrieval basket is passed through the instrument channel of the choledochoscope, passed beyond the stone, opened, and gently and slowly pulled back to ensnare the stone. Once caught in the basket, it is closed under direct vision, and the choledochoscope and basket are removed from the common bile duct. The older rigid

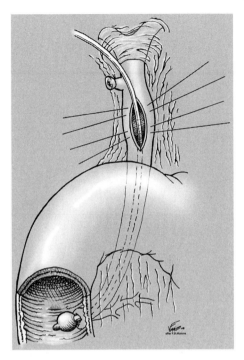

Fig. 4. After flushing, an initial attempt to dislodge a stone is done by passing a Fogarty balloon catheter though the choledochotomy into the duodenum. The balloon then is inflated and withdrawn until resistance is felt at the Sphincter of Oddi.

instruments, such as Randall stone forceps or scoops, have no place today, as they can cause injury to the bile duct and sphincter.

There may be instances where an impacted stone remains despite all of these described methods of dislodgement. In these difficult cases, intracorporeal electrohydraulic or laser lithotripsy can be attempted under direct vision, washing the fragments through into the duodenum. This is often not available, however; if it is, it must be done very cautiously, as it is easy to cause ductal injury.

If all of the previously mentioned maneuvers fail, the final step is to perform a transduodenal sphincterotomy. The duodenum is kocherized (dissected medially) and the area palpated to localize the stone. If the stone cannot be felt, a Fogarty catheter or probe can be placed through the choledochotomy and passed down toward the duodenum as a landmark for the sphincter. A 2 to 4 cm duodenotomy incision is made on the anterior wall of the second portion of the duodenum opposite the stone or probe. Internally, the ampulla should be visualized. Two traction sutures are placed in the duodenal mucosa at both ends of the incision so the duodenal wall can be everted and better exposure to the ampulla obtained. A sphincterotomy

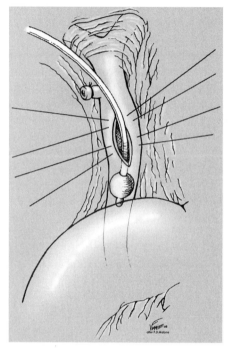

Fig. 5. When resistance is felt at the Sphincter of Oddi, the balloon is deflated, withdrawn a small amount and then reinflated. The balloon at this point should be positioned just above the sphincter. The Fogarty catheter then is withdrawn completely, bringing with it any stones it catches through the choledochotomy.

is performed at the 10 o'clock position, which should be directly opposite the most common position for the pancreatic duct [20]. The incision is made down onto the stone or probe. After the stone is extracted successfully, the sphincterotomy incision is matured with vicryl sutures to approximate the common bile duct mucosa with the duodenal mucosa. A catheter should be passed through the sphincter at the conclusion of this maneuver to verify its patency. The duodenotomy then is closed in two layers with vicryl and silk. Finally, a T-tube is place through the choledochotomy site, and the incision is closed with interrupted 4-0 vicryl sutures. Absorbable sutures always should be used in the bile duct, because the suture material can be lithogenic. The benefits of T-tube placement are maintaining ductal patency in the setting of edema and providing easy access for postoperative imaging.

In 2 to 3 weeks, a repeat cholangiogram is obtained through the T-tube. If this study is normal, the T-tube can be removed. An alternative treatment plan for a patient who has an impacted stone is to place a T-tube to drain the duct, and 4 weeks later, when the edema associated with the impaction has settled, the stones are extracted through the T-tube tract.

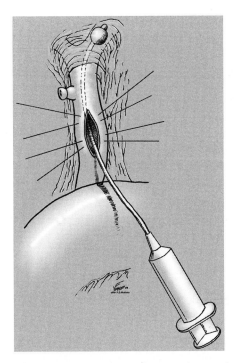

Fig. 6. After clearing the distal duct, the Fogarty catheter can be passed proximally to retrieve any proximal stones. Prior to this, some surgeons will flush the proximal ducts, but this frequently is avoided so that smaller stones will not be pushed up into small hepatic radicals. The catheter is withdrawn, hopefully pulling down any proximal stones out through the choledochotomy.

Laparoscopic common bile duct exploration

Because over 80% of gallbladders are removed laparoscopically, laparoscopic common bile duct exploration is being performed with increasing frequency. It is a difficult procedure, however, that requires a great deal of laparoscopic skill. Therefore it only is done by a select group of laparoscopic surgeons. The advantages are clear; the gallbladder and stones are taken care of simultaneously in a minimally invasive manner that leads to shorter hospital stays and less pain than the corresponding open procedure or laparoscopic cholecystectomy/ERCP combination. Still, laparoscopic common bile duct exploration has its own share of complications, and morbidity rates are quoted between 2% to 17%. Reported mortality rates are 1% to 5% [9]. Compared with the 4% to 20% mortality rates long quoted for open elective and emergency procedures in patients over 70 years old [21–24], there may be a great advantage if laparoscopic techniques are successful.

Laparoscopic common bile duct exploration can be achieved by means of two methods: transcystic or choledochotomy. If technically feasible, the transcystic approach is the preferred method, because it is the least invasive option, the quickest, and the least expensive. This approach, however, only will be successful for smaller stones and a duct that can be dilated to accept a 9 or 10 Fr diameter choledochoscope. Other factors that will dictate which approach is used include the presence and location of multiple stones, the anatomy of the cystic duct in relation to the common bile duct, the degree of inflammation in the surrounding areas, and the ability of the surgeon to complete a complex laparoscopic procedure that includes intracorporeal suturing of a small structure [8].

It is most important to first gather all of the equipment that may be needed during the procedure. The critical items include the following:

Second video camera
Cholangiogram catheter
Pneumatic dilators
4 or 5 Fr Fogarty balloon catheter
Stone extractor basket
T-tube
Flexible choledochoscope
Glucagon 1 mg

Most surgeons will use fluoroscopic imaging as their method of intraoperative imaging; however, percutaneous cholangiography and intraoperative ultrasonography also can be used. If fluoroscopic guidance will be used, it is also necessary to ensure a C-arm fluoroscope is in the operating room and a person capable of operating it is available.

The procedure starts with dilatation of the cystic duct if necessary. The cystic duct frequently already is dilated from the passage of stones into the common bile duct or small bowel. If not, a guidewire is placed through the cystic duct and advanced until it is in the common duct. Pneumatic dilators are inserted over the wire until the cystic duct is capable of accepting a 9 or 10 Fr choledochoscope, but not greater than 8 mm [25]. A 3 mm scope can be used for the procedure, but a 5 mm one is preferable because of better illumination and the access for larger instruments it provides.

If the transcystic approach is not going to provide adequate access, a choledochotomy is performed, provided that the common bile duct is dilated. This method of access is indicated for patients who have larger or multiple stones, proximally located stones, anatomy not conducive to the transcystic approach, or after a failed attempt transcystically. Two stay sutures on the common bile duct are optional [25]. An incision is made longitudinally, avoiding the common bile duct blood supply at the 3 and 9 o'clock positions. This can be performed using a laparoscopic scissors. The incision needs to be at least as long as the largest stone (usually approximately 1 cm). Care should be taken not to make the incision too large, as this will result in a longer and more difficult closure with intracorporeal suturing.

Whether through the cystic duct or the common bile duct, the remainder of the procedure is performed in a similar fashion. The first technique used to try to remove any stones is to irrigate the common bile duct using normal saline. This only will be successful for very small stones (<3 mm) or sludge. As an adjunct measure, the surgeon can ask the anesthesiologist to give the patient 1 mg of intravenous glucagon to relax the sphincter of Oddi and increase the chances of success [8]. Success or failure should be documented by choledochoscopy.

If the stones remain after flushing, the surgeon should proceed to trying to dislodge them using balloon Fogarty catheters. The balloon catheter is placed through the sleeve in the abdominal wall and inserted into the common duct, either by means of the cystic duct or through the choledochotomy. An endoscopic forceps can be used in the other hand to facilitate this step. The balloon catheter is advanced as far as possible, ideally into the duodenum. The balloon then is inflated and slowly withdrawn until resistance is felt. This should represent the balloon meeting the sphincter. At this point, the tension on the catheter should be released, the balloon deflated, the catheter withdrawn slightly, and the balloon reinflated to see if it is above the sphincter. This maneuver is repeated until the balloon is just above the sphincter and below a stone. With slow, deliberate withdrawal of the balloon catheter, small stones may be extracted through the cystic duct or choledochostomy.

If larger stones still remain despite these procedures, several other techniques may be employed. First, a choledochoscope may be used in combination with the balloon catheters, because direct visualization may increase the chance of success. Second, baskets can be used to try to capture the stones directly. The basket is inserted through the instrument channel or operating port of the choledochoscope into the common bile duct. The basket is advanced past the stone under direct vision, opened, and withdrawn to ensnare the stone. The basket is closed carefully to entrap the stone, and then the choledochoscope, basket, and stone are removed from the common bile duct. Confirmation of a clear duct should be made with choledochoscopic visualization.

If the stone is large or impacted, all of these maneuvers may fail, and lithotripsy can be tried or a T-tube placed and the stone removed postoperatively. Frequently, the choledochoscope will have limited usage through the cystic duct, because the anatomy will not allow the scope to turn and advance into the proximal duct. If this poses a problem, the incision in the cystic duct can be lengthened down to the junction of the cystic and common bile ducts. If the stone is visualized, a combination of flushing, balloon catheter use, and basket retrieval under direct visualization may be successful. There have been various attempts at the usage of lithotripsy at this juncture to destroy the stones and flush the fragments from the duct. This is difficult to do within a small duct, however, and has a relatively large risk of ductal damage; therefore it is not performed frequently [8].

Whenever it is felt that the common bile duct has been cleared of all stones, and no further manipulations are anticipated, it is important to shoot a completion cholangiogram documenting the free flow of contrast through the common bile duct into the duodenum, in addition to no new abnormalities in anatomy.

If a transcystic approach was used, the cystic duct needs to be ligated with clips and divided. If a choledochotomy was performed, it can be closed primarily with no drainage, or a biliary stent (T-tube), placed into the duodenum through the choledochotomy, can be used to protect the primary repair. Closure with T-tube drainage is the preferable and safer closure. The indications for T-tube drainage are [8]:

Decompression of the common bile duct if outflow obstruction due to residual stones or edema

Ability to obtain T-tube cholangiogram for postoperative visualization of ducts

Access for removal of residual stones

To place the T-tube, a small section of the back of the T is cut out, and the T-tube is placed into the common duct through the choledochotomy. The remainder of the common bile duct opening then is closed with a 4-0 or 5-0 absorbable suture with intracorporeal laparoscopic suturing and knot tying. It is important to use absorbable suture, because other sutures can be lithogenic. After placement of the T-tube, which is brought out through one of the trocar sites, a completion cholangiogram must be performed. The T-tube is tested by pushing fluid through it and verifying there is no leak. If a T-tube is not going to be used, the entire choledochotomy is closed primarily with the same suture. A T-tube cholangiogram is obtained before removing the tube 2 weeks after surgery.

The risks of T-tube placement include increased morbidity or mortality secondary to biliary infection, migration of the tube causing bile duct obstruction, or bile duct leaks or peritonitis after removal. To prevent the latter two complications, the T-tube must not be pulled up tightly to the abdominal wall, and the T-tube must not be removed for at least 2 weeks postoperatively. A 2007 Cochrane review found insufficient evidence to recommend T-tube drainage over primary closure or vice versa [26].

Laparoscopic common bile duct exploration has a high success rate, with rates reported from 83% to 96% in recent years (93.3% in 2008 Cochrane Review) [9]. The morbidity rate has been reported to be approximately 10% and includes minor complications such as: nausea, vomiting, diarrhea, fever, and urinary retention. Major complications, defined as those that require further procedures, include: wound infections, biliary leaks, abscess formation, subhepatic fluid collections, T-tube complications, and pulmonary, cardiac, or renal failure. Mortality rates are very low, at less than 1%.

References

[1] Williams EJ, Green J, Beckingham I, et al. Guidelines on the management of common bile duct stones. Gut 5 Mar 2008;57:1004–21.

[2] Neuhaus H, Feussner H, Ungeheuer A, et al. Prospective evaluation of the use of endoscopic retrograde cholangiography prior to laparoscopic cholecystectomy. Endoscopy 1992;23: 745–9.

[3] Saltzstein EC, Peacock JB, Thomas MD. Preoperative bilirubin, alkaline phosphatase, and amylase levels as predictors of common duct stones. Surg Gynecol Obstet 1982;154:381–4.

[4] Lacaine F, Corlette MB, Bismuth H. Preoperative evaluation of the risk of common bile duct stones. Arch Surg 1980;115:1114–6.

[5] Houdart R, Perniceni T, Darne B, et al. Predicting common bile duct lithiasis: determination and prospective validation of a model predicting low risk. Am J Surg 1995;170:38–43.

[6] Welbourn CR, Mehta D, Armstrong CP, et al. Selective preoperative endoscopic retrograde cholangiography with sphincterotomy avoids bile duct exploration during laparoscopic cholecystectomy. Gut 1995;37:576–9.

[7] Collins C, Maguire D, Ireland A, et al. A prospective study of common bile duct calculi in patients undergoing laparoscopic cholecystectomy: natural history of choledocholithiasis revisited. Ann Surg 2004;239:28–33.

[8] Petelin JB, Pruett CS. Common bile duct stones. In: Cameron JL, editor. Current surgical therapy. 8th edition. Philadelphia: Elsevier Mosby; 2004. p. 392–9.

[9] Martin DJ, Vernon DR, Toouli J. Surgical versus endoscopic treatment of bile duct stones. Cochrane Database Syst Rev 2006;(2). Art. No.: CD003327. 10.1002/14651858.CD003327.pub2.

[10] Onken JE, Brazer SR, Eisen GM, et al. Predicting the presence of choledocholithiasis in patients with symptomatic cholelithiasis. Am J Gastroenterol 1996;91:762–7.

[11] Trondsen E, Edwin B, Reiertsen O, et al. Prediction of common bile duct stones prior to cholecystectomy: a prospective validation of a discriminant analysis function. Arch Surg 1998; 133:162–6.

[12] Thornton JR, Lobo AJ, Lintott DJ, et al. Value of ultrasound and liver function tests in determining the need for endoscopic retrograde cholangiopancreatography in unexplained abdominal pain. Gut 1992;33:1559–61.

[13] Soto JA, Alvarez O, Munera F, et al. Diagnosing bile duct stones: comparison of unenhanced helical CT, oral contrast-enhanced CT cholangiography, and MR cholangiography. AJR Am J Roentgenol 2000;175:1127–34.

[14] Ishikawa M, Tagami Y, Toyota T, et al. Can three-dimensional helical CT cholangiography before laparoscopic cholecystectomy be a substitute study for endoscopic retrograde cholangiography? Surg Laparosc Endosc Percutan Tech 2000;10:351–6.

[15] Polkowski M, Palucki J, Regula J, et al. Helical computed tomographic cholangiography versus endosonography for suspected bile duct stones: a prospective blinded study in nonjaundiced patients. Gut 1999;45:744–9.

[16] Demartines N, Eisner L, Schnabel K, et al. Evaluation of magnetic resonance cholangiography in the management of bile duct stones. Arch Surg 2000;135:148–52.

[17] Varghese JC, Farrell MA, Courtney G, et al. A prospective comparison of magnetic resonance cholangiopancreatography with endoscopic retrograde cholangiopancreatography in the evaluation of patients with suspected biliary tract disease. Clin Radiol 1999;54:513–20.

[18] Mercer S, Singh S, Paterson I. Selective MRCP in the management of suspected common bile duct stones. HPB 2007;9:125–30.

[19] Morgenstern L. A history of choledochotomy. In: Berci G, Cuschieri A, editors. Bile ducts and bile duct stones. Philadelphia: WB Saunders; 1997. p. 3–8.

[20] Hutter MM, Rattner DW. Open common bile duct exploration: when is it indicated? In: Cameron JL, editor. Current surgical therapy. 8th edition. Philadelphia: Elsevier Mosby; 2004. p. 392–9.

[21] Lygidakis NJ. Operative risk factors of cholecystectomy–choledochotomy in the elderly. Surg Gynecol Obstet 1983;157:15–9.
[22] Siegel JH, Kasmin FE. Biliary tract diseases in the elderly: management and outcomes. Gut 1997;41:433–5.
[23] Gonzalez JJ, Sanz L, Grana JL, et al. Biliary lithiasis in the elderly patient: morbidity and mortality due to biliary surgery. Hepatogastroenterology 1997;44:1565–8.
[24] Hacker KA, Schultz CC, Helling TS. Choledochotomy for calculous disease in the elderly. Am J Surg 1990;160:610–2 [discussion: 3].
[25] Fried GM, Feldman LS, Klassen DR. Cholecystectomy and common bile duct exploration. In: Souba WW, Fink MP, Jurkovish GJ, editors. ACS Surgery: Principles & Practice. NY:WebMD, Inc.; 2005. p. 1–22.
[26] Gurusamy KS, Samraj K. Primary closure versus T-tube drainage after laparoscopic common bile duct stone exploration. Cochrane Database Syst Rev 2007;(1). Art. No.: CD005641. 10.1002/14651858.CD005641.pub2.

ELSEVIER
SAUNDERS

SURGICAL
CLINICS OF
NORTH AMERICA

Surg Clin N Am 88 (2008) 1329–1343

Iatrogenic Biliary Injuries: Classification, Identification, and Management

Kenneth J. McPartland, MD[a,b],
James J. Pomposelli, MD, PhD[a,b],*

[a]Division of Hepatobiliary Surgery and Liver Transplantation, Lahey Clinic Medical Center,
41 Mall Road, Burlington, MA 01805, USA
[b]Tufts University School of Medicine, 145 Harrison Avenue, Boston, MA 02111, USA

The biliary tract is a complex organ system that performs the simple though vital task of collecting, storing, and delivering bile to the gastrointestinal tract. Diseases of the biliary system can be extremely painful, debilitating, and occasionally life threatening. The complex development of the liver and biliary system in utero can result in multiple anatomic variations. An absolute knowledge of these anatomic variations with careful dissection and identification of structures at the time of surgery is a minimal requirement for the safe performance of any hepatobiliary operation. Because of the unforgiving nature of the biliary system, errors in technique or judgment can be disastrous to the patient, resulting in lifelong disability or death. For this reason, a high premium exists on performing the correct procedure, without technical misadventure, the first time. Equally important is the ability to recognize iatrogenic injury so that prompt repair or referral to a surgeon who has expertise in hepatobiliary surgery can be instituted. Positive outcome requires a balance between sound judgment, technical acumen, and attention to detail. Additionally, the hepatobiliary surgeon of today must be able to integrate surgical options with the broadening array of radiologic and endoscopic treatment options available in the management of patients who have hepatobiliary disorders.

This article examines the diagnosis, management, and outcome of bile duct injuries. Although there are many causes of bile duct injury, the diagnosis and management are essentially the same. Iatrogenic injury during gallbladder surgery, especially using the laparoscopic approach, is the most common and is the focus of this article.

---

* Corresponding author. Division of Hepatobiliary Surgery and Liver Transplantation, Lahey Clinic Medical Center, 41 Mall Road, Burlington, MA 01805.
E-mail address: james.pomposelli@lahey.org (J.J. Pomposelli).

0039-6109/08/$ - see front matter © 2008 Elsevier Inc. All rights reserved.
doi:10.1016/j.suc.2008.07.006 *surgical.theclinics.com*

Laparoscopic cholecystectomy was first introduced in the late 1980s and has become the gold standard for the management of benign gallbladder disease. Laparoscopic cholecystectomy has been associated with less morbidity, shorter hospital stay, earlier return to normal activity, less postoperative pain, and better cosmesis compared with laparotomy. It is estimated that more than 750,000 laparoscopic cholecystectomy procedures are performed annually in the United States, making it the most frequently performed abdominal procedure [1]. Despite the clear benefits of laparoscopic cholecystectomy, the rate of iatrogenic bile duct injury has increased from a rate of 0.1% to 0.2% during the era of open cholecystectomy [2,3] to between 0.4% and 0.6% during the era of laparoscopic cholecystectomy [1,4–6]. Of all types of biliary trauma, iatrogenic injury during laparoscopic cholecystectomy is the most common form. Unfortunately, iatrogenic bile duct injuries result in increased patient morbidity and mortality [7–10] and impart a huge increased financial burden in hospital resource use and excessive malpractice litigation [11].

Classification of biliary injuries

Various classification systems have been developed to anatomically describe bile duct injuries and to aid with treatment options. A major consequence of many bile duct injuries is an initial bile leak followed by the eventual development of stricture. Ligation of the proximal bile ducts with surgical clips can result in a worsening clinical condition with cholangitis and jaundice.

It is helpful to classify biliary injuries for documentation purposes and to help formulate prognosis after repair. A widely used system developed by Bismuth during the era of open cholecystectomy defines biliary strictures based on their anatomic location with respect to the hepatic bifurcation [12]. The Bismuth classification system (Table 1) is based on the most distal level at which healthy biliary mucosa is available for anastomosis during repair of a stricture or leak. This system was intended to help the surgeon choose the appropriate site for repair, and the degree of injury on this scale has been shown to correlate with outcomes after surgical repair [13].

McMahon and colleagues [14] devised a classification system that subdivided biliary injuries into bile duct laceration, transection, or excision, and stricture. The level of injury could then be further graded using Bismuth's classification system. In this schema, injuries are also subdivided into major and minor ductal injury, which has implications in the therapeutic approach to these injuries [14].

Biliary injuries that occur during laparoscopic cholecystectomy tend to be more severe than those encountered with open cholecystectomy. The reasons for this are varied but because laparoscopic cholecystectomy is generally performed in a retrograde fashion, the level of injury can be proximal and enter into the second- and third-order bile ducts well within the

Table 1
Bismuth classification of biliary stricture

Type	Criteria
1	Low common hepatic duct stricture with a length of common hepatic duct stump of >2 cm
2	Proximal common hepatic duct stricture with hepatic duct stump <2 cm
3	Hilar stricture, no residual common hepatic duct, but the hepatic ductal confluence is preserved
4	Hilar stricture with involvement of confluence and loss of communication between right and left hepatic duct
5	Involvement of an aberrant right sectorial duct alone or with concomitant stricture of the common hepatic duct

Adapted from Jarnagin WR, Blumgart LH. Benign biliary strictures. In: Blumgart LH, editor. Surgery of the liver, biliary tract, and pancreas. 4th edition. Philadelphia: Saunders; 2007. p. 634; with permission.

liver parenchyma. In an attempt to better characterize injury patterns seen with laparoscopic cholecystectomy, Strasberg and colleagues [3] modified the original Bismuth classification into a more comprehensive system (Table 2). This classification system stratifies injuries from type A to E, with type E injuries being further subdivided into E1 through E5 according to the Bismuth classification system (Fig. 1).

Several other authors have proposed classification systems to further cover the spectrum of possible biliary injuries [15–17]. The Stewart-Way classification (Fig. 2) is based primarily on the anatomic pattern and mechanism of a particular injury (Table 3) [18]. Unlike the earlier classification systems, both the Stewart-Way classification and a recently proposed classification by Lau and Lai include the presence of associated vascular injury [18,19]. Such vascular injuries have been associated with increased morbidity and occur more often with higher bile duct injuries [20,21].

Although several classification systems have been developed that help to better describe bile duct injuries, no system is without its shortcomings. The

Table 2
Strasberg classification of laparoscopic bile duct injury

Type	Criteria
A	Cystic duct leak or leak from small ducts in the liver bed
B	Occlusion of an aberrant right hepatic duct
C	Transection without ligation of an aberrant right hepatic duct
D	Lateral injury to a major bile duct
E1	Transection >2 cm from the hilum
E2	Transection <2 cm from the hilum
E3	Transection in the hilum
E4	Separation of major ducts in the hilum
E5	Type C injury plus injury in the hilum

Data from Strasberg SM, Hertl M, Soper NJ. An analysis of the problem of biliary injury during laparoscopic cholecystectomy. J Am Coll Surg 1995;180:101–25.

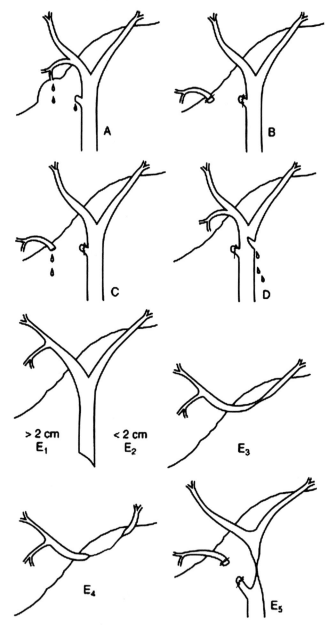

Fig. 1. Strasberg classification of laparoscopic bile duct injuries. Injuries stratified from type A to type E. Type E injuries further subdivided into E1 to E5 according to the Bismuth classification system (*From* Strasberg SM, Hertl M, Soper NJ. An analysis of the problem of biliary injury during laparoscopic cholecystectomy. J Am Coll Surg 1995;180:105; with permission.).

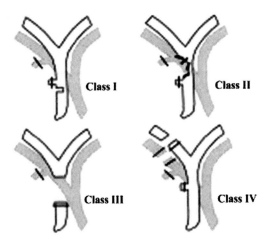

Fig. 2. Stewart-Way classification of laparoscopic bile duct injuries (*From* Way LW, Stewart L, Gantert W, et al. Causes and prevention of laparoscopic bile duct injuries. Ann Surg 2003;237:461; with permission.).

Strasberg and Bismuth classifications, the most commonly used systems, fail to incorporate key clinical information, such as the condition of the patient, vascular patency, timing of recognition of the injury, and the presence of sepsis, all of which greatly influence the management strategy used and the outcome.

Regardless of classification system used, a complete understanding of the anatomic level of injury and patency of the hepatic arterial and portal venous blood supply are the minimum requirements for safe biliary reconstruction. As with any operation, underlying sepsis or hemodynamic compromise should be corrected before attempting operative repair. To that end, prompt drainage of bile collections and initiation of broad-spectrum

Table 3
Stewart-Way classification of laparoscopic bile duct injury

Class	Criteria
I	CBD mistaken for cystic duct but recognized; cholangiogram incision of cystic duct extended into CBD
II	Lateral damage to common hepatic duct from cautery or clips placed on duct; associated bleeding, poor visibility
III	CBD mistaken for cystic duct, not recognized; CBD, CHD, RHD, LHD transected or resected
IV	RHD mistaken for cystic duct, RHA mistaken for cystic artery, RHD and RHA transected; lateral damage to the RHD from cautery or clips placed on ducts

Abbreviations: CBD, common bile duct; CHD, common hepatic duct; LHD, left hepatic duct; RHA, right hepatic artery; RHD, right hepatic duct.

Data from Way LW, Stewart L, Gantert W, et al. Causes and prevention of laparoscopic bile duct injuries. Ann Surg 2003;237:462; with permission.

antibiotics with appropriate volume resuscitation should be instituted before diagnostic intervention.

Mechanism of biliary injuries

The vast majority of bile duct injuries occur during laparoscopic cholecystectomy. Errors leading to bile duct injury during laparoscopic cholecystectomy most commonly result from surgeon misperception rather than from errors of skill, knowledge, or judgment [18]. Because bile duct anatomy is three-dimensional and projected in a two-dimensional format during laparoscopic cholecystectomy, misidentification of structures is more likely to occur than during an open procedure where visual and tactile cues are more readily apparent. The article by Way and colleagues [18], however, does not excuse all injuries. Lillemoe, in an editorial, emphasized that the Way article should not be used as a crutch to lean on in the case of a bile duct injury and that all cases of bile duct injury during laparoscopic cholecystectomy are not unavoidable [22].

The most common type of bile duct injury that occurs during laparoscopic cholecystectomy is the so-called "classical" laparoscopic bile duct injury. This injury occurs when a portion of the common bile duct is resected with the gallbladder [23]. Inflammation in the area of the triangle of Calot can result in close approximation of the cystic and common bile ducts. Excessive cephalad retraction on the gallbladder fundus or insufficient lateral retraction on the gallbladder infundibulum can also align the cystic and common bile ducts. In these cases, the common duct can be mistaken for the cystic duct, clipped, and divided, resulting in bile duct transection and injury. Because the surgeon was convinced that the cystic duct was conclusively identified, continued dissection results in the common bile duct being elevated and resected further, resulting in a more proximal injury.

Other factors that have been associated with bile duct injury during laparoscopic cholecystectomy include use of an end-viewing scope, excessive use of cautery, tenting of the common duct from excessive lateral retraction on the infundibulum resulting in a tear, and aberrant biliary anatomy [24]. A low insertion of the right posterior hepatic duct can easily be mistaken for the cystic duct or an accessory cystic duct. In these cases, failure to clip the duct results in persistent biliary leak, which may not be identified with endoscopic retrograde cholangiography (ERCP).

After the initial surge in laparoscopic cholecystectomy popularity, there was a concomitant increased incidence in iatrogenic bile duct injury. It was believed that surgeon inexperience was the primary reason for the increased complication rate [25]; however, subsequent studies have failed to confirm this learning curve effect [1,26]. A review of more than 1.6 million laparoscopic cholecystectomy procedures performed in Medicare patients between 1992 and 1996 showed a 0.5% incidence of bile duct injury, which did not decrease with increased surgeon experience [1].

Despite the lack of a relationship between surgeon experience and bile duct injury, several authors have recommended strategies to prevent bile duct injury during laparoscopic cholecystectomy [3,18,27]. Strasberg and colleagues [3] have championed the concept of meticulous dissection of the triangle of Calot to establish the "critical view of safety" before the division of any structures. This critical view technique involves retracting the fundus of the gallbladder superiorly and the infundibulum laterally, then clearing all the fat and connective tissue from the triangle of Calot until two structures are clearly seen connecting to the gallbladder. Unfortunately, these maneuvers are not always possible because of inflammation in the area, and overly aggressive dissection can also result in injury. Ideally, when two structures entering the gallbladder are clearly seen (cystic duct and cystic artery), safe clipping and division can be performed [3]. Other methods that may aid in the identification of the cystic duct include use of intraoperative cholangiography, or dissection of the cystic duct–common duct junction [28]. Intraoperative cholangiogram is an effective means to delineate the biliary anatomy, but its role in the prevention of bile duct injury is controversial. Although some studies have suggested that routine use of intraoperative cholangiogram reduces biliary injuries [1,29,30], other studies fail to support such a benefit [31]. There is evidence that use of intraoperative cholangiogram may lead to a higher rate of identification of bile duct injuries when they occur, which can result in decreased cost of treatment and shorter hospital stay [11,32–34]. It has not been our practice to use intraoperative cholangiogram in most cases.

As with any surgical procedure, prevention of complications through careful dissection and identification of structures before transection is the best means of a favorable outcome. Whenever the anatomy of the triangle of Calot cannot be clearly defined, conversion to an open procedure is indicated and should not be viewed as a failure or a complication, but as an expected outcome.

Identification of biliary injuries

Several large studies have demonstrated that less than one third of iatrogenic biliary injuries are detected at the time of laparoscopic cholecystectomy [10,35]. When a bile duct injury is identified at the time of the initial operation, measures should be taken to try to define the extent of the injury. If the level of the injury is clearly defined and the surgeon is comfortable with biliary reconstruction, immediate repair can be performed. If there is any question that the anatomy of the injury is not clearly defined, however, the patient should be drained and consultation with a hepatobiliary surgeon obtained. Proper evaluation of the extent of the injury preoperatively optimizes the chances for favorable outcome.

Obvious intraoperative signs of bile duct injury are sudden unexpected leakage of bile from the liver or soft tissue adjacent to the porta hepatis or persistent bile leakage after transection of an apparent cystic duct. Encountering a second duct during cholecystectomy requiring clipping cannot be ignored as a benign accessory duct because this may represent a right posterior duct. If there is any question of biliary anatomy, intraoperative cholangiogram should be performed but may not always be helpful in preventing injury. Conversion to an open laparotomy procedure simply to confirm an obvious bile duct injury is not indicated if immediate repair is not going to be performed. Referral to a hepatobiliary surgeon who has experience in the repair of bile duct injuries is indicated and may reduce liability.

An important but often neglected part of the evaluation of any bile duct injury is the identification of the patency of vascular structures. Intraoperative Doppler ultrasound should be performed to evaluate vascular integrity because 12% to 32% of patients who have laparoscopic cholecystectomy–associated bile duct injury have a concomitant arterial injury and vascular injury significantly increases morbidity and mortality and may increase the incidence of later stricture formation [8,9,20,21,36].

Most biliary injuries that occur during laparoscopic cholecystectomy are diagnosed in a delayed fashion. Patients often present with nonspecific symptoms, such as vague abdominal pain, nausea and vomiting, and low-grade fever, usually resulting from uncontrolled bile leakage into the peritoneal cavity. Some patients may present with sepsis from severe bile peritonitis, jaundice or intra-abdominal abscess. Patients who have ligation or early stricture formation may also present with cholangitis and jaundice.

Any patient who has an atypical course following cholecystectomy should be suspected of having a bile duct injury and be worked up accordingly.

Imaging techniques, such as ultrasound and CT, are extremely valuable during the initial evaluation of a patient suspected of having a biliary injury. Presence of fluid collections or ascites in the peritoneal cavity suggests a bile leak. Percutaneous drainage confirms the presence of bile in the collection and is the mainstay of initial treatment.

Hepatobiliary iminodiacetic acid (HIDA) scanning can be helpful in the diagnosis of a bile leakage but this study lacks specificity to accurately define biliary anatomy or the level of the leak. One useful role for a HIDA scan is in the symptomatic patient shortly after cholecystectomy in whom imaging fails to demonstrate any significant abdominal fluid to suggest a bile leak. In such patients, HIDA scan can confirm the presence of a bile leak and prompt further evaluation and potential treatment with ERCP. ERCP can confirm the presence of a biliary injury and provides a means for definitively managing many injuries with temporary internal stents. If complete disruption or occlusion of the proximal bile duct is present, prompt evaluation with percutaneous transhepatic cholangiography (PTC) is necessary to define the biliary anatomy and decompress the biliary system. Occlusion or transection of an aberrant right hepatic duct (Strasberg type B and C) may be difficult to diagnose. Endoscopic retrograde cholangiography may fail to identify the obstruction or leak and be interpreted as "normal." Careful examination of the films is required to look for a subtle "missing" duct appearance from failure to opacify the posterior segments of the right lobe [37]. In the case of a bile leak from an aberrant right hepatic duct not in communication with the common duct (Strasberg type C), a retrograde contrast study by way of a percutaneously placed drain may reveal the injured duct. When these injuries are identified, reconstruction of the isolated segment can be performed with Roux-n-Y hepaticojejunostomy.

Noninvasive imaging techniques, such as magnetic resonance cholangiopancreatography (MRCP) and CT cholangiography, can be used to evaluate bile duct injuries. Several small clinical studies have indicated that MRCP can be used postoperatively to classify bile duct injuries, potentially obviating the need for invasive procedures, such as ERCP or PTC [38,39]. CT cholangiography has also been shown to be an effective means of imaging the biliary tree, but the role of this modality in the evaluation of bile duct injury needs further evaluation [40]. Although noninvasive studies are appealing, MRCP and CT cholangiography do not allow for intervention of the biliary tract, thereby potentially delaying treatment.

Management of biliary injuries

Initial management

The initial management of biliary injuries includes appropriate volume resuscitation and the initiation of antibiotics after cultures have been obtained. Ultrasound or CT should be obtained to identify abdominal collections and to determine if intrahepatic biliary dilatation is present. The presence of obstructed bile within the liver or subhepatic collection requires prompt drainage. The final phase in the management of bile duct injury includes defining biliary anatomy and re-establishing biliary enteric communication. Through careful planning and management, it is hoped that further complications of continued bile leakage, cholangitis, and stricture formation can be avoided. Bile duct injuries that include a vascular injury can result in acute hepatic necrosis, abscess formation, or secondary biliary cirrhosis, and in rare cases liver transplantation may be required [18].

The best treatment of a particular injury depends on not only the extent and location of the injury but also the time frame in which the injury is recognized. Injuries diagnosed after a delay may significantly worsen the clinical condition of the patient and require immediate volume resuscitation, drainage collections and obstructed bile, and antibiotic therapy before repair should be performed. Some surgeons advocate waiting up to 6 weeks before repair to allow for the inflammation to settle down and infection to resolve [10,41,42]. In our experience, this approach results in the formation of dense adhesions in the area and may make repair more difficult. We therefore tend to repair injuries during the hospitalization of initial presentation as long as abdominal sepsis is resolved. Regardless of approach, every effort should be made to fully define the extent of the injury and to delineate the biliary anatomy before repair [43]. Initial repair by a qualified hepatobiliary surgeon who has expertise in the bile duct reconstruction provides the best opportunity for favorable outcome [1,11,21,44,45]. Salvage repair for secondary stricture after initial reconstruction has worse outcome [46], which places a premium on performing the correct operation, using the best possible technique, the first time.

Surgical repair

The extent of injury determines the operative course of action. A simple leak from the cystic duct stump found during laparoscopic cholecystectomy can usually be corrected with placement of an additional clip or a suture ligature loop, often without conversion to laparotomy. Complex biliary injuries usually require laparotomy, although successful laparoscopic repair of type C and D ductal injuries has been reported [47]. Laparoscopic approach to these injuries should only be undertaken by those who have experience in performing advanced laparoscopic surgery on the biliary system and should not be performed by the inexperienced surgeon attempting to minimize the event.

Lateral ductal injuries (Stasberg type D) that do not result in complete transaction can be repaired primarily over an adjacently place T-tube as long as there is no evidence of significant ischemia or cautery damage at the site of injury. A Kocher maneuver to mobilize to duodenum can help alleviate tension on the repair.

More extensive Strasberg type D and E injuries require biliary enteric anastomosis for reconstruction. We favor Roux an-Y hepaticojejunostomy over a 5-F pediatric feeding tube to serve as a biliary stent (Fig. 3A). A right subcostal incision with vertical midline extension is routinely used. Bisubcostal chevron incisions are generally not used and may contribute to increased morbidity. After entering the abdomen, complete examination for injuries is performed. Surgical clips in the hepatic hilum are removed and the bile ducts are examined with a biliary probe. Palpation and Doppler ultrasound examination of the hepatic artery is performed to document patency. Concomitant hepatic artery injury has been reported in up to one third of patients who have laparoscopic-related bile duct injury [9,21,48].

After the proximal ducts are identified, necrotic or infected tissue is débrided and a Roux-en-Y limb of at least 40 cm is created using either a hand-sewn or staple technique. Hepaticojejunostomy is performed using a single layer 5-0 absorbable suture in an interrupted fashion (Fig. 3B, C). The presence of multiple bile ducts observed with proximal injuries requires separate anastomoses (Strasberg type E4). Primary repair of complete bile duct transection over a T-tube should be discouraged given the high rate of stricture formation [49]. Postoperatively, routine cholangiography is

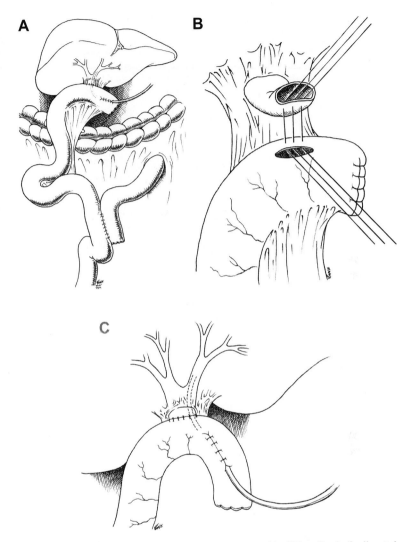

Fig. 3. (*A*) Completed Roux-en-Y hepaticojejunostomy with 5-F pediatric feeding tube as biliary stent. (*B*) Close-up view of hepaticojejunostomy using interrupted 5-0 PDS absorbable suture. Note back wall knots on inside of anastomosis. (*C*) Biliary stent secured with Witzel tunnel and used for imaging postoperatively. Omission of stent is acceptable.

performed by way of the biliary stent (Fig. 4), which is left in place for 6 to 8 weeks if no biliary complications are present.

Outcomes following repair of biliary injuries

Patients who undergo repair of bile duct injury following laparoscopic cholecystectomy have been shown to have an increased morbidity and

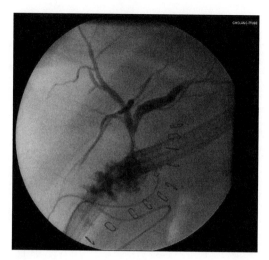

Fig. 4. Postoperative cholangiogram obtained by way of percutaneous biliary stent should show no leak and prompt (within 10 minutes) emptying after imaging. Failure to empty after 10 minutes with patient upright is consistent with stricture.

mortality [7–10]. In a large series from Johns Hopkins Hospital, morbidity rate after bile duct reconstruction was 43% but most complications were minor [10]. Mortality rates ranging from 1.7% to 9% have also been reported [7–10]. Postoperative stricture formation with long-term follow-up occurs in 10% to 19% of patients [50,51]. Most strictures can be effectively managed with transhepatic dilatation and stent placement, although some will require surgical revision [42,52]. The single factor most associated with development of biliary stricture following repair is the level of injury. One third of patients who have an injury proximal to the bifurcation develop stricture post-repair [51,53–55]. The rate of chronic liver disease following bile duct repair has been reported to be between 6% and 22% [51,55,56]. Lifelong surveillance and early intervention for suspected stricture is therefore indicated. Patient education is the best form of surveillance. Typically, patients who have recurrent biliary stricture complain of shaking chills and rigors followed by high fever. Right upper quadrant pain may or may not be present. Laboratory studies may suggest liver inflammation but also may remain normal. Absence of ductal dilatation on imaging is common and not reassuring. A high index of clinical suspicion is needed and initial episodes can be treated conservatively with antibiotics. Recurrent bouts of rigor and fever or obvious cholangitis need intervention with PTC and dilatation. Despite increased morbidity, need for long-term follow-up, and potential for litigation surrounding bile duct injuries, the rate of successful repair of these injuries as demonstrated by long-term follow-up in the hands of experienced hepatobiliary surgeons is greater than 90% [42,51].

Summary

Biliary injuries are complex problems requiring a multidisciplinary approach with surgeons, radiologists, and gastroenterologists knowledgeable in hepatobiliary disease. Mismanagement can result in lifelong disability and chronic liver disease. Given the unforgiving nature of the biliary tree, favorable outcome requires a well–thought-out strategy and attention to detail.

Acknowledgments

We thank Mr. Vinald Francis from the Lahey Clinic Art and Photography department for his artistic expertise in preparing figures 3A–C.

References

[1] Flum DR, Cheadle A, Prela C, et al. Bile duct injury during cholecystectomy and survival in Medicare beneficiaries. JAMA 2003;290(16):2168–73.

[2] Roslyn JJ, Binns GS, Hughes EF, et al. Open cholecystectomy. A contemporary analysis of 42,474 patients. Ann Surg 1993;218(2):129–37.

[3] Strasberg SM, Hertl M, Soper NJ. An analysis of the problem of biliary injury during laparoscopic cholecystectomy. J Am Coll Surg 1995;180(1):101–25.

[4] Adamsen S, Hansen OH, Funch-Jensen P, et al. Bile duct injury during laparoscopic cholecystectomy: a prospective nationwide series. J Am Coll Surg 1997;184(6):571–8.

[5] Ooi LL, Goh YC, Chew SP, et al. Bile duct injuries during laparoscopic cholecystectomy: a collective experience of four teaching hospitals and results of repair. Aust N Z J Surg 1999;69(12):844–6.

[6] Waage A, Nilsson M. Iatrogenic bile duct injury: a population-based study of 152 776 cholecystectomies in the Swedish Inpatient Registry. Arch Surg 2006;141(12):1207–13.

[7] Dolan JP, Diggs BS, Sheppard BC, et al. Ten-year trend in the national volume of bile duct injuries requiring operative repair. Surg Endosc 2005;19(7):967–73.

[8] Frilling A, Li J, Weber F, et al. Major bile duct injuries after laparoscopic cholecystectomy: a tertiary center experience. J Gastrointest Surg 2004;8(6):679–85.

[9] Mathisen O, Soreide O, Bergan A. Laparoscopic cholecystectomy: bile duct and vascular injuries: management and outcome. Scand J Gastroenterol 2002;37(4):476–81.

[10] Sicklick JK, Camp MS, Lillemoe KD, et al. Surgical management of bile duct injuries sustained during laparoscopic cholecystectomy: perioperative results in 200 patients. Ann Surg 2005;241(5):786–92 [discussion: 793–5].

[11] Savader SJ, Lillemoe KD, Prescott CA, et al. Laparoscopic cholecystectomy-related bile duct injuries: a health and financial disaster. Ann Surg 1997;225(3):268–73.

[12] Jarnagin WR, Blumgart LH. Benign biliary strictures. In: Blumgart LH, editor. Surgery of the liver, biliary tract, and pancreas. 4th edition. Philadelphia: Saunders, 2007. p. 628–54.

[13] Bismuth H, Majno PE. Biliary strictures: classification based on the principles of surgical treatment. World J Surg 2001;25(10):1241–4.

[14] McMahon AJ, Fullarton G, Baxter JN, et al. Bile duct injury and bile leakage in laparoscopic cholecystectomy. Br J Surg 1995;82(3):307–13.

[15] Bergman JJ, van den Brink GR, Rauws EA, et al. Treatment of bile duct lesions after laparoscopic cholecystectomy. Gut 1996;38(1):141–7.

[16] Csendes A, Navarrete C, Burdiles P, et al. Treatment of common bile duct injuries during laparoscopic cholecystectomy: endoscopic and surgical management. World J Surg 2001; 25(10):1346–51.

[17] Neuhaus P, Schmidt SC, Hintze RE, et al. [Classification and treatment of bile duct injuries after laparoscopic cholecystectomy]. Chirurg 2000;71(2):166–73 [in German].

[18] Way LW, Stewart L, Gantert W, et al. Causes and prevention of laparoscopic bile duct injuries: analysis of 252 cases from a human factors and cognitive psychology perspective. Ann Surg 2003;237(4):460–9.

[19] Lau WY, Lai EC. Classification of iatrogenic bile duct injury. Hepatobiliary Pancreat Dis Int 2007;6(5):459–63.

[20] Alves A, Farges O, Nicolet J, et al. Incidence and consequence of an hepatic artery injury in patients with postcholecystectomy bile duct strictures. Ann Surg 2003;238(1):93–6.

[21] Stewart L, Robinson TN, Lee CM, et al. Right hepatic artery injury associated with laparoscopic bile duct injury: incidence, mechanism, and consequences. J Gastrointest Surg 2004; 8(5):523–30 [discussion: 530–1].

[22] Lillemoe KD. To err is human, but should we expect more from a surgeon? Ann Surg 2003; 237(4):470–1.

[23] Branum G, Schmitt C, Baillie J, et al. Management of major biliary complications after laparoscopic cholecystectomy. Ann Surg 1993;217(5):532–40 [discussion: 540–1].

[24] Baker MS, Lillemore KD. Benign biliary strictures. In: Cameron JL, editor. Current surgical therapy. 9th edition. Philadelphia: Mosby; 2008. p. 420–5.

[25] A prospective analysis of 1518 laparoscopic cholecystectomies. The Southern Surgeons Club. N Engl J Med 1991;324(16):1073–8.

[26] Calvete J, Sabater L, Camps B, et al. Bile duct injury during laparoscopic cholecystectomy: myth or reality of the learning curve? Surg Endosc 2000;14(7):608–11.

[27] Hugh TB. New strategies to prevent laparoscopic bile duct injury–surgeons can learn from pilots. Surgery 2002;132(5):826–35.

[28] Strasberg SM. Biliary injury in laparoscopic surgery: part 1. Processes used in determination of standard of care in misidentification injuries. J Am Coll Surg 2005;201(4):598–603.

[29] Ferguson CM, Rattner DW, Warshaw AL. Bile duct injury in laparoscopic cholecystectomy. Surg Laparosc Endosc 1992;2(1):1–7.

[30] Ludwig K, Bernhardt J, Steffen H, et al. Contribution of intraoperative cholangiography to incidence and outcome of common bile duct injuries during laparoscopic cholecystectomy. Surg Endosc 2002;16(7):1098–104.

[31] Fletcher DR, Hobbs MS, Tan P, et al. Complications of cholecystectomy: risks of the laparoscopic approach and protective effects of operative cholangiography: a population-based study. Ann Surg 1999;229(4):449–57.

[32] Archer SB, Brown DW, Smith CD, et al. Bile duct injury during laparoscopic cholecystectomy: results of a national survey. Ann Surg 2001;234(4):549–58 [discussion: 558–9].

[33] Gigot J, Etienne J, Aerts R, et al. The dramatic reality of biliary tract injury during laparoscopic cholecystectomy. An anonymous multicenter Belgian survey of 65 patients. Surg Endosc 1997;11(12):1171–8.

[34] Z'Graggen K, Wehrli H, Metzger A, et al. Complications of laparoscopic cholecystectomy in Switzerland. A prospective 3-year study of 10,174 patients. Swiss Association of Laparoscopic and Thoracoscopic Surgery. Surg Endosc 1998;12(11):1303–10.

[35] Lillemoe KD, Martin SA, Cameron JL, et al. Major bile duct injuries during laparoscopic cholecystectomy. Follow-up after combined surgical and radiologic management. Ann Surg 1997;225(5):459–68 [discussion 468–71].

[36] Deziel DJ, Millikan KW, Economou SG, et al. Complications of laparoscopic cholecystectomy: a national survey of 4,292 hospitals and an analysis of 77,604 cases. Am J Surg 1993; 165(1):9–14.

[37] Perini RF, Uflacker R, Cunningham JT, et al. Isolated right segmental hepatic duct injury following laparoscopic cholecystectomy. Cardiovasc Intervent Radiol 2005;28(2): 185–95.

[38] Bujanda L, Calvo MM, Cabriada JL, et al. MRCP in the diagnosis of iatrogenic bile duct injury. NMR Biomed 2003;16(8):475–8.

[39] Ragozzino A, De Ritis R, Mosca A, et al. Value of MR cholangiography in patients with iatrogenic bile duct injury after cholecystectomy. AJR Am J Roentgenol 2004;183(6): 1567–72.

[40] Hirano Y, Tatsuzawa Y, Shimizu J, et al. Efficacy of multi-slice computed tomography cholangiography before laparoscopic cholecystectomy. ANZ J Surg 2006;76(8):693–5.

[41] Lillemoe KD. Current management of bile duct injury. Br J Surg 2008;95(4):403–5.

[42] Lillemoe KD, Melton GB, Cameron JL, et al. Postoperative bile duct strictures: management and outcome in the 1990s. Ann Surg 2000;232(3):430–41.

[43] Strasberg SM. Biliary injury in laparoscopic surgery: part 2. Changing the culture of cholecystectomy. J Am Coll Surg 2005;201(4):604–11.

[44] Carroll BJ, Birth M, Phillips EH. Common bile duct injuries during laparoscopic cholecystectomy that result in litigation. Surg Endosc 1998;12(4):310–3 [discussion: 314].

[45] de Reuver PR, Grossmann I, Busch OR, et al. Referral pattern and timing of repair are risk factors for complications after reconstructive surgery for bile duct injury. Ann Surg 2007; 245(5):763–70.

[46] Heise M, Schmidt SC, Adler A, et al. [Management of bile duct injuries following laparoscopic cholecystectomy]. Zentralbl Chir 2003;128(11):944–51 [in German].

[47] Tantia O, Jain M, Khanna S, et al. Iatrogenic biliary injury: 13,305 cholecystectomies experienced by a single surgical team over more than 13 years. Surg Endosc 2008;22(4): 1077–86.

[48] Chapman WC, Halevy A, Blumgart LH, et al. Postcholecystectomy bile duct strictures. Management and outcome in 130 patients. Arch Surg 1995;130(6):597–602 [discussion: 602–4].

[49] Stewart L, Way LW. Bile duct injuries during laparoscopic cholecystectomy. Factors that influence the results of treatment. Arch Surg 1995;130(10):1123–8 [discussion: 1129].

[50] Murr MM, Gigot JF, Nagorney DM, et al. Long-term results of biliary reconstruction after laparoscopic bile duct injuries. Arch Surg 1999;134(6):604–9 [discussion: 609–10].

[51] Schmidt SC, Langrehr JM, Hintze RE, et al. Long-term results and risk factors influencing outcome of major bile duct injuries following cholecystectomy. Br J Surg 2005;92(1):76–82.

[52] Misra S, Melton GB, Geschwind JF, et al. Percutaneous management of bile duct strictures and injuries associated with laparoscopic cholecystectomy: a decade of experience. J Am Coll Surg 2004;198(2):218–26.

[53] Al-Ghnaniem R, Benjamin IS. Long-term outcome of hepaticojejunostomy with routine access loop formation following iatrogenic bile duct injury. Br J Surg 2002;89(9):1118–24.

[54] Mercado MA, Chan C, Orozco H, et al. Prognostic implications of preserved bile duct confluence after iatrogenic injury. Hepatogastroenterology 2005;52(61):40–4.

[55] Walsh RM, Vogt DP, Ponsky JL, et al. Management of failed biliary repairs for major bile duct injuries after laparoscopic cholecystectomy. J Am Coll Surg 2004;199(2):192–7.

[56] Nordin A, Halme L, Makisalo H, et al. Management and outcome of major bile duct injuries after laparoscopic cholecystectomy: from therapeutic endoscopy to liver transplantation. Liver Transpl 2002;8(11):1036–43.

ELSEVIER
SAUNDERS

SURGICAL
CLINICS OF
NORTH AMERICA

Surg Clin N Am 88 (2008) 1345–1368

Complications of Gallstones: The Mirizzi Syndrome, Gallstone Ileus, Gallstone Pancreatitis, Complications of "Lost" Gallstones

Jill Zaliekas, MD, J. Lawrence Munson, MD*

*Department of General Surgery, Lahey Clinic Medical Center,
Tufts University Medical School, 41 Mall Road, Burlington, MA 01805, USA*

Mirizzi syndrome (MS) is a form of obstructive jaundice, first described by Mirizzi [1] in 1948 caused by a stone or stones impacted in the neck of the gallbladder or the cystic duct, such that the common hepatic duct is narrowed. Depending upon the degree of impingement and the chronicity of the condition, there may be a cholecysto–choledochal fistula. This rare complication of gallstones occurs in about 0.1% to 0.7% of patients who have gallstones [2,3]. There is also a greater risk of gallbladder cancer found in these patients, upwards of 25% [4]. The condition was classified by McSherry and colleagues [5] into types 1 and 2 in 1982, and reclassified by Csendes and colleagues [6] in 1989 into classes 1 through 4. There must be four components for the syndrome to occur:

1. Anatomy placing the cystic duct parallel to the common hepatic duct
2. Impaction of a stone in the cystic dust or gallbladder neck
3. Obstruction of the common hepatic duct from the stone itself, or from the resultant inflammatory response
4. Intermittent or constant jaundice occasionally causing cholangitis, and with longstanding obstruction, biliary cirrhosis [7]

The McSherry classification of Mirizzi syndrome based on endoscopic retrograde cholangiopancreatography (ERCP) is broken down into:

Type 1: external compression of the common hepatic duct by calculus in the cystic duct or Hartmann's pouch

---

* Corresponding author.
E-mail address: john.l.munson@lahey.org (J.L. Munson).

Type 2: a cholecysto–choledochal fistula is present, caused by calculus eroding partially or completely into the bile duct [5]

The Csendes classification of Mirizzi syndrome (Fig. 1) is broken down as follows:

Type 1: external compression of the common bile duct
Type 2: a cholecystobiliary fistula is present involving less than one third the circumference of the bile duct
Type 3: a fistula is present involving up to two thirds the circumference of the bile duct
Type 4: a fistula is present with complete destruction of the wall of the bile duct [6]

Diagnosis of Mirizzi syndrome

Symptoms of MS are essentially those of cholecystitis or choledocholithiasis. Most patients present with epigastric or right upper quadrant pain, jaundice, and elevated liver function tests [8]. They may have episodic pain like biliary colic, or manifest systemic symptoms of fever, chills, tachycardia, and anorexia. The condition may be intermittent and relapsing, or fulminant, presenting as cholangitis. Imaging is, thus, essential to preoperative diagnosis, and in a literature search, the correct diagnosis was made in 8% to 62% of patients until ERCP was used regularly [9]. Most patients

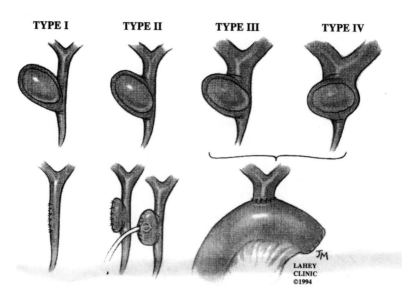

Fig. 1. Classification of Mirizzi's syndrome (*upper panel*). Bile duct reconstruction options are shown (*lower panel*). (*Courtesy of* Lahey Clinic, Burlington, MA; with permission.)

who have suspected biliary tract disease undergo ultrasound as a first test, with MRI or CT often following. Cholangiography, either percutaneous, or endoscopic, is performed when liver function tests are sufficiently abnormal [10,11]. The most sensitive test for MS is ERCP, which has allowed 100% correct preoperative diagnosis to Yeh's group (Figs. 2 and 3) [12].

In addition to making the diagnosis, the endoscopist also can palliatively stent the jaundiced patient to allow planned exploration in a more stable patient (Fig. 4). The authors' belief is that any patient presenting with gallstones and altered liver function should have some imaging of the biliary tree before exploration.

When the diagnosis is made, there should be a planned open procedure. When the condition is encountered during laparoscopic cholecystectomy, the challenges inherent in the dissection of Calot's triangle in an inflamed, fibrotic field mandate open conversion in most cases. The diagnosis of a cholecysto–choledochal fistula made intraoperatively also is handled best in an open fashion, unless an expert and experienced laparoscopic surgeon is present [13].

When one considers that this syndrome occurs in 0.1% to 0.7% of patients who have symptomatic gallstones, the average general surgeon will encounter MS only a few times during his or her career. Although reports continue to surface of managing MS laparoscopically, one cannot help but speculate why the incidence of major biliary operative injury mirrors the incidence of MS itself [14,15]. When one then factors in the incidence of biliary injuries occurring during laparoscopy as still being twice the incidence of those occurring during open surgery, there seems little

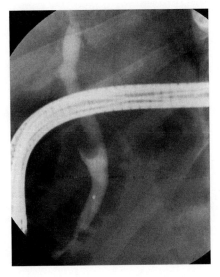

Fig. 2. Csendes type 3 Mirizzi, arrow showing stone greater than two thirds impacting duct wall.

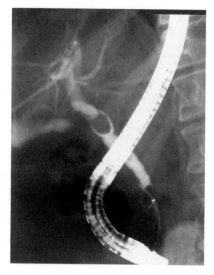

Fig. 3. Mirizzi type 4 with complete cholecysto–choledochal fistula.

justification in trying to manage the situation in a laparoscopic manner. As in any difficult laparoscopic case, open conversion in the face of a tough dissection adjacent to the common hepatic duct or common bile duct is well advised, as the minimal additional discomfort of a right upper quadrant

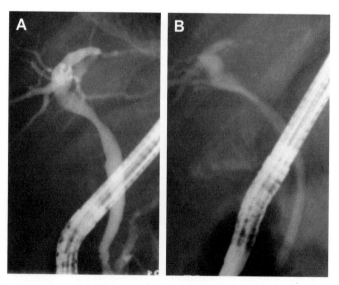

Fig. 4. (A) Mirizzi type 1 with stone impacting lateral duct wall. (B) Same patient with preoperative stent.

incision is far less than the morbidity of a major biliary injury created laparoscopically [7,9,16–18].

Treatment of MS may consist of cholecystectomy, partial cholecystectomy with stone extraction, use of the remnant of the gallbladder to close a cholecysto–choledochal fistula, or Roux-Y hepaticojejunostomy in the face of inflammatory destruction of the common hepatic duct. For type 1 (in either classification scheme), cholecystectomy alone performed in a fundus-down manner is the best treatment. If the phlegmon or fibrous reaction in the area of Calot's triangle is dense, a partial cholecystectomy with stone extraction and closure of the remnant is sufficient and safe. In all cases, a frozen section of the gallbladder wall should be done to rule out coexistent cancer [19]. For the types 2 and above, simple repair of a fistula over a T-tube, or the creation of a choledochoduodenal fistula is not advised. Use of the remnant gallbladder wall to repair a fistula with placement of a T-tube distally in the common duct may be used if the tissue appears healthy. Roux-Y reconstruction is the safest alternative in the face of compromised ductal tissue from compression of the 9-o'clock vessels of the common duct. Viability of the bilio-enteric anastomosis is secured from retrograde perfusion of the proximal common hepatic duct and from the jejunal vessels to the Roux-en-Y loop.

If the diagnosis of MS is suspected by preoperative imaging, and the condition of the patient is not pressing urgently for operation, the surgeon must decide if he or she is capable of, and comfortable with, major biliary repair. Data from the Accreditation Council for Graduate Medical Education (ACGME) (resident case logs from 2006 to 2007) [20] reveal that graduating chief residents average only one open common bile duct exploration and two bilio-enteric anastomoses in their training. If satisfactory experience is not present, serious consideration should be given to transferring the patient to a tertiary care center familiar with bilio-enteric anastomoses. This is especially important for Csendes types 2 through 4, where injuries to the right hepatic duct, common hepatic duct, right hepatic artery, and replaced right hepatic artery can occur with difficult dissection in the hepatocystic triangle.

The prognosis of MS is very good for type 1 lesions, as simple cholecystectomy is all that is necessary for cure. In treating more serious types with fistulous destruction of the common duct, postoperative morbidity rises, with 10% or more biliary fistulae, biliary stricturing requiring dilation or reoperation, or hepatic abscesses requiring drainage [8,16].

Gallstone ileus

Bartholin [21] first described a cholecystointestinal fistula with a gallstone within the gastrointestinal (GI) tract in 1654. Courvoisier published the first series of 131 cases of gallstone ileus in 1890 [21]. Gallstone ileus has remained a rare entity in the general population, accounting for 1% to 3% of all mechanical obstructions [22]; however, it is mainly a disease of the elderly and of women. Gallstone ileus accounts for 25% of all small bowel obstructions in patients age 65 or older [23]. Because of the advanced age in this group, medical comorbidities contribute to the high morbidity and mortality that is associated with gallstone ileus. Early data reported mortality of 40% to 70% [21], which has decreased in recent years to approximately 15% to 18% [23]. Because this remains a lethal process, clinical suspicion for this entity must exist for proper diagnosis and timely management.

Pathogenesis

Gallstone ileus is a result of fistula formation from the biliary tract to the intestine. This is often a consequence of an episode of cholecystitis, causing inflammation of the gallbladder, adhesions to adjacent bowel, with subsequent pressure and ischemia causing a gallstone to erode into the bowel, resulting in fistula formation. Most fistulas occur in the duodenum, because of its proximity to the gallbladder; however, fistulas also occur to the stomach, colon, and jejunum [24].

Most gallstones that enter the intestinal tract are passed without consequence, but obstruction may result if the stone is of large enough size, usually greater than 2 to 2.5 cm. The point of obstruction is most often in the terminal ileum because of its smaller diameter, but it can occur throughout the GI system [24]. Bouveret syndrome, as first described in 1896, is a gastric outlet obstruction secondary to proximal migration of a gallstone from a cholecystoduodenal fistula lodging in the proximal duodenum [24,25].

Presentation

Gallstone ileus is actually a mechanical obstruction, rather than a true ileus. Its presentation can vary depending on the site of obstruction; however, the symptoms of nausea, vomiting, pain, and constipation are commonly present [26]. Symptoms often can be intermittent in nature, caused by a tumbling phenomenon. This is a result of a stone intermittently obstructing, then traveling through the GI tract until it passes or becomes impacted in the intestine [24]. Patients usually present in a delayed fashion, and diagnosis often is made 3 to 8 days after onset of symptoms [27]. Approximately half of all patients who present with gallstone ileus have a prior history of biliary disease; however, biliary symptoms immediately preceding gallstone ileus are rare [21,22].

Diagnosis

The diagnosis of gallstone ileus is often difficult to make clinically because of its nonspecific symptoms. Throughout the literature, reports of correct preoperative diagnosis are infrequent, ranging from 20% to 50% [21,26]. Historically, the plain abdominal radiograph was the gold standard diagnostic test. Rigler, Borman, and Noble in 1941 described the classic radiologic findings of gallstone ileus, known as Rigler's triad: (1) partial or complete intestinal obstruction, (2) pneumobilia, and (3) aberrant gallstone in the intestine (Fig. 5) [24,28,29]. The presence of all three findings, however, is only reported between 17% and 35% in the literature [28–30]. Several studies advocate the use of ultrasound in combination with abdominal films to increase the sensitivity of diagnosis. Ultrasound techniques are more sensitive at detecting pneumobilia and ectopic gallstones. Combining the two modalities has increased the sensitivity of diagnosis of gallstone ileus to 74% [28].

More recent studies report CT findings of gallstone ileus to be more sensitive than plain abdominal films or ultrasound. Rigler's triad is detected more frequently using CT examinations [29–31]. Sensitivity of diagnosing gallstone ileus using CT is reported up to 93% [30]. CT examinations can be useful for detecting ectopic gallstones and the presence of pneumobilia, and for helping assess of the degree of inflammation around the site of the cholecystointestinal fistula (Figs. 6–8) [31]. Although symptoms are nonspecific, one should have a higher index of suspicion in elderly patients without a prior surgical history or other obvious cause for a mechanical obstruction. The radiographic studies can augment clinical findings to make the correct preoperative diagnosis of gallstone ileus.

Treatment

Although gallstone ileus was described nearly 400 years ago, great controversy still exists on the proper surgical management of this disease. The main therapeutic goal of surgery is to relieve the intestinal obstruction.

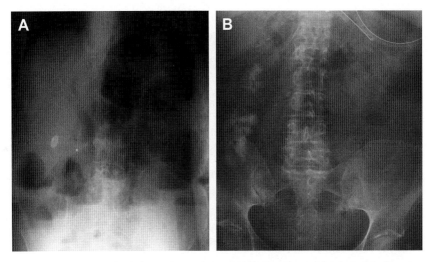

Fig. 5. (*A, B*) Intestinal obstruction and pneumobilia found on abdominal plain films.

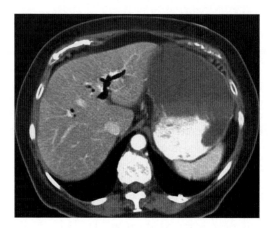

Fig. 6. Pneumobilia found on abdominal CT.

Preoperatively, efforts are made to resuscitate the patient, who often has metabolic derangements from intestinal obstruction and delayed presentation, as well as pre-existing comorbidities. The gold standard procedure is exploratory laparotomy and enterolithotomy (Fig. 9). A longitudinal incision is made proximal to the impacted gallstone; the stone is extracted, and the enterotomy is closed in two layers. The entire length of the bowel then should be examined to evaluate for other potential stones [21].

The high mortality rates associated with gallstone ileus, often secondary to the comorbidities of the affected population, historically prompted surgeons to solely address removal of the obstructing stone. There was no attempt at the initial operation to treat the cholecystoenteric fistula or remove the gallbladder [21]. Holz [32] in 1929 and Welch in 1957, however,

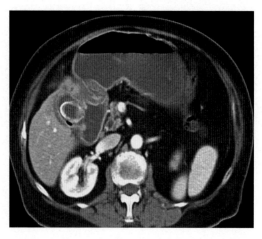

Fig. 7. Gallstone and cholecystoenteric fistula depicted on abdominal CT.

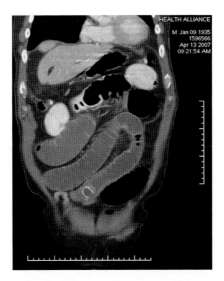

Fig. 8. Intestinal obstruction and intraluminal gallstone illustrated on abdominal CT.

described a one-stage procedure with cholecystectomy, closure of the chol-ecystoenteric fistula, and enterolithotomy to prevent future recurrence. This has been the topic of debate in the literature over the ensuing years.

In the largest review of the literature of by Reisner [23], citing over 1000 cases, the one-stage procedure had a 16.9% mortality rate compared with 11.7% for enterolithotomy alone. Eighty-percent of patients were treated with enterolithotomy alone. Proponents of the one-stage procedure argue that it prevents future biliary complications, recurrent gallstone ileus, and persistent fistula [32,33]. Interestingly, the recurrence rate of gallstone ileus

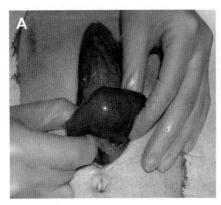
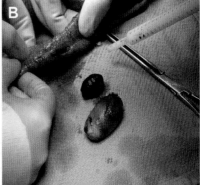

Fig. 9. Intraluminal gallstone (*A*) and enterotomy with stone extraction (*B*) found at time of exploratory laparotomy.

in those treated only with enterolithotomy was less than 5% to 9% in the literature [22,23]. Additionally, only 10% of patients required reoperation for persistent biliary symptoms [3]. It is also thought that the remaining fistula can close spontaneously once the obstruction has been resolved, and complications related to persistent fistula are rare [24,33,34].

A recent study published by Doko and colleagues compared the management of gallstone ileus either by enterolithotomy with a one-stage procedure consisting of enterolithotomy and cholecystectomy with fistula repair. This retrospective review included 30 patients and showed no statistical difference between the two groups in terms of age, America Society of Anesthesiologists (ASA) score and duration of symptoms. There was a statistically significant difference in the operating time, with the duration of surgery 100 minutes longer in the one-stage group. The in-hospital mortality was 9% for the enterolithotomy group and 11% for the one-stage group. In logistic regression analysis, the one-stage procedure group had significantly higher complication rate (odds ratio [OR] 12). The authors concluded from their data that one-stage procedure should be reserved only for select groups of patients with acute cholecystitis, gangrenous gallbladder, or residual gallstones at the time of operation [33].

Tan and colleagues [34] also reviewed their series of 19 patients who had the one-stage procedure versus enterolithotomy alone. The one-stage procedure was performed in those patients who had lower ASA class, and operative times were significantly longer (100 minutes greater) in the one-stage group. There were no complications in the group having enterolithotomy alone in their follow-up period. They had no significant difference in morbidity between the groups, and they had no mortality in either group. A review of the literature thus defends the one-stage procedure in the ideal patient, however with potentially significant morbidity and mortality. For those patients who are hemodynamically unstable or have significant inflammation or dense adhesions, enterolithotomy alone should be performed [33–35].

The final treatment option is a two-stage procedure, where the enterolithotomy is performed as the initial emergency procedure, and subsequent cholecystectomy and fistula closure are performed 4 to 6 weeks later. The results of recent literature reveal the low recurrence rates of gallstone ileus and few complications in patients managed expectantly after enterolithotomy. Therefore, the two-stage procedure with scheduled follow-up biliary surgery is not common [23,27,34].

The evolution of laparoscopy has prompted some surgeons to attempt enterolithotomy laparoscopically. A few authors have reported small series; however, this is should not be considered the gold standard of treatment. There is greater difficulty examining the entire length of the small bowel and identifying the gallstone; the operative times are longer, and performing laparoscopic surgery on patients who have dilated bowel secondary to intestinal obstruction can be technically challenging. This technique only should be considered with extremely experienced surgeons in highly selected patients [27].

Conclusion

Gallstone ileus should be suspected in the elderly population, especially in women who present with signs of bowel obstruction without another cause for mechanical obstruction. Radiographic findings that may assist in the preoperative diagnosis include pneumobilia, intestinal dilation with air/fluid levels, and intraluminal gallstone(s). Urgent laparotomy is required, and the standard operation performed is enterolithotomy. A one-stage procedure including cholecystectomy with fistula repair should be reserved for select cases, in otherwise healthy patients without serious phlegmonous changes in the right upper quadrant. This single-stage procedure adds to the operative time and can increase morbidity and mortality. Enterolithotomy alone may suffice for patients who have major comorbidities. A two-stage procedure should be considered in younger patients who remain at risk for future biliary complications.

Gallstone pancreatitis

In 1901, Opie proposed a theory for pancreatitis that involved gallstone migration and obstruction in the distal common bile duct with subsequent impairment of pancreatic secretion and reflux of bile into the pancreatic duct. Acute pancreatitis is responsible for more than 200,000 hospitalizations per year in the United States. The most common causative agents of pancreatitis are gallstones and alcohol abuse. Approximately 80% of cases of gallstone pancreatitis are mild and self-limiting. Twenty percent of cases, however, can be severe and cause significant morbidity and mortality [36].

Pathophysiology

The exact mechanism of pancreatitis is somewhat controversial; however, the key components include elements of Opie's common channel theory and duodenal reflux theory, whereby obstruction of the pancreatic duct and reflux of duodenal contents into the pancreatic duct cause an activation of trypsinogen to trypsin in the pancreas and stimulation of inflammatory mediators, specifically interleukin (IL)-1, IL-6, IL-8, and tumor necrosis factor α (TNF-α). Additionally, permeability of endothelial cells contributes to pancreatic gland destruction and inflammation [36,37].

Diagnosis

Acute pancreatitis presents with severe, constant epigastric or right upper quadrant pain that radiates to the back. Nausea and vomiting often are associated symptoms. Patients can present with varying severity of symptoms from mild to severe, with associated hypotension, tachycardia, and abdominal distension. Two clinical examination findings that can aid in the diagnosis, although not often seen, are Cullen's sign, which is a blue discoloration around the umbilicus, and Grey Turner's sign, which is a blue discoloration of the flanks. These findings are a result of severe hemorrhagic pancreatitis with blood tracking along these areas [37].

The laboratory findings associated with gallstone pancreatitis include elevated amylase, often three times normal values, elevated lipase, and often elevated alanine aminotransferase (ALT). Studies have shown that when the ALT is elevated three times normal, the positive predictive value is 95% for gallstone pancreatitis [38]. The presence of leukocytosis suggests a more severe clinical picture involving pancreatic necrosis or cholangitis [37]. The initial radiologic workup of pancreatitis involves ultrasound examination to identify gallstones as a potential source. Abdominal CT can be used to examine the pancreas for degree of inflammation, perfusion of the gland, and presence of abscess or pseudocyst (Fig. 10). Alternatively, MRI can be obtained, which can provide better detail of the pancreatic duct and degree of inflammation [36].

There are several grading criteria that are used to assess disease severity and aid in determining prognosis. The most widely used system is Ranson's criteria, which assess five criteria on admission, and six criteria 48 hours after admission. Ranson's criteria are subdivided further into nonbiliary and biliary pancreatitis (Table 1). The presence of three criteria is characteristic of mild disease. More than three criteria herald severe pancreatitis, and the presence of five criteria is predictive of severe pancreatitis with associated mortality greater than 40% [38]. Other scales that have been used to assess prognosis include Acute Physiology and Chronic Health Evaluation (APACHE) II score, Sequential Organ Failure Assesment (SOFA) score, and Glasgow Scale. Organ failure, respiratory insufficiency, and renal failure are markers of severe disease [36–38]. These prognostic indicators, unfortunately, do not tell exactly how to manage pancreatitis; however, anyone who has severe pancreatitis probably requires an admission to the ICU.

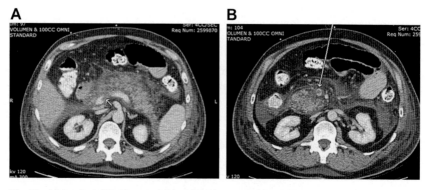

Fig. 10. Abdominal CT of pancreatitis (A) and pancreatitis with thrombosed superior mesenteric veiu (B).

Table 1
Ranson's criteria

	Nonbiliary pancreatitis	Biliary pancreatitis
Admission		
Age	> 55	> 70
White blood cell count (mm3)	> 16,000	> 18,000
Glucose (mg/dL)	> 200	> 220
Lactose dehydrogenase (IU/L)	> 350	> 400
Aspartate aminotransferase (IU/L)	> 250	> 250
Within 48 hours		
Serum urea nitrogen rise (mg/dL)	> 5	> 2
P_{AO_2} (mm Hg)	< 60	< 60
Serum calcium (mg/dL)	< 8	< 8
Hematocrit decrease (points)	> 10	> 10
Base deficit (mEq/L)	> 4	> 5
Fluid sequestration (L)	> 6	> 4

Management

The initial treatment of pancreatitis is supportive with bowel rest, aggressive intravenous fluid resuscitation, pain control, antiemetics, and oxygen supplementation. Most cases of pancreatitis are mild and self-limiting without complication. In severe cases of pancreatitis, intensive care monitoring and support are required [36]. Several complications specific to the pancreas can occur, including pancreatic pseudocyst (Fig. 11), necrosis (Fig. 12), and abscess formation (Fig. 13). The surgical and endoscopic management of acute gallstone pancreatitis and its complications have been controversial and are ongoing topics for research and discussion. The following section presents some of the most current thoughts on ERCP, cholecystectomy, and the treatment of the complications of pancreatitis.

Endoscopic retrograde cholangiopancreatography

The role of ERCP and endoscopic sphincterotomy in the management of gallstone pancreatitis has evolved over the years. The absolute indications for early ERCP and sphincterotomy are cholangitis and obstructive jaundice. The value of ERCP in other cases of gallstone pancreatitis has been the topic of significant review There has been great variation in study design and inclusion or exclusion criteria in the published studies, making it difficult to derive a consensus on management. The American Gastroenterology Association 2007 Guidelines recognize that the data at present are too controversial to provide definitive recommendations for the use of early ERCP. Several recommendations, however, have been proposed on the use of ERCP for gallstone pancreatitis from a review of the literature [39]. Neoptolemos was the first to study the role of early ERCP versus conventional therapy for gallstone pancreatitis in his randomized–control trial in 1988. He

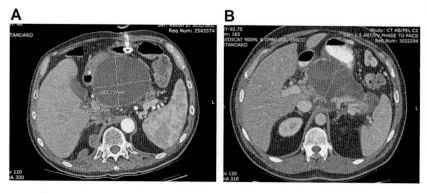

Fig. 11. (*A, B*) Abdominal CT with pancreatitis complicated with pseudocyst formation.

found no difference in mortality; however, overall complications were decreased in the ERCP group compared with conventional therapy [40]. Subsequent studies in the 1990s also found a decrease in complications in the ERCP group in those who had severe disease; however, no difference in mortality was found. Recommendations at that time were that early ERCP was safe, resulted in diminished sepsis, and decreased complications for severe pancreatitis; however, ERCP was of no benefit for cases of mild pancreatitis [38].

The use of ERCP postoperatively, after identification of a common bile duct stone on intraoperative cholangiogram, has been evaluated. Chang and colleagues [41] conducted a prospective randomized trial comparing preoperative versus postoperative use of ERCP to determine if ERCP should be used routinely preoperatively. The results demonstrated that selective postoperative ERCP was associated with shorter hospitalization, less cost, and no increased complications.

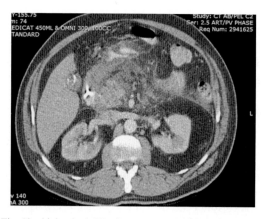

Fig. 12. Abdominal CT of severe pancreatitis with necrosis.

A   B

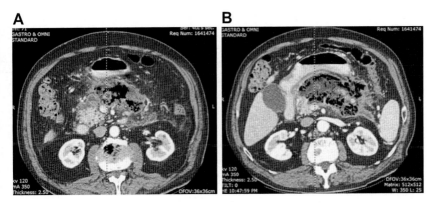

Fig. 13. (*A, B*) Abdominal CT representing pancreatitis with infected necrosis/abscess.

Oria, in 2007, performed a randomized–control trial that specifically included patients who had biliary obstruction but omitted those with cholangitis. These patients were randomized to early ERCP or conservative treatment. This trial showed no difference in the mortality, morbidity, or complications between the two groups [42]. The meta-analysis done by Petrov and colleagues and the review by Behrns and colleagues [39,40], both in 2008, concluded that that early ERCP does not improve mortality or complications, especially in mild disease and is not a necessary procedure for acute gallstone pancreatitis. The use of ERCP therefore should be limited to those who have cholangitis, biliary obstruction that has not improved with conservative treatment, and the elderly patient for whom surgical risk is too great.

Cholecystectomy

Because the presumptive cause for pancreatitis in the setting of gallstones is the passage of gallstones down the common bile duct, cholecystectomy must be the key to preventing recurrences. The timing of cholecystectomy is related in part to the severity of pancreatitis, the patient's health, and the surgeon's preference. In the group of patients who have mild pancreatitis, it is accepted that cholecystectomy with intraoperative cholangiogram should be performed during the first admission to prevent recurrent pancreatitis [43,44]. The rate of recurrence of gallstone pancreatitis when the gallbladder remains is reported between 50% and 90% [45]. Most surgeons delay surgery until amylase and lipase values have normalized or are trending toward normal values. A prospective study was conducted by Rosing and colleagues [44] to evaluate early cholecystectomy (within 48 hours of admission) in patients who had mild-to-moderate gallstone pancreatitis. The study revealed that there was no increase in morbidity or mortality in the early group, and there was a shorter hospitalization with early cholecystectomy.

The timing of cholecystectomy for severe pancreatitis is still controversial. This group of patients often has complications of pancreatitis including acute pseudocyst formation or pancreatic necrosis, which makes the operation more challenging. Several authors have examined timing of cholecystectomy for severe pancreatitis, and it is apparent that early cholecystectomy is not indicated and can have increased morbidity. Recommendations are for delayed cholecystectomy for 4 to 6 weeks after the acute attack of pancreatitis. At this point, if there are residual pseudocysts, they may be mature enough to treat surgically at the time of cholecystectomy. Additionally, the inflammation from the acute attack has had a chance to resolve [46]. In order to protect against the potential risk of recurrent pancreatitis, some have advocated ERCP with sphincterotomy on initial hospitalization. Sanjay and colleagues [47] demonstrated that initial sphincterotomy with interval cholecystectomy for patients with severe pancreatitis had minimal morbidity and low readmission rates, making this a safe alternative in the management of acute pancreatitis. In patients who have significant comorbidities where cholecystectomy is too high a risk, ERCP with sphincterotomy has been shown to be a viable option. Sphincterotomy has been tolerated well, with low rates of recurrent pancreatitis [45,48].

Surgical management of the complications of pancreatitis

The scope of operative management of acute gallstone pancreatitis is limited to treating the complications associated with it. Surgery is indicated for those patients who have infected necrosis, hemorrhage from bleeding pseudoaneurysms of the pancreas, and perforated viscus from ischemic necrosis. Those patients with sterile necrosis who have progressive multisystem organ failure unresponsive to medical management should be considered for operative intervention; however, no consensus exists. In the early phase of pancreatitis, the release of proinflammatory mediators stimulates a systemic inflammatory response and development of SIRS (systemic inflammatory response syndrome). This can occur without active infection being present. Operating during this time period can accelerate the progression of the inflammatory response and can become more detrimental than beneficial to the patient. Mortality rates up to 65% have been reported in patients who were operated on early in the course of severe pancreatitis [49,50].

Once there is infected necrosis in the face of acute pancreatitis, mortality rates approach 100% without operative intervention. The distinction between sterile and infected necrosis is integral to the proper management. This is determined by fine needle aspiration (FNA), which can be completed by CT or ultrasound guidance. An FNA should be performed in a patient who has worsening organ failure, leukocytosis, or deteriorating clinical status, which often occurs by day 10 to 14 of the disease course [51]. Even with proper surgical and antibiotic treatment, the mortality rate for infected pancreatic necrosis approaches 50% [49].

There are several surgical options for managing pancreatic necrosis, each with the goal of controlling the focus of infection and limiting the amount of pancreatic tissue loss. Surgical options include necrosectomy, combined with open packing, planned staged relaparotomy with repeated lavage, or closed continuous lavage using drainage. Mortality rates have been reported between 15% and 25% [49]. More recently, minimally invasive techniques have been attempted for debridement, including video-assisted retroperitoneal drainage, laparoscopic transperitoneal necrosectomy, and endoscopic drainage. The evidence in the literature is scant, such that no recommendations can be made to support or refute their use at this point [52]. This should be in the realm of extremely proficient and experienced laparoscopic surgeons.

Pseudocyst formation is a result of disruption of the pancreatic duct secondary to increased pressure and extravasation of pancreatic fluid. This is encapsulated by a reactive fibrous wall, which matures over a 4- to 6-week period to its maximal strength. Pseudocysts less than 6 cm have caused few complications and can be observed. Those 6 cm or greater, however, may require operative drainage. Large pseudocysts left untreated can cause chronic abdominal pain, biliary or gastroduodenal obstruction, or hemorrhage from pseudoaneurysms in the wall of the pseudocyst. Therefore, after a period of 6 weeks, which allows the cyst wall to mature, definitive operative treatment can be undertaken. Management can be through endoscopic transgastric drainage if the pseudocyst is simple, small, and without debris. Surgical created enteric drainage is preferred for pseudocysts large in size or associated with pancreatic necrosis, multiple loculations, or considerable debris. Operative options include cystgastrostomy, cystduodenostomy, Roux-en-Y cystjejunostomy, or lateral pancreaticojejunostomy, depending on the location of the pseudocyst. Surgical drainage has an associated morbidity of 20% to 30% and mortality of 2% to 6%. Recurrences are rare, occurring in 5% of patients [53,54].

Conclusion

Acute gallstone pancreatitis is often mild and self-limiting. In a significant number of patients, however, the disease can be severe, with high rates of morbidity and mortality. The data presented in the literature illustrate the controversies in management and the constant evolution of practice. There are few conclusions, however, that can be made with support by the literature in regards to the management of gallstone pancreatitis. First, for mild gallstone pancreatitis, there is no indication for early ERCP. Management should involve laparoscopic cholecystectomy with intraoperative cholangiogram on admission, and subsequent ERCP and sphincterotomy if an obstructing stone is found. Second, in cases of severe pancreatitis, surgical intervention is indicated for infected pancreatic necrosis, hemorrhage, or intestinal perforation. The management of the late complications of pancreatitis should be delayed as long as the patient is clinically stable. Such intervention, such as pseudocyst drainage, should be delayed for at least 4 to 6 weeks to allow for the cyst wall to mature. A concomitant cholecystectomy can be performed at the same time. Third, in those patients who deteriorate clinically, and who have progressive organ dysfunction despite aggressive medical management, surgery may be indicated. FNA and cultures should be obtained with signs of sepsis or clinical deterioration. Surgery is indicted for those who develop infected necrosis or late pancreatic abscess. Finally, in those patients who have severe pancreatitis, or high surgical risk secondary to multiple comorbidities, an ERCP with sphincterotomy can be performed in an attempt to reduce recurrent episodes of pancreatitis and to relieve biliary obstruction.

Lost gallstones

When open cholecystectomy was the only option available to patients, a mark of excellence was to complete a cholecystectomy without opening the gallbladder and spilling stones. To a resident in surgery, it was a badge of merit to be able to perform this operation in such a manner. In reality, there were no grave consequences to spilled stones and bile as they were irrigated out and retrieved easily. In performance of open cholecystectomy, the right upper quadrant is packed off routinely and Morrison's pouch occluded with a laparotomy pad, so that spillage from the gallbladder cannot migrate from the area. During laparoscopy, spillage of bile is still relatively benign; however, the loss of gallstones may carry considerable morbidity. Stones quickly can become disseminated in the abdominal cavity, though most settle quickly by irrigation and gravity into the retrohepatic recess (Morrison's pouch) or above and lateral to the liver. A stone then may act as a nidus for inflammation, and in the face of infected bile, a focus of fistulization or abscess formation.

Perforation of the gallbladder and spillage of bile and stones are the most common complications of laparoscopic cholecystectomy. Reviewing the literature reveals an incidence of perforation of 20% to 40% [55,56]. Risk factors for perforation include acute cholecystitis, age of patient, presence of pigment stones, number of gallstones, (>15), and performance of the operation by residents [57,58]. The loss of gallstones may occur during a difficult dissection, or during extraction of the gallbladder not contained within a retrieval pouch.

The spectrum of complications associated with lost gallstones includes: wound infection, fibrosis, small bowel obstruction, intra-abdominal abscess formation, fevers, fistulas, weight loss, and cutaneous sinuses [56,59]. Fistulas can occur as bilio-cutaneous, colocutaneous, bilio colocutaneous, and bilio-enteric in nature (Fig. 14) [60]. Gallstones settling into Morrison's pouch may develop a chronic abscess that can necessitate posteriorly and present externally out the lumbar and flank areas (Fig. 15). Stones settling

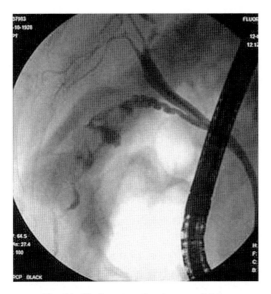

Fig. 14. Cholecysto–colocutaneous fistula.

into the gastrocolic omentum can result in painful, fibrotic masses ultimately requiring exploration (Fig. 16) [61]. Chronic irritation from a stone adjacent to the bowel ultimately can result in enteric fistulization and gallstone ileus (Fig. 17) [62].

These complications can be divided further into immediate and delayed in occurrence. The immediate problems are the easiest to diagnose. Patients may present soon after surgery with trocar site infections associated with

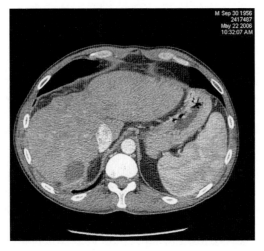

Fig. 15. Abscess in retrohepatic recess.

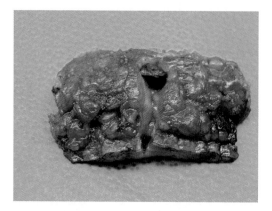

Fig. 16. Omental mass encasing dropped gallstone.

stone debris. Some may have fevers in the early postoperative period without evidence of other sites of infection.

Delays of up to 8 years have been reported between cholecystectomy and the appearance of new symptoms [62]. Because of the delay of months to years before the appearance of abscesses or fistulas, these new problems often are not linked to the prior, seemingly minor, procedure [63]. The population mobility and changing health care providers and hospitals put temporal and geographic distance between the cholecystectomy and the presentation with new symptoms. Documentation may be poor, even when the patient remains in the same health care system, since surgeons may be reluctant to provide evidence in the operative note that the gallbladder was perforated, or that stones were spilled.

Diagnostic workup for these patients may involve CT scanning, endoscopy, barium studies, and ultrasound. The last may be most helpful in determining the etiology, as it is best at imaging stones. CT scanning will diagnose abscesses and some fistulae. Contrast studies can diagnose enterocutaneous and enterocolonic fistulae. ERCP may be necessary to find bilio-enteric fistulae, although retrograde barium studies also may show these [60].

Management of the complications of lost stones may be as simple as opening a trocar site and evacuating debris. For cases of chronic intra-abdominal abscess with cutaneous fistulas, treatment requires an open anterior approach for drainage and debridement, with removal of all stone debris (Fig. 18). For a chronic, posterior, necessitating abscess, posterior drainage by means of a 12th rib approach may avoid a difficult anterior exposure to debride behind the liver. Treatment of bilio-cutaneous, bilio-enteric, and bilio-colonic fistulae mandates removal of the stone debris and closure of the biliary fistula and resection of the involved portion of bowel. Gallstone ileus requires enterotomy and removal of the gallstone(s).

The consequences of lost gallstones during laparoscopic cholecystectomy can reach far from the actual operation. Perhaps the greatest difficulty in

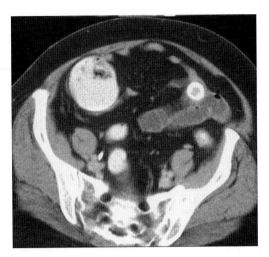

Fig. 17. CT of gallstone causing obstruction, gallstone ileus.

diagnosis and management of these conditions is the frequent inability to associate a remote and routine outpatient procedure with chronic and often, severe, intra-abdominal problems. Absolute documentation by the operating surgeon that the gallbladder was ruptured, stones spilled, and whether they were retrieved, will help prevent diagnostic delay. The actual number of complications of lost gallstones is impossible to document, because quite often, patients come from other institutions, from which obtaining knowledge of the total number of cholecystectomies performed is extremely difficult. Memon and colleagues' [56] documentation of a single surgeon's experience over 7 years with 856 patients, perhaps gives the best insight. He reported 106 gallbladder perforations with four short-term complications and one long-term complication. What can be done to prevent lost

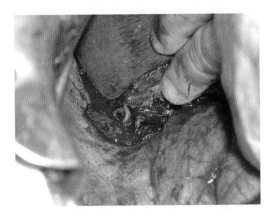

Fig. 18. Lost gallstones retrieved at laparotomy.

gallstones? Faced with an acutely inflamed gallbladder, the surgeon should perform early decompression with a large bore suction device, and suture or clip the opening of the gallbladder wall. During a difficult dissection, perhaps the attending surgeon should take over that part of the operation. And if the gallbladder is ruptured, early placement of a retrieval pouch below the gallbladder can allow the surgeon to milk the stones out of the gallbladder into the bag. What should the surgeon do then, when a perforation with spillage occurs? Based on all the available data, the best option is to make every attempt to retrieve lost gallstones, irrigate extensively, consider short-term antibiotics, and document the perforation in the operative note. Lost gallstones do not mandate open conversion, although massive contamination with pigment stones may warrant it.

References

[1] Mirizzi PL. Syndrome del conducto hepatico. J Int Chir 1948;8:731–77.
[2] Kok KY, Goh PY, Ngoi SS. Management of Mirizzi's syndrome in the laparoscopic era. Surg Endosc 1998;12(10):1242–4.
[3] Hazzan D, Golijanin D, Reissman P, et al. Combined endoscopic and surgical management of Mirizzi syndrome. Surg Endosc 1999;13(6):618–20.
[4] Redaelli CA, Buchler MW, Schilling MK, et al. High coincidence of Mirizzi syndrome and gallbladder cancer. Surgery 1997;121(1):58–63.
[5] McSherry CK, Fertenberg H, Virshup M. The Mirizzi syndrome: suggested classification and surgical therapy. Surg Gastroenterol 1982;1(3):219–25.
[6] Csendes A, Diaz JC, Burdiles P, et al. Mirizzi syndrome and cholecystobiliary fistula: a unifying classification. Br J Surg 1989;76(11):1139–43.
[7] Johnson LW, Sehon JK, Lee WC, et al. Mirizzi's syndrome: experience from a multi-institutional review. Am Surg 2001;67(1):11–4.
[8] Waisberg J, Corona A, de Abreu IW, et al. Benign obstruction of the common hepatic duct (Mirizzi syndrome):diagnosis and operative management. Arq Gastroenterol 2005;42(1): 13–8.
[9] Lai EC, Lau WY. Mirizzi syndrome: history, present, and future development. ANZ J Surg 2006;76(4):251–7.
[10] Bower TC, Nagorney DM. Mirizzi syndrome. HPB Surg 1988;1(1):67–74.
[11] Toursarkissian B, Holley DT, Kearney PA, et al. Mirizzi's syndrome. South Med J 1994; 87(4):471–5.
[12] Yeh CN, Jan YY, Chen MF. Laparoscopic treatment for Mirizzi syndrome. Surg Endosc 2003;17(10):1573–8.
[13] Berta R, Pansini GC, Zamboni P, et al. Laparoscopic treatment of Mirizzi's syndrome. Minerva Chir 1995;50(6):547–52.
[14] Frilling A, Li J, Weber F, et al. Major bile duct injuries after laparoscopic cholecystectomy: a tertiary center experience. J Gastrointest Surg 2004;8(6):679–85.
[15] MacFadyen BV Jr, Vecchio R, Ricardo AE, et al. Bile duct injury after laparoscopic cholecystectomy: the United States experience. Surg Endosc 1998;12(4):315–21.
[16] Moser JJ, Baer HU, Glatti A, et al. Mirizzi syndrome—a contraindication for laparoscopic surgery. Helv Chir Acta 1993;59(4):577–80.
[17] Desai DC, Smink RD Jr. Mirizzi syndrome type II: is laparoscopic cholecystectomy justified? JSLS 1997;1(3):237–9.
[18] Peterli R, Geering P, Huber AK. Mirizzi syndrome: preoperative diagnosis and therapeutic management. Swiss Surg 1995;6:298–303.

[19] Gomez G. Mirizzi syndrome. Curr Treat Options Gastroenterol 2002;5(2):95–9.

[20] General Surgery Case Logs, Accreditation Council for Graduate Medical Education, 2007.

[21] Deckoff SL. Gallstone ileus: a report of 12 cases. Ann Surg 1955;142(1):52–65.

[22] Cooperman AM, Dickson ER, ReMine WH. Changing concepts in the surgical treatment of gallstone ileus. Ann Surg 1968;167(3):377–83.

[23] Reisner RM, Cohen JR. Gallstone ileus: a review of 1001 reported cases. Am Surg 1994; 60(6):441–6.

[24] Masannat Y, Masannat Y, Shatnawel A. Gallstone ileus: a review. Mt Sinai J Med 2006; 73(8):1132–4.

[25] Masannat YA, Caplin S, Brown T. A rare complication of a common disease: bouveret syndrome, a case report. World J Gastroenterol 2006;12(16):2620–1.

[26] Chou JW, Hsu CH, Liao KF, et al. Gallstone ileus: report of two cases and review of the literature. World J Gastroenterol 2007;13(8):1295–8.

[27] Ayantunde AA, Agrawal A. Gallstone ileus: diagnosis and management. World J Surg 2007; 31:1292–7.

[28] Ripolles T, Miguel-Dasit A, Errando J, et al. Gallstone ileus: increased diagnostic sensitivity by combining plain film and ultrasound. Abdom Imaging 2001;26:401–5.

[29] Lassandro F, Gagliardi N, Scuderi M, et al. Gallstone ileus analysis of radiological findings in 27 patients. Eur J Radiol 2004;50:23–9.

[30] Yu CY, Lin CC, Shyu RY, et al. Value of CT in the diagnosis and management of gallstone ileus. World J Gastroenterol 2005;11(14):2142–7.

[31] Lassandro F, Romano S, Ragozzino A, et al. Role of helical CT in diagnosis of gallstone ileus and related conditions. AJR Am J Roentgenol 2005;185:1159–65.

[32] Warshaw AL, Bartlett MK. Choice of operation for gallstone intestinal obstruction. Ann Surg 1966;164(6):1051–5.

[33] Doko M, Zovak M, Kopljar M, et al. Comparison of surgical treatments of gallstone ileus: preliminary report. World J Surg 2003;27(4):400–4.

[34] Tan YM, Wong WK, Ooi LL. A comparison of two surgical strategies for the emergency treatment of gallstone ileus. Singapore Med J 2004;45(2):69–72.

[35] Pavlidis TE, Atmatzidis KS, Papaziogas BT, et al. Management of gallstone ileus. J Hepatobiliary Pancreat Surg 2003;10:299–302.

[36] Frossard JL, Steer ML, Pastor CM. Acute pancreatitis. Lancet 2008;371:143–52.

[37] West DM, Adrales GL, Schwartz RW. Current diagnosis and management of gallstone pancreatitis. Curr Surg 2002;59(3):296–8.

[38] Barkun AN. Early endoscopic management of acute gallstone pancreatitis—an evidence-based review. J Gastrointest Surg 2001;5(3):243–50.

[39] Petrov MS, van Santvoort HC, Besselik MG, et al. Early endoscopic retrograde cholangiopancreatography versus conservative management in acute biliary pancreatitis without cholangitis: a meta-analysis of randomized trials. Ann Surg 2008;247(2):250–7.

[40] Behrns KE, Ashley SW, Hunter JG, et al. Early ERCP for gallstone pancreatitis: for whom and when? J Gastrointest Surg 2008;12:629–33.

[41] Chang L, Lo S, Stabile BE, et al. Preoperative versus postoperative endoscopic retrograde cholangiopancreatography in mild-to-moderate gallstone pancreatitis. Ann Surg 2000; 231(1):82–7.

[42] Oria A, Cimmino D, Ocampo C, et al. Early endoscopic intervention versus early conservative management in patients with acute gallstone pancreatitis and biliopancreatic obstruction. Ann Surg 2007;245(1):10–7.

[43] Aiyer MK, Burdick JS, Sonnenberg A. Outcome of surgical and endoscopic management of biliary pancreatitis. Dig Dis Sci 1999;44(8):1684–90.

[44] Rosing DK, deVirgilio C, Yaghoubian A, et al. Early cholecystectomy for mild-to-moderate gallstone pancreatitis shortens hospital stay. J Am Coll Surg 2007;205(6):762–6.

[45] Kaw M, Al-Antably Y, Kaw P. Management of gallstone pancreatitis: cholecystectomy or ERCP and endoscopic sphincterotomy. Gastrointest Endosc 2002;56(1):61–5.

[46] Nealon WH, Bawduniak J, Walser EM. Appropriate timing of cholecystectomy in patients who present with moderate-to-severe gallstone-associated acute pancreatitis with peri-pancreatic fluid collections. Ann Surg 2004;239(6):741–51.

[47] Sanjay P, Yeeting S, Whigham C, et al. Endoscopic sphincterotomy and interval cholecystectomy are reasonable alternatives to index cholecystectomy in severe acute gall-stone pancreatitis. Surg Endosc 2007 [Epub ahead of print].

[48] Canlas KR, Branch MS. Role of endoscopic retrograde cholangiopancreatography in acute pancreatitis. World J Gastroenterol 2007;13(47):6314–20.

[49] Hartwig W, Werner J, Muller CA, et al. Surgical management of severe pancreatitis including sterile necrosis. J Hepatobiliary Pancreat Surg 2002;9:429–35.

[50] Reber HA, McFadden DW. Indications for surgery in necrotizing pancreatitis. West J Med 1993;159(6):704–7.

[51] Jamdar S, Siriwardena A. Contemporary management of infected necrosis complicating severe acute pancreatitis. Crit Care 2006;10:1–3.

[52] Bradley EL, Howard TJ, van Sonnenberg E, et al. Intervention in necrotizing pancreatitis: an evidence-based review of surgical and percutaneous alternatives. J Gastrointest Surg 2008; 12:634–9.

[53] Behrns KE, Ben-David K. Surgical therapy of pancreatic pseudocysts. J Gastrointest Surg 2008 [Epub ahead of print].

[54] Cheruvu CVN, Clarke MG, Prentice M, et al. Conservative treatment as an option in the management of pancreatic pseudocyst. Ann R Coll Surg Engl 2003;85:313–6.

[55] Gerlizani S, Tos M, Gornati R, et al. Is the loss of gallstones during laparoscopic cholecystectomy an underestimnated complication? Surg Endosc 2000;14(4):373–4.

[56] Memon MA, Deeik RK, Maffi TR, et al. The outcome of unretrieved gallstones in the peritoneal cavity during laparoscopic cholecystectomy. Prospective analysis. Surg Endosc 1999; 13(9):848–57.

[57] Barrat C, Champault A, Matthyssens L, et al. Iatrogenic perforation of the gallbladder during laparoscopic cholecystectomy does not influence prognosis. Prospective study. Ann Chir 2004;129(1):25–9.

[58] Brockmann JG, Kocher T, Senninger NJ, et al. Complications due to gallstones lost during laparoscopic cholecystectomy. Surg Endosc 2002;16(8):1226–32.

[59] Zehetner J, Shamiyeh A, Wayand W. Lost gallstones in laparoscopic cholectectomy: all possible complications. Am J Surg 2007;193(1):73–8.

[60] McDonald MP, Munson JL, Sanders L, et al. Consequences of lost gallstones. Surg Endosc 1997;11(7):774–7.

[61] Zulfikaroglu B, Ozalp N, Mahir Ozmen M, et al. What happens to the lost gallstone during laparoscopic cholecystectomy? Surg Endosc 2003;17(1):158.

[62] Habib E, Khoury R, Elhadad A, et al. Digestive complications of biliary gallstone lost during laparoscopic cholecystectomy. Gastroenterol Clin Biol 2002;26(10):930–4.

[63] Loffeld RJ. The consequences of lost gallstones during laparoscopic cholecystectomy. Neth J Med 2006;64(10):364–6.

ELSEVIER
SAUNDERS

SURGICAL
CLINICS OF
NORTH AMERICA

Surg Clin N Am 88 (2008) 1369–1384

Bile Duct Cysts

Marc Mesleh, MD, Daniel J. Deziel, MD*

*Department of General Surgery, Rush Medical College, Rush University Medical Center,
1653 West Congress Parkway, Chicago, IL 60612, USA*

Although relatively uncommon, cystic lesions of the bile ducts are more than a surgical curiosity. The clinical presentation may include several hepatic, biliary, and pancreatic conditions. The association of bile duct cysts with anomalous junctions between the common bile duct and the main pancreatic duct and with hepatobiliary cancers has important surgical implications. Concepts about the pathogenesis, diagnosis, and surgical treatment of bile duct cysts have evolved over several decades. Surgeons who treat biliary tract disease, in either adult or pediatric patients, should be familiar with the current evaluation and treatment of individuals who have these anomalies.

Epidemiology

The incidence of bile duct cysts ranges between 1 in 13,000 to 1 in 2 million births [1]. The disease is two to four times more frequent in females than in males [2,3]. About 25% to 45% of cases are diagnosed in neonates or infants and two thirds of cases are identified during the first decade of life. Some 20% to 25% of cases are not discovered until adulthood, however [3,4]. There is a preponderance of cases from the Far East, particularly from Japan, compared with other parts of the world. Even in Western series, a substantial proportion of patients are of Asian descent [5].

Etiology

Cysts of the bile ducts are believed to originate from the embryonic proximal liver anlage. This origin is in contradistinction to simple hepatic cysts derived from the distal liver anlage, which are not connected to the ductal system [6].

* Corresponding author.
E-mail address: daniel_j_deziel@rush.edu (D.J. Deziel).

0039-6109/08/$ - see front matter © 2008 Elsevier Inc. All rights reserved.
doi:10.1016/j.suc.2008.07.002
surgical.theclinics.com

Several theories have been proposed to explain the development of bile duct cysts. The general mechanisms involve distal bile duct obstruction and structural weakness of the wall of the ducts. Although no one theory has been conclusively established, the most widely accepted current understanding is that these ductal changes are related to an anomalous connection between the biliary and pancreatic ductal systems referred to as abnormal pancreatic-biliary junction (APBJ).

The etiologic role of APBJ in bile duct cysts was first proposed by Babbitt in 1969 [7]. The anomaly described was an early junction of the pancreatic duct and common bile duct outside of the duodenal wall (Fig. 1). This arrangement results in a common pancreaticobiliary channel that could allow pancreatic exocrine secretions to reflux into the biliary system. Pancreatic secretory pressure exceeds hepatic secretory pressure and, in the presence of a common channel, there is no sphincter mechanism to prevent pancreaticobiliary reflux. It is theorized that refluxed pancreatic juice raises intraductal pressure, causes irritation and inflammation, and inflicts structural damage to the duct wall, thereby resulting in cystic degeneration. Obstruction of the distal bile duct because of the anomalous junction itself or caused by protein plugs from pancreatic acinar cells may also be a contributory factor [8,9]. Supportive evidence for the reflux theory includes demonstration of high amylase content in aspirated cyst contents, a positive pressure gradient between the pancreatic duct and cyst, and observed

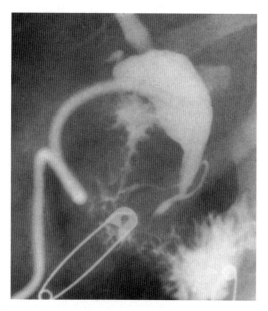

Fig. 1. Abnormal pancreaticobiliary junction. Type I bile duct cyst with long common channel after joining main pancreatic duct. (*From* Deziel DJ, Rossi RL, Munson JL, et al. Cystic disease of the bile ducts: surgical management and reoperation. Problems in General Surgery 1985;22(4):467–80; with permission).

inflammatory reaction in the cyst wall [10,11]. The reported prevalence of APBJ in patients who have bile duct cysts is approximately 60% to 90% [1,12].

Additional theories have been proposed to account for the occurrence of bile duct cysts in patients who have normal pancreaticobiliary junctional anatomy. Most of these alternative theories implicate distal obstruction as the cause of elevated intraluminal pressure. Cystic dilatation of the bile ducts has been produced experimentally in infant animals by duct occlusion [9,13,14]. Congenital webs in the distal bile duct or abnormal sphincter of Oddi function with spasm could also cause obstruction [12].

Fewer ganglion cells have been found in the ducts of some patients who have bile duct cysts. A viral infection has been proposed to lead to the destruction of the ganglion cells based on elevated levels of reoviral RNA that have been observed in the bile ducts of patients who have cysts [15].

Yotuyanagi, in 1936 [16], suggested that bile duct cysts resulted from an unequal distribution of epithelial cells during embryologic maturation. Initially, the embryonic bile ducts are a cord of solid tissue. Proliferation of epithelial elements within the cord leads to vacuolization and canalization. The relative development of more epithelial cells in the proximal duct system and fewer cells in the distal segment could produce cystic dilatation with distal stenosis at the time of canalization.

Caroli's disease, a subset of bile duct cyst disease, is believed to originate from incomplete and faulty remodeling of the embryonic ductal plate [17]. This remodeling results in abnormalities of the intrahepatic bile ducts with segmental and communicating dilatations.

The role of genetic factors in the formation of bile duct cysts is uncertain. There are a few familial cases described with variable cyst types [12]. Caroli's disease may be autosomal recessively inherited [18]. Most patients, however, do not have a known genetic link.

Classifications

Alonso-Lej and colleagues [19] first proposed a classification scheme for bile duct cysts in 1959. This scheme was modified by Todani and colleagues in 1977 [2] to the classification most commonly used today (Figs. 2 and 3). Type I cysts are a dilatation of the extrahepatic bile duct (Fig. 4). These are the most common, found in 75% to 85% of cases [3,4]. Type I cysts may be further described as cystic (IA), focal (IB), or fusiform (IC). Type II cysts are a saccular diverticulum of the common bile duct. Type III represents cystic dilatation of the common bile duct within the wall of the duodenum (Fig. 5). These lesions are also known as choledochoceles. Type II and III cysts are uncommon, occurring in only 3% to 4% of cases each. Type IV disease refers to multiple cysts. Type IVA lesions involve both the intra- and extrahepatic portions of the bile ducts and type IVB are multiple cysts limited to the extrahepatic bile ducts. Type IV cysts account for 10% to

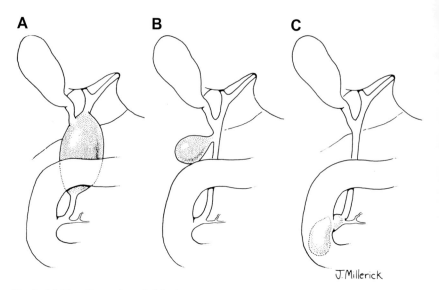

Fig. 2. (*A*) Type I, extrahepatic bile duct cyst. (*B*) Type II, diverticulum of common bile duct. (*C*) Type III, choledochocele. (*From* Deziel DJ, Rossi RL, Munson JL, et al. Cystic disease of the bile ducts: surgical management and reoperation. Problems in General Surgery 1985;22(4):468; with permission).

40%, although Type IVB disease is uncommon [1]. Type V cysts involve the intrahepatic bile ducts. These are usually multiple (Caroli's disease) (Fig. 6) and occasionally solitary (Fig. 7). Type V cysts are reported in less than 1% of patients in most series. Intrahepatic bile duct cysts may be bilobar or unilobar, with 90% of unilobar cysts occurring on the left side [17]. The frequency of type V cysts is higher in series using modern imaging techniques for diagnosis [20].

The distribution of cyst types may vary somewhat between adult and pediatric populations. Although type I cysts are the most common in patients of all ages, type IVA cysts may be more prevalent in adults [1,21]. This difference can potentially be explained by progression of asymptomatic type I disease in childhood, but there are no conclusive data.

More recently, it has been suggested that the classification of congenital bile duct cysts be modified to exclude diverticula (type II), choledochoceles (type III), and Caroli's disease [22]. These varieties may have distinctly different causes and clinical considerations. Type II cysts may be a form of gallbladder duplication or acquired inflammatory diverticulum related to stone disease. Choledochoceles are lined with duodenal mucosa and may be a type of duodenal duplication or web. Caroli's disease arises from ductal plate malformation and is associated with hepatic fibrosis. It has also been observed that the intrahepatic bile ducts are never entirely normal in patients believed only to have extrahepatic disease. The distinction between types I and IV cysts may therefore be arbitrary.

A B

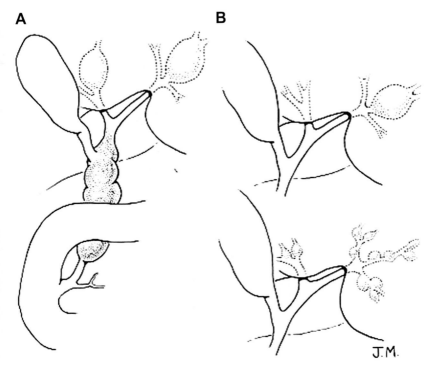

Fig. 3. (*A*) Type IV, combined intrahepatic and extrahepatic bile ducts. (*B*) Type V cysts demonstrating isolated and diffuse cystic dilatation of the intrahepatic ducts. (*From* Deziel DJ, Rossi RL, Munson JL, et al. Cystic disease of the bile ducts: surgical management and reoperation. Problems in General Surgery 1985;22(4):469; with permission).

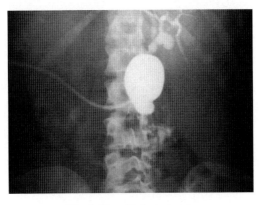

Fig. 4. Type I bile duct cyst.

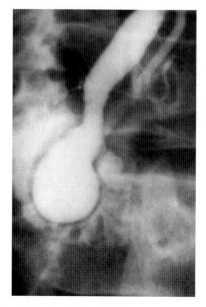

Fig. 5. Type III bile duct cyst (choledochocele).

Histologically, the wall of bile duct cysts is composed of dense fibrous tissue with inflammatory reaction. Some smooth muscle fibers may be present. The mucosa may be absent or only consist of scattered patches of columnar epithelium interspersed amid granulation tissue and ulcerations.

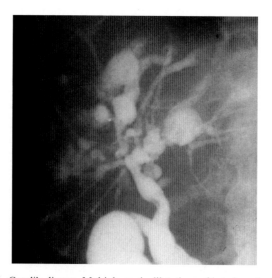

Fig. 6. Caroli's disease. Multiple cystic dilatations of intrahepatic ducts.

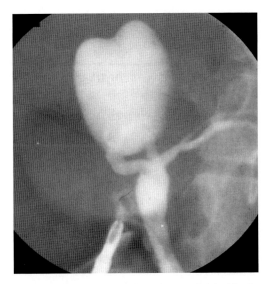

Fig. 7. Type V, isolated intrahepatic cyst of right bile duct.

This inconsistency in the mucosa is believed to be responsible for the high rate of anastomotic failure between cysts and small bowel.

Clinical Presentation

The classic symptom triad for choledochal cysts is abdominal pain, jaundice, and a right upper quadrant abdominal mass. Although this was originally described in most patients, in reality the triad is rarely seen, occurring in only 5% to 10% of pediatric patients and in virtually none of the adult patients [20,21,23]. Tables 1 and 2 summarize the clinical symptoms reported in pediatric and adult populations from representative series.

In pediatric patients, abdominal pain is the most common presenting symptom. Although few present with the full triad, approximately 85% of children show at least two of the symptoms. Jaundice, which is the presenting symptom in 27% to 57% of these patients, is more common than cholangitis or pancreatitis.

Abdominal pain is also the most common presenting symptom in adults, followed by jaundice and cholangitis. Other presenting symptoms include nausea or vomiting, weight loss, pruritus, or gastrointestinal bleeding. An abdominal mass is distinctly uncommon in adults, reported in only 3% of patients [24]. Adults who have choledochal cysts may present with vague symptoms or they may be completely asymptomatic. Consequently, diagnosis may be delayed.

Several important hepatobiliary and pancreatic conditions can coexist with bile duct cysts and influence the clinical presentation and management. These include lithiasis, cholangitis, pancreatitis, cirrhosis, hepatic fibrosis,

Table 1
The prevalence of presenting symptoms in studies of pediatric populations

Series, year	No. of patients	Abdominal pain (%)	Jaundice (%)	Abdominal mass (%)	Weight loss (%)	Nausea/vomiting (%)	Cholangitis (%)	Pancreatitis (%)
Chaudhary et al, 1996 [21]	22	91	27	18	NR	NR	9	NR
DeVries et al, 2002 [20]	42	76	57	17	23	45	35	17
Singham et al, 2007 [23]	19	79	32	16	11	42	NR	21

Abbreviation: NR, not reported.

Table 2
The prevalence of presenting symptoms in studies of adult populations

Series	No. of patients	Abdominal pain (%)	Jaundice (%)	Weight loss (%)	Nausea/ vomiting (%)	Cholangitis (%)	Pancreatitis (%)
Deziel, et al [24]	31	86	45	10	24	NR	6
Chaudhary, et al [21]	27	89	70	NR	NR	37	7
Visser, et al [22]	39	92	13	11	NR	21	16
Singham, et al [23]	51	88	39	NR	63	37	11
Bois, et al [25]	68	81	21	NR	NR	18	NR

Abbreviation: NR, not reported.

ampullary stenosis, portal hypertension, and malignancy [24]. Commonly, adult patients develop pancreatitis, which is believed to be caused by the abnormal activation of pancreatic enzymes related to the APBJ. The risk for pancreatitis is also related to cyst size, suggesting that the cyst may mechanically cause an obstruction of the pancreatic duct. Secondary biliary cirrhosis can develop with advanced disease. Intraoperative liver biopsies have revealed the presence of bile duct proliferation, cholestasis, parenchymal damage, inflammatory infiltrates, and fibrosis. The severity of associated conditions impacts the outcome of operative intervention and prognosis. Biliary stones are often found in adult patients who have bile duct cysts and are attributed to stasis [26]. Stones can occur in the gallbladder, in the cysts themselves, and in the hepatic ducts proximal to stenotic areas. Symptoms of biliary lithiasis, such as pain, cholangitis, jaundice, and sepsis may be the primary manifestation of cystic disease. Rarely, large cysts may rupture, resulting in bile peritonitis.

Diagnostic imaging

Bile duct cysts are typically diagnosed by hepatobiliary imaging. Advances in imaging modalities over the years have greatly improved the recognition and characterization of these anomalies. Cystic lesions are most frequently first suspected based on findings from transabdominal ultrasonography or CT scanning. The sensitivity of transabdominal ultrasonography ranges from 70% to 97% [27]. Ultrasound is less accurate for the specific diagnosis of bile duct cysts in adults who have more secondary causes for bile duct dilatation. Ultrasound and CT are reliable for detecting cystic right upper abdominal lesions and for assessing their size and extent but they may not always be able to precisely identify that the cyst originates from the bile duct.

Magnetic resonance cholangiopancreatography (MRCP) is the best method for noninvasive imaging of bile duct cysts [1,12]. MRCP may not demonstrate the junctional anatomy of the bile duct and pancreatic duct as clearly as direct endoscopic cholangiography, however. Traditionally, MRCP has also not been as useful in pediatric patients who are not able to cooperate with the requisite breath holds. The development of newer single-shot fast spin echo sequences may overcome some of this limitation [28].

Direct cholangiography by endoscopic retrograde cholangiopancreatography (ERCP) or percutaneous transhepatic cholangiography (PTC) provides accurate anatomic detail to characterize the configuration and extent of bile duct cysts. The relationship of the pancreatic duct and bile ducts is least demonstrated by ERCP. PTC is usually reserved for situations in which ERCP cannot be accomplished or is unable to visualize the intrahepatic ducts sufficiently because of more proximal obstruction.

Cancer and bile duct cysts

Bile duct cysts are premalignant lesions. Since first described by Irwin and Morison in 1944, the association of bile duct cysts and cancer has been well recognized [29–33]. The overall frequency of hepatobiliary malignancy in adult patients who have bile duct cysts ranges from 10% to 30% [1,24,34,35]. The relative risk has been estimated to be twenty to thirty times higher than that of the general population. Most individuals have been adults when diagnosed and the risk for cancer increases with age [36]. Cancer has occurred in children who have bile duct cysts also [2].

Cancer has been described in association with all types of bile duct cysts but most commonly with type I and type IV disease (Fig. 8). The vast majority of cancers are cholangiocarcinomas. Squamous cell cancer and anaplastic or undifferentiated malignancies have also been reported. Although many cancers have occurred in the cysts themselves, the entire biliary tract is at risk, including other bile duct sites (whether dilated or non-dilated), the gallbladder, and the pancreas. Cancers may be diagnosed synchronously when the cyst is detected or metachronously years after total excision, partial excision, or anastomotic drainage of benign cysts. The high incidence observed in patients previously treated by internal drainage gave impetus to cyst resection as the preferred treatment. Unfortunately, even complete excision of benign choledochal cysts does not necessarily prevent the development of cancer in the intrahepatic bile ducts later [37,38].

The pathogenesis of malignant cyst degeneration is believed to be related to the carcinogenic effects of chronic mucosal irritation and exposure to refluxed pancreatic enzymes and bile. K-ras and p-53 mutations have been identified in the biliary epithelium of patients who have APBJ and cysts [39]. Premalignant proliferative histologic changes have been reported in one third of benign cysts [40]. The risk for malignant transformation in bile duct cysts or in the gallbladder is higher in the presence of an APBJ.

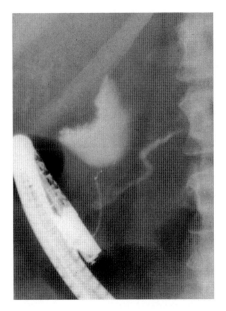

Fig. 8. Adenocarcinoma in bile duct cyst. ERCP demonstrates type I cyst with large irregular filling defect.

The risk for cancer in bile duct cysts can be considered a field effect that jeopardizes the entire biliary epithelium. Because cancer can occur in even nondilated ducts years after complete cyst excision long-term follow-up for these patients is important. Surveillance is particularly important for those who have type I or type IV cysts, APBJ, or any residual cystic component. Although the rate of metachronous cancer may be low, cholangiocarcinoma has a poor prognosis. The median survival of individuals who have cholangiocarcinoma associated with bile ducts cysts is 6 to 21 months and 2-year survival is 5% or less [12,34,35,40].

Surgical management

The preferred treatment of bile duct cysts is complete surgical excision with cholecystectomy and reconstruction by Roux-en-Y hepaticojejunostomy. In former years, patients were often treated without excision by anastomosing the cyst to the jejunum, duodenum, or stomach. Such internal drainage procedures resulted in high rates of stenosis, lithiasis, cholangitis, and reoperation and failed to address the premalignant nature of these lesions. In the current time, cyst excision can be accomplished with low morbidity and mortality rates compared with outdated operations for internal drainage [21,24,34,35,41]. Unfortunately, when the cystic process involves multiple intrahepatic and extrahepatic sites, complete excision may not be feasible. Under these circumstances, partial excision combined with drainage of the residual abnormal ducts may be the only solution.

Type I cysts are exposed by mobilizing the hepatic flexure of the colon downward and Kocherizing the duodenum. The location of the hepatic artery and of any replaced right hepatic artery originated from the superior mesenteric artery is identified. Intrahepatic fluorocholangiography is performed to verify the anatomy of the proximal ducts and of the pancreatico-biliary junction. Cholangiography can be obtained by way of the cystic duct or by direct cyst puncture, or, if the cyst is large, with the cyst open by placing appropriately sized balloon catheters for injection of the proximal and distal duct. Intraoperative biliary endoscopy can be useful for examination of the proximal bile ducts in search of stenoses or debris. In some patients, intrahepatic stenoses may be caused by intraluminal membranes that can be excised [42].

A type I cyst should be excised in total (Fig. 9). The surgeon should resist the temptation to leave too much residual proximal or distal duct. Distally, the resection is carried down into the pancreas and there are two notes of caution. If the resection is taken too far, the main pancreatic duct can be injured. It is not usually possible to visualize the pancreatic duct and the cyst often narrows considerably near its termination. Second, the distal bile duct should be oversewn to prevent a postoperative pancreatic fistula, which is prone to occur if the patient has an abnormal early pancreaticobiliary junction [24]. The distal duct may be tiny and imprecise suture placement may occlude the pancreatic duct, however. Drains are advisable.

The proximal extent of resection should be to normal mucosa. An anastomosis to granulated or ulcerated mucosa will result in stricture. Leaving a proximal rim of residual cyst so that the anastomosis will be wider or easier to construct is an incorrect concept. Both the right hepatic duct and, in particular, the left hepatic duct can be incised (after the hilar plate is opened) to provide a perfectly adequate length for anastomosis.

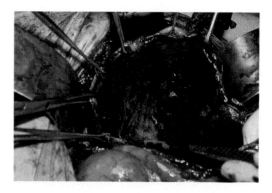

Fig. 9. Intraoperative view of opened extrahepatic bile duct cyst.

Although the entire cyst wall can usually be dissected off of the portal vein and hepatic artery, the presence of pronounced fibrosis may occasionally make this more difficult. Under these circumstances, an intraluminal plane of dissection has been used [43], which permits excision of the diseased cyst lining while protecting nearby vascular structures. The anterior, medial, and lateral cyst walls are divided and the posterior plane of dissection is developed, leaving the fibrotic outer cyst wall in place.

The standard reconstruction after cyst excision is by Roux-en-Y hepaticojejunostomy with a 40- to 60-cm Roux limb. The Roux limb is shorter for infants (15–20 cm) or children (30–40 cm) [44]. Other methods of reconstruction have been described in an attempt to reduce the risk for postoperative enterobiliary reflux. Experience with these approaches has largely been limited to pediatric patients. Techniques have included creation of an intussuscepted valve in the small intestinal limb and interposition of a conduit between the bile duct and duodenum consisting of an isolated small bowel segment, the appendix, or a segment of terminal ileum and cecum with the ileocecal valve [44].

Type II cysts are uncommon. When encountered, treatment has been by cyst excision. If an anomalous pancreaticobiliary junction is present, biliary diversion by Roux-en-Y hepaticojejunostomy may be necessary to prevent continued pathogenetic pancreaticobiliary reflux.

Type III cysts (choledochoceles) are also a rarity and are approached transduodenally. Because there is not uniformity as to the pathogenesis, classification, anatomy, and clinical presentation of this entity, the treatment is individualized. Endoscopic division and sphincterotomy may be sufficient for some patients who have smaller cysts without duodenal obstruction. Otherwise, transduodenal excision with sphincteroplasty or duct reimplantation has been performed.

Type IV cysts involve multiple duct sites. Those confined to the extrahepatic ducts are treated by complete excision, similar to type I cysts. Type IV cysts that involve both the intrahepatic and extrahepatic bile ducts are problematic because complete excision may not be possible short of total hepatectomy. These are usually treated by resection of the extrahepatic component with Roux-en-Y hepaticojejunostomy at the hepatic hilum. Intrahepatic strictures can be dilated. If the intrahepatic disease is limited to one lobe, then hepatic resection can be done.

The surgical treatment of patients who have type V disease involving the intrahepatic bile ducts must also be individualized depending on anatomic extent and hepatic function [17,18]. Unilobar involvement is effectively managed by hepatic resection. Hepatic transplantation is the definitive therapy for those who have diffuse disease, hepatic cirrhosis, or associated malignancy. For those who do not have cirrhosis, drainage by biliary-enteric anastomosis, transhepatic stenting, and combinations may help control symptoms.

Laparoscopic and robotic-assisted operations for bile duct cysts have been described [45,46]. Because these lesions are uncommon to begin with, experience with minimally invasive techniques is limited. These cases have presented a technical challenge but feasibility has been demonstrated. The outcome of cyst excision and hepaticoenterostomy in children can be excellent. In a series of 180 patients followed for a mean of 11 years, only 2.3% developed late complications of cholangitis or ductal stones [47].

In experienced hands, cyst excision in adults can be performed with negligible mortality, although morbidity rates are 20% or greater [24,25,34,35,41]. Following complete excision, about 10% of adult patients have recurrent cholangitis, pancreatitis, or chronic liver disease, and there is a small but finite risk for future malignancy. For these reasons, long-term follow-up is advisable.

References

[1] Soreide K, Korner H, Havnen J, et al. Bile duct cysts in adults. Br J Surg 2004;91(12): 1538–48.
[2] Todani T, Watanabe Y, Narusue M, et al. Congenital bile duct cysts: classification, operative procedures, and review of thirty-seven cases including cancer arising from choledochal cyst. Am J Surg 1977;134(2):263–9.
[3] Flanigan DP. Biliary cysts. Ann Surg 1975;182:635–43.
[4] Yamaguchi M. Congenital choledochal cyst. Analysis of 1,433 patients in the Japanese literature. Am J Surg 1980;140:653–7.
[5] Wiseman K, Buczkowski AK, Chung SW, et al. Epidemiology, presentation, diagnosis, and outcomes of choledochal cysts in adults in an urban environment. Am J Surg 2005;189(5): 527–31.
[6] Longmire WP, Mandiola SA, Gordon HE. Congenital cystic disease of the liver and biliary system. Ann Surg 1971;174(4):711–26.
[7] Babbitt DP. Congenital choledochal cysts: new etiological concept based on anomalous relationships of the common bile duct and the pancreatic bulb. Ann Radiol (Paris) 1969; 12(3):231–40.
[8] Kaneko K, Ando H, Seo T, et al. Proteomic analysis of protein plugs: causative agent of symptoms in patients with choledochal cyst. Dig Dis Sci 2007;52(8):1979–86.
[9] Miyano T, Suruga K, Chen SC. A clinicopathologic study of choledochal cyst. World J Surg 1980;4(2):231–8.
[10] Babbitt DP, Starshak RJ, Clemett AR. Choledochal cyst: a concept of etiology. Am J Roentgenol Radium Ther Nucl Med 1973;119(1):57–62.
[11] Tanaka M, Ikeda S, Kawakami K, et al. The presence of a positive pressure gradient from pancreatic duct to choledochal cyst demonstrated by duodenoscopic microtransducer manometry: clue to pancreaticobiliary reflux. Endoscopy 1982;14:45–7.
[12] Metcalfe MS, Wemyss-Holden SA, Maddern GJ. Management dilemmas with choledochal cysts. Arch Surg 2003;138(3):333–9.
[13] Ohkawa H, Sawaguchi S, Yamazaki Y, et al. Experimental analysis of the ill effect of anomalous pancreaticobiliary ductal union. J Pediatr Surg 1982;17(1):7–13.
[14] Deziel DJ, Rossi RL, Munson JL, et al. Cystic disease of the bile ducts: surgical management and reoperation. Problems in General Surgery: Secondary Procedures 1985;2(4): 467–79.
[15] Tyler KL, Sokol RJ, Oberhaus SM, et al. Detection of reovirus RNA in hepatobiliary tissues from patients with extrahepatic biliary atresia and choledochal cysts. Hepatology 1998; 27(6):1475–82.
[16] Yotuyanagi S. Contribution to etiology and pathology of idiopathic cystic dilatation of the common bile duct with report of 3 cases. Gann 1936;30:601–8.

[17] Ulrich F, Pratschke J, Pascher A, et al. Long-term outcome of liver resection and transplantation for Caroli disease and syndrome. Ann Surg 2008;247(2):357–64.
[18] Lendoire J, Schelotto PB, Rodriguez JA, et al. Bile duct cyst type V (Caroli's disease): surgical strategies and results. HPB (Oxford) 2007;9:281–4.
[19] Alonso-Lej F, Rever WB Jr, Pessagno DJ. Congenital choledochal cyst, with a report of 2 and an analysis of 94, cases. Int Abstr Surg 1959;108(1):1–30.
[20] DeVries JS, DeVries S, Aronson DC, et al. Choledochal cysts: age of presentation, symptoms, and late complications related to Todani's classification. J Pediatr Surg 2002;37(11): 1568–73.
[21] Chaudhary A, Dhar P, Sachdev A, et al. Choledochal cysts—differences in children and adults. Br J Surg 1996;83(2):186–8.
[22] Visser BC, Suh I, Way LW, et al. Congenital choledochal cysts in adults. Arch Surg 2004; 139(8):855–62.
[23] Singham J, Schaeffer D, Yoshida E, et al. Choledochal cysts: analysis of disease pattern and optimal treatment in adult and pediatric patients. HPB (Oxford) 2007;9:383–7.
[24] Deziel DJ, Rossi RL, Munson JL, et al. Management of bile duct cysts in adults. Arch Surg 1986;121(4):410–5.
[25] Bois JP, Kendrick ML, Farnell MB, et al. Choledochal cysts: risk of malignancy and outcome in 68 patients undergoing surgical management at a single institution. Poster presented at the Society for Surgery of the Alimentary Tract, San Diego, CA, May 2008.
[26] Matsumoto Y, Uchida K, Nakase A, et al. Congenital cystic dilatation of the common bile duct as a cause of primary bile duct stone. Am J Surg 1977;134(3):346–52.
[27] Sato M, Ishida H, Konno K, et al. Choledochal cyst due to anomalous pancreaticobiliary junction in the adult: sonographic findings. Abdom Imaging 2001;26(4):395–400.
[28] Kim MJ, Han SJ, Yoon CS, et al. Using MR cholangiopancreatography to reveal anomalous pancreaticobiliary ductal union in infants and children with choledochal cysts. AJR Am J Roentgenol 2002;179(1):209–14.
[29] Irwin ST, Morison JE. Congenital cyst of the common bile-duct containing stones and undergoing cancerous change. Br J Surg 1944;32:319–21.
[30] Flanigan DP. Biliary carcinoma associated with biliary cysts. Cancer 1977;40:880–3.
[31] Bloustein PA. Association of carcinoma with congenital cystic conditions of the liver and bile ducts. Am J Gastroenterol 1977;67(1):40–6.
[32] Todani T, Tabuchi K, Watanabe Y, et al. Carcinoma arising in the wall of congenital bile ducts. Cancer 1979;44:1134–41.
[33] Bismuth H, Krissat J. Choledochal cyst malignancies. Ann Oncol 1999;10(Suppl 4):94–8.
[34] Stain SC, Guthrie CR, Yellin AE, et al. Choledochal cyst in the adult. Ann Surg 1995;222(2): 128–33.
[35] Liu CL, Fan ST, Lo CM, et al. Cysts in adults. Arch Surg 2002;137(4):465–8.
[36] Voyles CR, Smadja C, Shanda WC, et al. Carcinoma in choledochal cycts: age related incidence. Arch Surg 1983;118:986–8.
[37] Watanabe Y, Toki A, Todani T. Bile duct cancer developed after cyst excision for choledochal cyst. HPB (Oxford) 1999;6(3):207–12.
[38] Kobayashi S, Asano T, Yamasaki M, et al. Risk of bile duct carcinogenesis after excision of extrahepatic bile ducts in pancreaticobiliary maljunction. Surgery 1999;126(5):939–44.
[39] Nagai M, Watanabe M, Iwase T, et al. Clinical and genetic analysis of noncancerous and cancerous biliary epithelium in patients with pancreaticobiliary maljunction. World J Surg 2002;26(1):91–8.
[40] Rossi RL, Silverman ML, Braasch JW, et al. Carcinomas arising in cystic conditions of the bile ducts. A clinical and pathologic study. Ann Surg 1987;205(4):377–84.
[41] Chaudhary A, Dhar P, Sachdev A. Reoperative surgery for choledochal cysts. Br J Surg 1997;84(6):781–4.
[42] Ando H, Kaneko K, Ito F, et al. Operative treatment of congenital stenoses of the intrahepatic bile ducts in patients with choledochal cysts. Am J Surg 1997;173(6):491–4.

[43] Lilly JR. The surgical treatment of choledochal cyst. Surg Gynecol Obstet 1979;149(1): 36–42.

[44] Martin LW, Ziegler MM. Operative treatment for choledochal cyst. In: Baker RJ, Fischer JE, editors. Master of surgery. 4th edition. Philadelphia: Lippincott Williams & Wilkins; 2001. p. 1206–12.

[45] Abbas HM, Yassin NA, Ammori BJ. Laparoscopic resection of type I choledochal cyst in an adult and Roux-en-Y hepaticojejunostomy: a case report and literature review. Surg Laparosc Endosc Percutan Tech 2006;16(6):439–44.

[46] Meehan JJ, Elliott S, Sandler A. The robotic approach to complex hepatobiliary anomalies in children: preliminary report. J Pediatr Surg 2007;42(12):2110–4.

[47] Miyano T, Yamataka A, Kato Y, et al. Hepaticoenterostomy after excision of choledochal cyst in children: a 30-year experience with 180 cases. J Pediatr Surg 1996;31(10):1417–21.

ELSEVIER
SAUNDERS

SURGICAL
CLINICS OF
NORTH AMERICA

Surg Clin N Am 88 (2008) 1385–1407

Primary Sclerosing Cholangitis

Fredric D. Gordon, MD[a,b]

[a]Lahey Clinic Medical Center, Hepatobiliary and Liver Transplantation, 41 Mall Road,
4 West, Burlington, MA 01805, USA
[b]Department of Medicine, Tufts Medical School, 145 Harrison Avenue, Boston,
MA 02111, USA

Sclerosing cholangitis is a clinical syndrome characterized by recurrent fever, pain, and jaundice resulting from fibrosing and inflammatory obstruction of the bile ducts caused by primary or secondary abnormalities of the biliary system.

Primary sclerosing cholangitis (PSC) is a chronic cholestatic syndrome of unknown etiology characterized by diffuse fibrosing inflammation of the intra- and extrahepatic biliary ductal systems. The disease is usually progressive, albeit at an unpredictable rate, advancing to biliary cirrhosis, portal hypertension, and, unless intervention with liver transplantation is accomplished, premature death from liver failure. The diagnosis of PSC usually is based on a combination of clinical, biochemical, histologic and radiologic abnormalities. In the past, PSC often was diagnosed in its late stages after the patient became jaundiced and cachectic. More recently, increased physician awareness and accessibility of endoscopic retrograde cholangiography (ERCP) allow earlier recognition of the disease, in the asymptomatic stage. It often is seen in association with inflammatory bowel disease (IBD).

Primary sclerosing cholangitis must be distinguished from secondary sclerosing cholangitis, a syndrome with similar clinical characteristics but resulting from identifiable causes (Box 1). The term primary sclerosing cholangitis indicates that this form of sclerosing cholangitis is idiopathic but also associated with induration of the bile ducts that results from chronic inflammation and fibrous connective tissue as a result of inflammation of the bile ducts.

Lahey Clinic Medical Center, Hepatobiliary and Liver Transplantation, 41 Mall Road,
West, Burlington, MA 01805, USA.
E-mail address: fredric_d_gordon@lahey.org

Box 1. Sclerosing cholangitis

Primary
Intrahepatic and extrahepatic
Intrahepatic
Extrahepatic
Small duct

Secondary
Choledocholithiasis
Trauma
Ischemic
Chemical toxicity
Infection
Eosinophilic cholangitis
AIDS cholangiopathy
Congenital anomaly
Malignancy
Amyloidosis

Epidemiology

PSC once was considered a medical curiosity; indeed fewer than 100 cases had been reported in the English-language literature between Delbert's first description in 1924 and 1980. This situation has changed dramatically, and recent experience indicates that PSC and primary biliary cirrhosis (PBC) represent the two most common adult chronic cholestatic liver diseases. Moreover, PSC is now one of the most common indications for liver transplantation in adults [1]. Without question, the frequency of diagnosis of PSC has increased dramatically in the last 20 years. This increase likely reflects increased clinical awareness and use of ERCP rather than a true increase in the incidence of the disease.

There are no good data regarding the overall prevalence of PSC; thus, crude estimates are necessary. In the United States and Northern Europe, the estimated incidence of PSC is 0.9 to 1.3 cases per 100,000 population [2–5]. The prevalence in these areas ranges from 8 to 14 per 100,000 population but is far less in southern Europe and Asia. The frequency of PSC in United States minority populations is unknown. It appears to be rare among native Alaskans [6].

PSC is predominantly a disease of young and middle-aged men. Approximately 67% of patients are male, and the mean age at the time of diagnosis is 40 years. In Northern Europe and the United States, 70% to 80% of patients with PSC will have or develop IBD. Alternatively, in Western countries, 2.4% to 4% of patients with IBD will have primary sclerosing cholangitis [7–9].

Chronic ulcerative colitis (CUC) affects both sexes equally, and no major differences between male and female CUC patients with PSC have been identified.

Diagnosis

The diagnosis of PSC is based on selection and exclusion criteria. A persistent twofold or greater elevation of the serum alkaline phosphatase level is typical. Aminotransferase levels are often less than twice the upper limit of normal, and hyperbilirubinemia may be present. Although there are no unequivocally specific, biochemical markers for PSC, perinuclear antineutrophil cytoplasmic antibodies (pANCA) are present in the serum of 80% of patients who have PSC [10]. A positive pANCA is highly suggestive of the syndrome but not specific.

The radiologic inclusion criteria include the presence of multifocal, diffusely distributed strictures of the biliary system seen on cholangiography. Such strictures often are associated with tortuosity and irregularity of the extrahepatic or intrahepatic ductal systems (Fig. 1). Additionally, the cystic duct and pancreatic duct can be involved.

Hepatic histologic abnormalities seen in PSC can be categorized, as suggested by Ludwig [11], as follows: cholangitis or portal hepatitis (stage 1); periportal hepatitis or periportal fibrosis (stage 2); necrosis, septal fibrosis, or both extending beyond the limiting plate (stage 3); and biliary cirrhosis

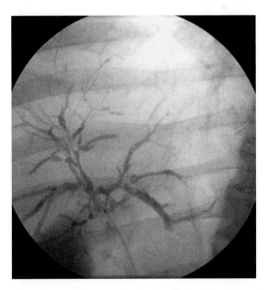

Fig. 1. Cholangiogram with features typical of primary sclerosing cholangitis including intrahepatic stricturing with poststricture dilatation.

(stage 4). Technically, a patient should not be considered as having PSC if he or she has had:

Prior bile duct surgery other than simple cholecystectomy
Documented choledocholithiasis before the development of symptoms
The documentation of biochemical, radiologic, and histologic abnormalities

Additionally, sclerosing cholangitis should not be called primary if identifiable causes, such as those listed in Box 1, are apparent.

Modes of presentation

Until recently, the sine qua non for the diagnosis of PSC was an abnormal cholangiogram. Indeed, under most circumstances, this is still the case. Additionally, a small duct variety of PSC has been recognized in which cholangiographic abnormalities may not be present, but the liver histology most often shows the finding of pericholangitis with fibro-obliterative duct damage in a patient who has associated IBD or appropriate clinical symptoms (Table 1).

PSC usually begins insidiously, making it difficult to accurately determine the onset of the disease. Nevertheless, most patients with symptoms have had them for an average of 12 to 24 months before the diagnosis is made (Table 2). The gradual onset of progressive fatigue and pruritus followed by jaundice represents the most frequent symptom complex that leads to the diagnosis of PSC.

Patients who have PSC present clinically in a variety of ways:

Asymptomatic, with abnormal liver tests;
Pruritus, fatigue, jaundice;
Recurrent cholangitis;
Complications of chronic liver disease;
Incidental discovery at laparotomy.

Most commonly, patients who have PSC will present without any symptoms or signs, but with a cholestatic biochemical profile identified during

Table 1
Terminology of the bile duct disease in primary sclerosing cholangitis

Diagnostic term	Cholangiopathy	Liver biopsy
Classic primary sclerosing cholangitis (PSC)	Combined large and small duct involvement	Typical
Intrahepatic duct PSC	Intrahepatic duct involvement only	Typical
Extrahepatic duct PSC	Large duct involvement only	Not diagnostic
Small duct PSC	Normal	Typical

Table 2
Symptoms and signs at diagnosis of primary sclerosing cholangitis

Symptom or sign	Frequency (%)
Fatigue	75
Pruritus	70
Jaundice	65
Weight loss	40
Fever	35
Hepatomegaly	55
Splenomegaly	30
Hyperpigmentation	25
Xanthomas	4

routine examination. Often, these individuals have associated IBD for which they have been followed on a regular basis. A cholangiogram should be performed to confirm the suspected diagnosis. Alternatively, a patient may develop pruritus and fatigue, which may be associated with dark urine, light stools, and jaundice. This constellation of symptoms and signs, particularly in a young male who has IBD, often warrants cholangiography with or without liver biopsy.

Patients who have PSC also may present with episodes of fever and abdominal pain with or without associated jaundice. Such episodes of recurrent bacterial cholangitis occur more commonly in PSC patients who have had previous biliary tract surgical procedures, such as choledocho-enterostomy.

On occasion, the first symptoms of PSC may reflect complications of advanced liver disease, such as ascites or upper gastrointestinal bleeding from gastroesophageal varices.

Finally, a patient may undergo diagnostic laparotomy for other reasons such as exploration for malignancy or obesity surgery. The diagnosis of PSC may be suspected at laparotomy, because the common bile duct upon palpation is rope-like and hard. An operative cholangiogram then will show changes characteristic of PSC.

Several extremely uncommon modes of presentation of PSC deserve mention including:

A patient who has recurrent fever and septicemia of unknown etiology;

A patient who has a remote proctocolectomy and ileostomy and presents with peristomal variceal bleeding;

A patient who has steatorrhea and weight loss caused by either complicating pancreatic exocrine insufficiency or associated celiac sprue;

A patient who has IBD and a previous diagnosis of chronic idiopathic or autoimmune chronic active hepatitis that does not respond to standard immunosuppressive therapy.

Associated diseases

Various diseases have been seen in association with PSC (Box 2). IBD is the most common and most important disease associated with PSC. The most common form of IBD associated with PSC is CUC; Crohn's colitis or Crohn's ileocolitis is associated much less often. Of interest are the observations that CUC associated with PSC most commonly involves a major portion of the colon, is frequently but associated with rectal sparing, and is more likely to be found in male than in female patients who have PSC. Additional features of this association include:

No difference between patients who have PSC alone and PSC with associated IBD with respect to hepatobiliary symptoms and signs, standard biochemical tests, cholangiography, and hepatic histology;

The diagnosis of IBD usually precedes the diagnosis of PSC, but diagnosis of PSC may precede that of IBD. PSC may develop after proctocolectomy for IBD, and PSC and IBD may be diagnosed simultaneously;

The IBD associated with PSC is usually symptomatically quiescent or mild; however, some patients who have PSC and CUC require

---

Box 2. Diseases associated with primary sclerosing cholangitis

IBD
Celiac sprue
Sarcoidosis
Chronic pancreatitis
Rheumatoid arthritis
Retroperitoneal fibrosis
Thyroiditis
Sjogren's syndrome
Autoimmune hepatitis
Systemic sclerosis
Lupus erythematosus
Vasculitis
Peyronie's disease
Membranous nephropathy
Bronchiectasis
Autoimmune hemolytic anemia
Idiopathic thrombocytopenic purpura
Histiocytosis X
Cystic fibrosis
Eosinophilia

colectomy for colitic symptoms, premalignant changes, or malignant changes.

It should be mentioned that the association of celiac sprue with PSC is of importance, because it adds credence to the hypothesis of that, like IBD and celiac sprue, PSC is likely a disease of altered immunity. Other autoimmune diseases associated with PSC include rheumatoid arthritis, thyroiditis, Sjogren's syndrome, autoimmune hepatitis, vasculitis, and eosinophilia.

Complications

As itemized in Box 3, the complications of PSC can be categorized under two major headings: general complications (ie, those that are common to other forms of chronic liver disease) and specific complications (ie, those that are to be more specific to PSC). Liver failure and portal hypertension occur in PSC as they do in other forms of chronic liver disease. Hepatic osteodystrophy, specifically osteoporosis, is common in PSC. Approximately 50% of patients with PSC have bone mineral density levels below the fracture threshold [12]. Vitamin levels, hormone levels, and severity of PSC and CUC do not correlate with the severity of bone disease. Despite active investigation, the pathogenesis remains unclear. Finally, malabsorption of fat and fat-soluble vitamins occurs in PSC usually on the basis of intraluminal bile acid deficiency caused by cholestasis, or less commonly caused by associated celiac sprue or chronic pancreatitis. The management of these complications is similar to their management in other forms of chronic liver disease.

In contrast, the complications that appear to be peculiar to PSC pose unique and challenging management problems. Although PSC most

---

Box 3. Complications of primary sclerosing cholangitis

General complications
Liver failure
Portal hypertension
Hepatic osteodystrophy
Steatorrhea
Fat-soluble vitamin deficiency

Specific complications
Dominant stricture
Cholelithiasis/choledocholithiasis
Adenocarcinoma of the bile duct
Peristomal varices

commonly involves the entire biliary system, the presence of a dominant stricture (ie, a high-grade, localized area of narrowing) (Fig. 2) may result in the rapid worsening of jaundice and in recurrent clinical episodes of bacterial cholangitis. Moreover, benign dominant strictures may be difficult to distinguish from a high-grade stricture because of adenocarcinoma of the bile duct. Cholelithiasis appears to occur more commonly in patients who have PSC than in the general population; indeed, using ultrasound screening, approximately 25% of patients with PSC have gallstones [13]. Because most of these patients are young men, among whom gallstones are uncommon, this likely represents an increased frequency of cholelithiasis. Choledocholithiasis related to pigment stones also may complicate PSC.

Finally, patients with PSC who have undergone proctocolectomy for associated CUC with traditional or continent ileostomy frequently develop varices around the stoma as a manifestation of portal hypertension. These varices are painful, frequently bleed such that transfusions are necessary, and can be reversed only by alleviating the portal hypertension, ideally by orthotopic liver transplantation or transjugular intrahepatic portosystemic shunt [14].

Cholangiocarcinoma

Currently adenocarcinoma of the bile duct represents the most lethal and devastating complication of PSC. Clinical observations have established unequivocally that cholangiocarcinoma arises in the biliary system of patients who have pre-existing primary sclerosing cholangitis. In fact, most consider PSC to be a premalignant lesion much the same as CUC is considered to be a premalignant lesion of the colon. The frequency of cholangiocarcinoma is acknowledged to be increased relative to the general population; however, absolute numbers vary. Autopsy studies suggest a frequency of somewhere

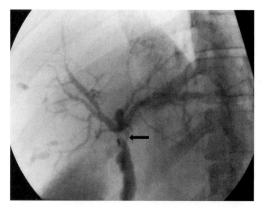

Fig. 2. Dominant stricture (*arrow*) at the biliary hilum.

between 20% and 43%, whereas clinical reviews, including experience with PSC patients undergoing orthotopic liver transplantation, suggesting a frequency closer to 10% [15]. The risk factors for the development of adenocarcinoma of the bile ducts in patients who have PSC include IBD, alcohol use, smoking, and diabetes [16,17]. Patients who have both PSC and adenocarcinoma of the bile ducts usually, but not always, have cirrhosis, portal hypertension, and long-standing CUC; they generally will be older at the time of diagnosis of PSC and may show progressive changes on cholangiography. Nevertheless, young patients with early PSC also have been identified with this devastating complication. Cholangiocarcinoma should be a primary consideration in any PSC patient who experiences a sudden, rapid decline in clinical or biochemical status. The diagnostic use of the tumor marker CA19-9 was evaluated in PSC patients. Using a lower cutoff value of 100 U/mL, the sensitivity and specificity of CA19-9 in detecting cholangiocarcinoma were 75% and 80%, respectively [18]. Significant elevations in CA19-9 can be seen in patients before the clinical diagnosis of cholangiocarcinoma. This observation implies that the tumor may be identified while it is at an occult and potentially treatable stage. A normal CA19-9 level in a patient who has PSC does not exclude the diagnosis of cholangiocarcinoma, however.

Patients with PSC have an increased risk of developing cholangiocarcinoma. Approximately 0.6% to 1.5% of patients per year will develop superimposed adenocarcinoma of the bile duct, resulting in a 20% lifetime risk [19,20]. The management of a suspected or established cholangiocarcinoma superimposed on PSC is complicated and largely ineffective. Diagnosis may be established by ERCP, although cytologic brushings are often inconclusive. If the lesion is surgically resectable, and the patient is not a candidate for transplantation, an attempt at surgical resection is warranted, although surgical margins are often positive, and cure is rare. Five-year survival rates range from 9% to 28% [21]. Survival after liver transplantation for cholangiocarcinoma is extremely poor, with 3-year survival rates ranging from 0% to 39% [22–24]. Recurrence of the malignancy is nearly universal. Even cholangiocarcinoma discovered incidentally on explanted liver from PSC patients receiving transplantation have shown a propensity to recur.

Diagnosis

Biochemical tests

Virtually all patients who have PSC will have an elevated serum alkaline phosphatase level, usually greater than three times the upper limit of normal (Table 3). Rarely, the serum alkaline phosphatase level may be normal. Similarly, most patients will have an increase in serum aspartate or alanine aminotransferase levels, usually only to a mild-to-moderate degree. At the time of diagnosis, one half to two thirds of patients who have PSC will have an

Table 3
Biochemical tests in primary sclerosing cholangitis at diagnosis

Test	Percent of patients with abnormal results
Serum alkaline phosphatase	99
Serum transaminases	95
Serum bilirubin	65
Serum albumin	20
Prothrombin time	10
Serum copper	50
Serum ceruloplasmin	75
Urinary copper	65

increase in their total serum bilirubin. Bilirubin levels may fluctuate considerably, with high levels suggesting disease progression or the development of complications such as a benign dominant stricture or superimposed adenocarcinoma of the bile duct. Abnormalities in serum albumin and prothrombin levels at the time of diagnosis are uncommon; however, with advanced disease, these values become abnormal in most patients. Serum copper and serum ceruloplasmin levels are increased commonly, and urine copper excretion is accelerated. Moreover, hepatic copper levels may be increased in most patients who have PSC, frequently in the range seen in Wilson's disease. The abnormalities in copper metabolism reflect the cholestatic nature of the syndrome. Until recently, there were no serologic markers in the serum that strongly suggested the syndrome of PSC. For example, tests for antimitochondrial antibody usually are negative; if positive, the antibody is present in only low titer. Similarly, smooth muscle antibodies and antinuclear antibodies (50%) are occasionally positive [10]. Although the serum IgM levels may be increased in PSC, they rarely reach the levels seen in PBC. Recently, it has been demonstrated that perinuclear antineutrophil cytoplasmic antibodies (pANCA) occur in 80% of patients who have PSC [10]. Disease activity does not correlate with pANCA positivity or titer, although one study has reported a worse prognosis among pANCA-positive PSC patients as compared with pANCA-negative patients. Although the sensitivity of pANCA is high, the specificity is much lower, as it has been found in patients who have CUC, Crohn's disease, autoimmune chronic active hepatitis, and several other hepatobiliary conditions. After liver transplantation, pANCA often persists. Other laboratory abnormalities occasionally are noted in PSC. For example, eosinophilia of a mild-to-moderate degree rarely may be observed.

Cholangiography

The increased frequency of diagnosis of PSC is because of the availability of endoscopic and transhepatic cholangiographic techniques. Indeed, in most cases, the diagnosis of PSC requires a characteristic cholangiogram. The radiologic features most commonly seen in the syndrome include:

Diffusely distributed, multifocal annular strictures with intervening segments of normal or slightly ectatic ducts (see Fig. 1);
Short band-like strictures;
Diverticulum-like outpouchings.

Cholangiographic abnormalities may be limited to the intrahepatic and proximal extrahepatic ducts. Other diffuse diseases—metastases, advanced cirrhosis, polycystic liver disease, and lymphoma—also may produce narrowing and deformity of bile duct cholangiographically. These abnormalities, however, rarely are difficult to distinguish from the characteristic constellation of radiographic abnormalities present in PSC. Additionally, the pancreatic main pancreatic duct and cystic duct may be involved.

In the past few years, magnetic resonance technology has improved significantly, and magnetic resonance cholangiopancreatography (MRCP) offers the potential for a noninvasive diagnostic test [25,26]. MRCP allows not only the visualization of the intra-and extrahepatic biliary tree, but also ducts proximal to tight strictures, which may not be visualized adequately during ERCP. Additional advantages of MRCP include the avoidance of radiation, the risk of pancreatitis, conscious sedation, and invasive diagnostic testing. MRCP, however, does not permit intervention such as bile duct brushing, balloon dilatation, or stenting. Therefore, it is reasonable to perform MRCP initially and then proceed to ERCP if necessary.

Liver biopsy

The main features on liver biopsy specimens include concentric periductal fibrosis (onion skinning) and inflammation, bile duct proliferation alternating with ductal obliteration, and ductopenia (Fig. 3). A staging system

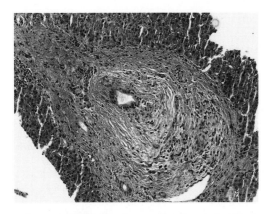

Fig. 3. Liver biopsy from a patient with primary sclerosing cholangitis demonstrating onion skin fibrosis surrounding a bile duct.

developed by Ludwig is shown in Table 4. Most if not all patients with PSC have a fibrooliterative cholangitis (chronic nonsuppurative obliterative cholangitis) on biopsy. This near diagnostic lesion is, unfortunately, often not seen on liver biopsy specimens in patients who have PSC. Nevertheless, accumulating experience with liver biopsies in patients who have PSC suggests that the other histologic findings noted in Table 4 can be strongly suggestive of the syndrome.

From a histologic viewpoint, abnormalities seen in liver biopsy from patients who have PSC must be differentiated from those seen in specimens from patients who have PBC, prolonged extrahepatic obstruction, and autoimmune hepatitis. Indeed, PBC has many histologic features on biopsy specimens that overlap with those seen in PSC, including periportal cholestasis, copper deposition, and granulomas. Nevertheless, the classic florid duct lesion is not seen in PSC and is nearly pathognomonic of PBC. Conversely, fibrous obliterative cholangitis, the hallmark of PSC, is not observed in PBC.

Changes showing pleomorphic or fibrous cholangitis also may be present in biopsy specimens from patients who have idiopathic or autoimmune hepatitis, and cholangiography may be necessary to help with biopsy interpretation.

Etiology

The cause of PSC is unknown; genetic factors, acquired factors, or both may be involved. Factors include:

Portal bacteremia;
Absorbed colonic toxins;
Toxic bile acids;
Copper toxicity;
Viral infection;
Genetic predisposition;
Immunologic mechanisms;
Ischemic arteriolar injury.

Table 4
Hepatic histology in primary sclerosing cholangitis Ludwig staging system

Portal stage (stage 1)	Portal hepatitis, bile duct abnormalities, or both; fibrosis or edema may be present; abnormalities do not exist beyond the limiting plate
Periportal stage (stage 2)	Periportal fibrosis with or without inflammation extending beyond the limiting plate; piecemeal macros may be present
Septal stage (stage 3)	Septal fibrosis, bridging necrosis, or both
Cirrhotic stage (stage 4)	Biliary cirrhosis

Currently, the pathogenesis of PSC is linked most closely with alterations in immune mechanisms. For example, PSC is associated with CUC and, to a lesser extent, with celiac sprue, two diseases thought to result from alterations in the immune system. Moreover, HLA B8 frequently is noted to be present in autoimmune diseases, occur with greater frequency in PSC than in the general population. Other more direct lines of evidence supporting immunologic basis for the disease include the inhibition of leukocyte migration by biliary antigens, elevated IgM levels, the presence of circulating immune complexes, decreased clearance of immune complexes, and increased complement catabolism. Additionally, cells involved in the destruction of bile ducts in PSC have been shown recently to be T lymphocytes. Enhanced autoreactivity of suppressor/cytotoxic T lymphocytes from the peripheral blood of patients who have PSC also has been reported [27].

The most likely scenario for the etiopathogenesis of PSC involves the exposure of a genetically predisposed individual to an acute insult to the biliary system, perhaps a transient viral infection. It is proposed that an alteration in the bile ducts that marks them as foreign then results and leads to their destruction by autoimmune mechanisms.

The diagnosis of PSC is usually not difficult, assuming the clinician is aware of the syndrome. PSC should be the major working diagnosis in a male with chronic cholestatic liver test abnormalities and IBD. In such a patient, the first major diagnostic study should be a cholangiogram (either MRCP or ERCP). Generally, a suitable cholangiogram in the appropriate clinical setting is all that is required for diagnosis. A liver biopsy also may be useful to provide diagnostic confirmation; however, its primary value is for accurate histologic staging and prognosis.

Natural history

Information regarding the natural history of PSC is currently in evolution. Given the lack of knowledge of the pathogenesis of PSC and the sometimes variable and often unpredictable nature of the syndrome, defining the natural history and prognosis of PSC is difficult. Nevertheless, based on various recent studies, most would agree that PSC is usually a progressive syndrome leading to significant complications related to chronic cholestasis. The largest of several studies addressing this issue analyzed data on 174 patients who had PSC. During the study, 34% died as a result of underlying liver disease or the development of cholangiocarcinoma; an additional 10% were referred for liver transplantation. Median survival from the time of diagnosis was 12 years [28]. A subgroup of 45 patients with asymptomatic PSC has been followed for over 6 years. During this period, 66% had histologic progression of disease; 29% developed portal hypertension, and 31% had liver failure resulting in death or need for liver transplantation. Both symptomatic and asymptomatic patients had reduced survival when compared with age-, sex-, and race-matched

United States population [29]. Another report on over 100 patients who had PSC and followed retrospectively for a mean of 6 years indicated that 16% of patients died secondary to liver failure, and an additional 21% underwent transplantation for advanced liver disease. The estimated median survival in the group was 12 years [30]. These and other studies strongly suggest that PSC is a progressive disease that frequently leads to death from liver failure.

Other studies have suggested that PSC may follow a more benign course. In one retrospective study based on historical data from 42 patients who had PSC and followed for a mean of 56 months, the investigators estimated 75% 9-year survival [31]. In several studies from Scandinavia, authors estimated a mean survival time of 17 years for patients who had PSC [32]. Thus, a body of data suggests that PSC has a relatively good prognosis.

Recently, a group of 83 patients who had well-characterized small duct PSC were compared with a game-matched cohort of patients who had large duct PSC. Twenty-three percent of the patients who had small duct PSC progressed to large duct PSC in a median of 7.4 years. One (1.2%) small duct PSC patient who progressed to large duct PSC developed cholangiocarcinoma. This compares favorably with12% of large duct PSC patients who developed cholangiocarcinoma. In addition, patients with small duct PSC had a significantly longer transplant-free survival period compared with their large duct PSC counterparts (13 years versus 10 years) [33].

Several possibilities for these differences regarding the natural history of PSC are apparent, including inherent disease variability, small patient numbers, clinically silent progression, short follow-up, incomplete data, retrospective analysis, and design deficiencies (eg, lead time bias, backdating of diagnosis, variable referral patterns, and length bias). Nevertheless, even if these differences are taken into account, the weight of current evidence indicates that PSC is a progressive disease. Assuming that PSC evolves into a ductopenic syndrome affecting large and small bile ducts, the overall result is that interlobular and septal bile ducts become obliterated and nonfunctional. When a critical number of ducts is lost, cholestasis and ultimately portal fibrosis and biliary cirrhosis occur.

One of the main purposes of analyzing the natural history of PSC is to more accurately determine its rate of progression and to be able to estimate survival for the individual patient at any particular point in the course of the patient's disease. Predicting survival based on clinical, biochemical, and histologic features of PSC is also very important for the timing of liver transplantation. Five major worldwide centers interested in PSC combined data to develop a prognosis model based on four independent variables from which risk scores could be calculated and translated into a survival curve for the individual patient at any time during the course of his or her disease. The variables identified include age, serum bilirubin, hepatic histologic stage, and the presence or absence of splenomegaly [34]. This and other models (Table 5) provide some objective evidence with regard to disease

Table 5
Independent clinical predictors used in prognostic models for primary sclerosing cholangitis

Multicenter [34]	Kings College [30]	Mayo model [28]	Swedish [35]	Revised Mayo [36]
Age	Age	Age	Age	Age
Bilirubin	Hepatomegaly	Bilirubin	Bilirubin	Bilirubin
Histologic stage	Histologic stage	Histologic stage	Histologic stage	Albumin
Hemoglobin	Splenomegaly	Splenomegaly	—	AST
IBD	Alkaline phosphatase	—	—	Variceal bleed

Abbreviations: AST, Aspartate aminotransferase; IBD, inflammatory bowel disease.

progression and estimation of survival, but require cross- validation and application assessment before their true utility can be ascertained.

Management

The management of PSC provides a challenge to the clinician given the array of symptoms and complications that can develop in the absence of effective, specific therapy for the underlying hepatobiliary disease. The first decision for the physician regarding management is whether any therapeutic intervention is needed in a patient who has newly diagnosed PSC. In the asymptomatic patient who has minimal liver test abnormalities and an early histologic lesion by liver biopsy, observation is a reasonable approach. Alternatively, experimental therapy might be considered in the context of a randomized, controlled trial. Such an approach may be modified in the future with additional progress in the understanding of the natural history of the syndrome. If a decision is made to intervene therapeutically, one needs to clearly identify the goals of treatment. Specifically, therapy can be directed toward relief of symptoms, the correction of complications, or the underlying hepatobiliary disease. For example, pruritus and fat-soluble vitamin deficiencies are common problems in patients who have PSC, and conventional approaches to their management are reasonable. Similarly, when complications such as variceal bleeding develop, appropriate interventions (eg, use of beta blockers, endoscopic variceal obliteration, or transjugular intrahepatic portosystemic shunt) should be considered.

Assuming intervention is contemplated; three categories of therapeutic options are available to the clinician for treating patients who have PSC, including medical treatment, mechanical manipulation, and surgical intervention. As mentioned earlier, complications of PSC include those that are relatively specific for this chronic cholestatic syndrome. Therapeutic approaches for the major specific complications are available, although their effectiveness is quite variable.

Medical

Medical approaches for treating the underlying hepatobiliary disease in PSC have focused principally on the use of choleretic, immunosuppressive, and antifiberogenic agents (Box 4).

Considerable recent interest has focused on the use of ursodeoxycholic acid (UDCA), the 7β epimer of chenodeoxycholic acid, for treating PSC. Although this agent is known to be choleretic and to dissolve cholesterol gallstones, its mechanism of action in PSC is unknown. Three potential mechanisms of action have been suggested:

Direct protection against hepatotoxicity endogenous bile salts;
Competitive inhibition of the absorption of hepatotoxic endogenous bile salts at the terminal ileum;
Suppression of the expression of abnormal HLA class 1 antigens on hepatocyte membranes.

UDCA has been shown to improve several biochemical parameters, including the serum bilirubin, alkaline phosphatase, and ALT, but not slow the course of illness or prolong survival [37]. A large, prospective, randomized–controlled trial from the United States demonstrated that UDCA at doses of 12 to 15 mg/kg/d had no effect on liver histology or transplant free survival [38]. A Scandinavian randomized–controlled trial using 17 to

---

Box 4. Therapeutic options in primary sclerosing cholangitis

Medical
  Supportive
  Possible definitive treatment
    Choleretic
      Ursodeoxycholic acid
    Immunosuppressive
      Prednisone
      Azathioprine
      Cyclosporine
      Methotrexate
    Antifibrogenic
      Colchicine
Mechanical
  Cholangioplasty
Surgical
  Reconstructive biliary tract procedures
  Proctocolectomy
  Liver transplantation

22 mg/kg/d of UDCA similarly showed no effect on quality of life or transplant-free survival, although this study may have been underpowered [39]. Small pilot studies have suggested that higher doses of UDCA (25 to 30 mg/kg/d) may be more effective than previously applied doses [40,41]. A large National Institutes of Health (NIH)-sponsored trial of high-dose UDCA therapy in PSC is underway [42]. At this time, UDCA cannot be recommended for treating primary sclerosing cholangitis outside of a controlled trial.

Various agents that may affect the immune system have been evaluated in uncontrolled trials. Corticosteroids have been used, both topically and systemically, in several small studies. A small controlled trial of biliary lavage with corticosteroids versus placebo showed no difference between drug and placebo [43]. Uncontrolled observations in a small number of patients who had a marked inflammatory component to their PSC showed impressive responses to orally administered corticosteroids; other uncontrolled trials have shown no beneficial effect. The risks of systemic corticosteroids in patients who have PSC are significant and include osteoporosis and an increased risk of infection. Other in-human modulating agents such as methotrexate, azathioprine, cyclosporine, tacrolimus, and pentoxifylline have failed to show efficacy in controlled trials [37,44]. A small double-blind, placebo-controlled, randomized study of 24 patients who had PSC and were treated with infliximab also showed no benefit [45].

The antifibrogenic agent, colchicine, has been evaluated for treating PSC. A randomized study of 84 patients treated with either colchicine or placebo showed no improvement in biochemical, clinical, or histologic parameters after 35 months of follow-up [46]. It is, therefore, unlikely that colchicine, alone or in combination with prednisone, will be an effective option for treating PSC.

Patients who have recurrent episodes of cholangitis without dominant stricture formation should be treated with broad-spectrum antibiotics [37]. Prophylactic antibiotics are favored by some in patients who have frequent episodes of cholangitis; this approach is reasonable, but its efficacy has not been established by randomized trials and carries the risk of the development of resistant organisms. In the 10% to 15% [9] of patients who develop dominant strictures in the biliary tract that lead to cholestatic symptoms, antibiotics are ineffective and can lead to a delay in diagnosis. Dilatation of critical biliary strictures (cholangioplasty) in an asymptomatic patient presents a dilemma; early intervention may prevent future episodes of cholangitis. Manipulation of the biliary tree, however, also can cause cholangitis. Indeed, a growing experience with stricture dilation in symptomatic patients who have PSC strongly suggests that balloon dilatation is effective in alleviating pruritus and in diminishing the frequency of cholangitis episodes caused by dominant strictures. Retrospective model analysis has shown that cholangioplasty improves survival [47]. The most prudent approach may be to perform cholangioplasty when jaundice or bacterial cholangitis develop or there is significant concern for cholangiocarcinoma.

Complications caused by cholestasis associated with PSC include pruritus, steatorrhea, fat-soluble vitamin deficiency, and osteoporosis. Pruritus can be particularly debilitating and does not correlate with disease progression. In fact, pruritus tends to diminish in later stages of disease. Various options for treating cholestatic pruritus are available, including cholestyramine, activated charcoal, phenobarbital, rifampin, plasmapheresis, opiate antagonists, and ondansetron. Controlled trials have demonstrated that UDCA is not effective for treating pruritus associated with PSC [38,39]. Steatorrhea and fat-soluble vitamin deficiency often coexist. Causes other than PSC, including pancreatitis and celiac sprue, should be considered. Supplementation of vitamins A, D, E, and K may be required. Finally, osteoporosis and subsequent compression fracture are common in PSC. Unfortunately, effect of therapy, apart from liver transplantation, has not been found.

Surgical

There are three surgical procedures considered of potential benefit for treating PSC: (1) biliary tract reconstructive procedures, (2) proctocolectomy in a patient who has PSC and CUC, and (3) orthotopic liver transplantation. The author considers biliary tract reconstructive procedures in the same category as balloon dilatation of a dominant structure; that is, it represents a palliative procedure whose objective is to alleviate symptoms rather than to affect the natural history of the underlying hepatobiliary disease. It must be mentioned, however, that some surgeons have encouraged an aggressive surgical approach to treating PSC itself, using various imaginative procedures for internal or external biliary drainage; to the author's knowledge, however, no controlled trials have been performed. Although such procedures might provide transient symptomatic benefit in the occasional patient who has jaundice and pruritus caused by a dominant structure, the same result almost always can be accomplished via a nonsurgical mechanical approach as described earlier. Thus, the author reserves hepatobiliary surgical drainage procedures for the very rare PSC patient who has severe pruritus and jaundice or recurrent bacterial cholangitis with a dominant extrahepatic narrowing and in whom balloon dilatation by means of percutaneous or endoscopic route is not feasible or has been tried unsuccessfully. In such cases, a choledochoduodenostomy may be appropriate.

Until the mid-1990s, the role of proctocolectomy for treating patients who had PSC with associated CUC was uncertain. The rationale for this procedure was that, by removing the colon, one may affect the progress of the underlying hepatobiliary disease beneficially in a patient with both PSC and CUC. This issue is an important one, not only because beneficial treatment for PSC is needed, but also because proctocolectomy in patients who have PSC and CUC may be associated with considerable morbidity. Proctocolectomy with a continent or conventional ileostomy results in development of varices around the ostomy stoma in at least 25% to 50% of patients who have PSC. In many of these patients, serious and often life-threatening bleeding can occur from these abdominal wall varices. This complication can be avoided by performing an ileal pouch–anal anastomosis rather than a conventional Brooke ileostomy. The Mayo Clinic group prospectively studied the effects of proctocolectomy on the progression of clinical, biochemical, cholangiographic, and hepatic histologic features in 53 patients who had PSC and CUC. Patients with both diseases who had undergone proctocolectomy (n = 23) were compared with those who had not (n = 30) over 4 years. New onset of complications, serial changes in biochemical tests, histologic progression of liver biopsy, and survival were not different in the two groups [48]. Based on these data, it appears that proctocolectomy for CUC is not beneficial for PSC in patients who have both diseases. Proctocolectomy is appropriate in a patient who has PSC and CUC for traditional colitis indications (eg, medical intractability, development of persistent high-grade dysplasia).

Liver transplantation

Orthotopic liver transplantation is a realistic consideration for patients who have any form of advanced liver disease, including PSC. Indeed, it remains the only life-saving therapeutic alternative and, in the judgment of most, the treatment of choice for patients who have advanced disease. Recent results suggest that the outcome of liver transplantation in patients who have PSC is no different and perhaps better than the outcome in patients who have other forms of noninfectious, nonmalignant chronic liver disease, with 5-year survival rates of 75% to 85% [49]. Using the PSC survival models in Table 5, it has been demonstrated that liver transplantation significantly prolongs survival in patients who have end-stage PSC. The Model of End-stage Liver Disease (MELD) scoring system has been validated in patients who have PSC [50].

Cholangiocarcinoma generally has been considered a contraindication to liver transplantation because of poor outcomes caused by recurrent disease. Recently, the Mayo Clinic group reported its experience in a highly selected population of patients who had cholangiocarcinoma measuring less than 3 cm in maximal diameter without evidence of extra hepatic spread. These patients received external beam radiation plus 5-fluorouracil intravenously followed by endoscopic brachytherapy and exploratory laparotomy. Patients who remain eligible for continuation within the protocol then received further chemotherapy and rapid liver transplantation. Five-year survival rates have been approximately 70%. These results have not been duplicated [51]. At this time, liver transplantation for cholangiocarcinoma can be recommended only within experimental protocols.

Despite excellent survival, special problems may occur after liver transplantation for patients who have PSC. For example, early postliver transplant surgical complications may be increased in patients who have PSC.

Moreover, diffuse biliary stricture occurs more frequently in PSC patients who undergo liver transplantation than it does in other liver diseases. Although biliary stricture after liver transplantation for PSC raises the question of recurrence of disease, other factors (eg, reflux of intestinal contents with associated chemical or bacterial cholangitis related to the Roux-en-Y biliary anastomosis; ductopenic rejection, which occurs more frequently in PSC patients) represent alternative etiologies for biliary stricture in PSC after transplantation. Finally, symptoms related to IBD usually improve or remain quiescent after liver transplantation in the patients who have PSC and IBD possibly because of the immunomodulatory and anti-inflammatory effects of the immunosuppressive agents. This effect is not universal, however. The incidence of colon cancer may be increased following liver transplantation in patients who have PSC and associated CUC, emphasizing the importance of continued annual colon cancer surveillance in these patients.

Summary

PSC is a generally progressive, sometimes fatal chronic hepatobiliary disorder for which no effective medical therapy now exists. The syndrome, which occurs mostly in young men, is characterized by frequent association with IBD, usually CUC, chronic cholestasis, a relative paucity of serologic markers, and characteristic abnormalities in some liver biopsy specimens and in virtually all cholangiograms. Although a definitive conclusion regarding natural history of the syndrome requires additional studies, the weight of evidence suggests that the disease progresses slowly and relentlessly over 5 to 15 years from an asymptomatic stage to a condition characterized by cholestasis and complicated by cirrhosis, portal hypertension, and, in perhaps 10% to 15% of patients, carcinoma of the bile ducts. Management first should involve a thoughtful decision to observe (which may be reasonable in some asymptomatic patients with early disease) or to intervene, particularly in patients who have symptoms, in the context of a randomized, controlled clinical trial. Before intervention is undertaken, however, therapeutic goals need to be defined and should focus on either alleviating symptoms dealing effectively with complications, or attempting to affect the underlying hepatobiliary disease. Symptomatic treatment and therapy for complications are similar to those employed in other chronic liver diseases. Additionally, balloon dilatation of dominant strictures is appropriate in selected, symptomatic patients. Current medical therapy directed at arresting the progression of the underlying hepatobiliary disease remains experimental and includes choleretic, antifibrogenic, and immunosuppressive agents. Although biliary tract reconstructive surgery may alleviate symptoms in a small number of selected patients who have PSC, its effect on the natural history of the syndrome has not yet been determined and may be deleterious. In contrast, orthotopic liver transplantation may prolong life for patients who have advanced disease and should be considered before potentially life-threatening complications occur.

References

[1] 2006 OPTN/SRTR Annual report. Table 9.4a. Available at: http://www.optn.org/AR2006/904a_rec-dgn_li.htm. Accessed March 12, 2008.

[2] Bahmba K, Kim WR, Talwalker J, et al. Incidence, clinical spectrum, and outcomes of primary sclerosing cholangitis in a United States community. Gastroenterology 2003;125: 1364–9.

[3] Shrumpf E, Boberg KM. Epidemiology of primary sclerosing cholangitis. Best Pract Res Clin Gastroenterol 2001;15:553–62.

[4] Boberg KM, Aadand E, Jahnsen J, et al. Incidence and prevalence of primary biliary cirrhosis, primary sclerosing cholangitis, and autoimmune hepatitis in a Norwegian population. Scand J Gastroenterol 1998;33:99–103.

[5] Kingham JG, Kochar N, Gravenor MB. Incidence, clinical pattern, and outcomes of primary sclerosing cholangitis in South Wales, United Kingdom. Gastroenterology 2004;126: 1929–30.

[6] Hurlbert KJ, McMahon BJ, Deubner H, et al. Prevalence of autoimmune liver disease and Alaska natives. Am J Gastroenterol 2002;97:2402–7.

[7] Rasmussen HH, Fallingborg JF, Mortensen PD, et al. Hepatobiliary dysfunction and primary sclerosing cholangitis in patients with Crohn's disease. Scand J Gastroenterol 1997; 32:604–10.

[8] Olsson R, Danielsson A, Jarnerot G, et al. Prevalence of primary sclerosing cholangitis in patients with ulcerative colitis. Gastroenterology 1991;100:1319–23.

[9] Lee YM, Kaplan MM. Primary sclerosing cholangitis. N Engl J Med 1995;332:924–33.

[10] Mulder AH, Horst G, Haagsma EB, et al. Prevalence and characterization of neutrophil cytoplasmic antibodies and autoimmune liver disease. Hepatology 1993;17:411–7.

[11] Ludwig J, Barham SS, LaRusso NF, et al. Morphologic features of chronic hepatitis associated with primary sclerosing cholangitis or chronic ulcerative colitis. Hepatology 1981;1: 632–40.

[12] Hay JE. Bone disease in cholestatic liver disease. Gastroenterology 1995;108:276–83.

[13] Said K, Glaumann H, Bergquist A. Gallbladder disease in patients with primary sclerosing cholangitis. J Hepatol 2008;48:598–605.

[14] Shibata D, Brophy D, Gordon F, et al. Portosystemic shunt for treatment of bleeding ectopic varices with portal hypertension. Dis Colon Rectum 1999;42:1581–5.

[15] Malhi H, Gores GJ. Cholangiocarcinoma: modern advances in understanding a deadly old disease. J Hepatol 2006;45:856–67.

[16] Donato F, Gelatti U, Tagger A, et al. Intrahepatic cholangiocarcinoma and hepatitis C and B virus infection, alcohol intake, and a lip bias: a case–control study in Italy. Cancer Causes Control 2001;12:959–64.

[17] Shaib YH, El-Serag HB, Davila JA, et al. Risk factors of intrahepatic cholangiocarcinoma in the United States: a case–control study. Gastroenterology 2005;128:620–6.

[18] Gores GJ. Early detection and treatment of cholangiocarcinoma. Liver Transpl 2000;6:S30–4.

[19] Bergquist A, Ekbom A, Olsson R, et al. Hepatic and extrahepatic malignancies in primary sclerosing cholangitis. J Hepatol 2002;36:321–7.

[20] Burak K, Angulo P, Pasha TM, et al. Incidence and risk factors for cholangiocarcinoma in primary sclerosing cholangitis. Am J Gastroenterol 2004;99:523–6.

[21] Iwatsuki S, Todo S, Marsh JW, et al. Treatment of hilar cholangiocarcinoma (Klatskin tumors) with hepatic resection or transplantation. J Am Coll Surg 1998;187:358–64.

[22] Meyer CG, Penn I, James L. Liver transplantation for cholangiocarcinoma: results in 207 patients. Transplantation 2000;69:1633–7.

[23] Lang H, Sotiropoulos GC, Domland M, et al. Extended hepatectomy before intrahepatic cholangiocellular carcinoma (ICC)—when is it worthwhile? Single-center experience with 27 receptions in 50 patients over a five-year period. Ann Surg 2005;241:134–43.

[24] Pichlmyer R, Weimann A, Klempnauer J, et al. Surgical treatment in proximal bile duct cancer: a single-center experience. Ann Surg 1996;224:628–38.

[25] Angulo P, Pierce DH, Johnson CD, et al. Magnetic resonance cholangiography in the evaluation of the biliary tree: its role in patients with primary sclerosing cholangitis. J Hepatol 2000;33:520–7.

[26] Vitellas KM, Enns RA, Keogan MT, et al. Comparison of MR cholangiopancreatographic techniques with contrast-enhanced cholangiography in the evaluation of sclerosing cholangitis. AJR Am J Roentgenol 2002;178:327–34.

[27] LaRusso NF, Shneider BL, Black D, et al. Primary sclerosing cholangitis: summary of a workshop. Hepatology 2006;44:746–64.

[28] Weisner RH, Grambsch PM, Dickson ER, et al. Primary sclerosing cholangitis: natural history, prognostic factors, and survival analysis. Hepatology 1989;10:430–6.

[29] Porayko MK, Weisner RH, LaRusso NF, et al. Patients with asymptomatic primary sclerosing cholangitis frequently have progressive disease. Gastroenterology 1990;98:1594–602.

[30] Farrant JM, Hayllar KM, Wilkinson ML, et al. Natural history and prognostic variables in primary sclerosing cholangitis. Gastroenterology 1991;100:1710–7.

[31] Helzberg JH, Petersen JM, Boyer JL. Improved survival with primary sclerosing cholangitis. A review of clinicopathologic features and comparison of symptomatic and asymptomatic patients. Gastroenterology 1987;92:1869–75.

[32] Aadland E, Schrumpf E, Fausa O, et al. Primary sclerosing cholangitis: a long-term follow-up study. Scand J Gastroenterol 1987;22:655–64.

[33] Bjornsson E, Olsson R, Bergquist A, et al. The natural history of small duct primary sclerosing cholangitis. Gastroenterol 2008;134:975–80.

[34] Dickson ER, Murtaugh PA, Wiesner RH, et al. Primary sclerosing cholangitis: refinement and validation of survival models. Gastroenterology 1992;103:1893–901.

[35] Broom U, Olsson R, Loof L, et al. Natural history and prognostic factors in 305 Swedish patients with primary sclerosing cholangitis. Gut 1996;38:610–5.

[36] Kim WR, Therneau TM, Wiesner RH, et al. A revised natural history model for primary sclerosing cholangitis. Mayo Clinic Proc 2000;75:688–94.

[37] Lee YM, Kaplan MM. ACG Practice Guidelines Committee. Practice guidelines for management of primary sclerosing cholangitis. Am J Gastroenterol 2002;97:528–34.

[38] Lindor KD, Mayo PSC/UDCA Study Group. Ursodiol for the treatment of primary sclerosing cholangitis. N Engl J Med 1997;336:691–5.

[39] Olsson R, Boberg KM, Schaffalitsky de Muckadell O, et al. High-dose ursodeoxycholic acid in primary sclerosing cholangitis: a 5-year multicenter randomized–controlled study. Gastroenterology 2005;129:1464–72.

[40] Mitchell SA, Bansi D, Hunt N, et al. A preliminary trial of high-dose ursodeoxycholic acid in primary sclerosing cholangitis. Gastroenterology 2001;121:900–7.

[41] Harnois DM, Angulo P, Jorgensen RA, et al. High-dose ursodeoxycholic acid in primary sclerosing cholangitis. Am J Gastroenterol 2001;96:1558–62.

[42] Hoofnagle JH. This month from the NIH: primary sclerosing cholangitis. Hepatology 2005; 41:955.

[43] Allison MC, Burroughs AK, Noone P, et al. Biliary lavage with corticosteroids in primary sclerosing cholangitis. A clinical, cholangiographic, and bacteriological study. J Hepatol 1986;3:118–22.

[44] Kaplan MM. Toward better treatment for primary sclerosing cholangitis. N Engl J Med 1997;336:719–21.

[45] Hommes DW, Erkelens W, Ponsioen C, et al. A double-blind, placebo-controlled, random-ized study of infliximab in primary sclerosing cholangitis. J Clin Gastroenterol 2008;42: 522–6.

[46] Olsson R, Broomé U, Danielsson A, et al. Colchicine treatment of primary sclerosing chol-angitis. Gastroenterology 1995;108:1199–203.

[47] Baluyut AR, Sherman S, Lehman GA, et al. Impact of endoscopic therapy on the survival of patients with primary sclerosing cholangitis. Gastrointest Endosc 2001;53:308–12.

[48] Cangemi JR, Wiesner RH, Beaver SJ, et al. Effect of proctocolectomy for chronic ulcerative colitis on the natural history of primary sclerosing cholangitis. Gastroenterology 1989;96: 790–4.

[49] Roberts MS, Angus DC, Bryce CL, et al. Survival after liver transplantation in the United States: a disease-specific analysis of the UNOS database. Liver Transpl 2004;10:886–97.

[50] Brandsaeter B, Broome U, Isoniemi H, et al. Liver transplantation for primary sclerosing cholangitis in the Nordic countries: outcome after acceptance to the waiting list. Liver Transpl 2003;9:961–9.

[51] Gores GJ, Nagorny DM, Rosen CB. Cholangiocarcinoma: is transplantation an option? For whom? J Hepatol 2007;47:455–9.

ELSEVIER
SAUNDERS

SURGICAL
CLINICS OF
NORTH AMERICA

Surg Clin N Am 88 (2008) 1409–1428

Proximal Biliary Malignancy

Mohamed Akoad, MD, FACS[a],
Roger Jenkins, MD, FACS[b],*

[a]Division of Hepatobiliary and Liver Transplantation, The Lahey Clinic Medical Center,
41 Mall Road, 4 West, Burlington, MA 01803, USA
[b]Division of Surgery, The Lahey Clinic Medical Center, Tufts University School of Medicine,
41 Mall Road, 4 West, Burlington, MA 01803, USA

Malignant strictures involving the proximal bile ducts present diagnostic and therapeutic challenges to all specialties involved in its management. They can result from metastatic spread of nonbiliary tumors (eg, pancreas, gallbladder, stomach, colon and rectum, lymphoma) to the hepatic hilum or from primary biliary cancer (cholangiocarcinoma). Cholangiocarcinoma comprises less than 10% of primary hepatic malignancies and can arise from the intrahepatic or extrahepatic bile ducts [1]. Although these tumors can occur at any level of the biliary tree, 67% occur at the bifurcation of the bile duct (hilar cholangiocarcinoma) [2], where they are often referred to as Klatskin tumors [3]. These tumors often invade major branches of the portal vein and the hepatic artery, making resection difficult.

Surgical resection with negative margins carries the only hope for long-term survival. Recently, innovative aggressive techniques combining hepatic resection and hilar vascular resection have increased the number of patients in whom resection with negative margins is achieved [4–7]. A protocol combining neoadjuvant therapy with liver transplantation is currently undergoing evaluation at several transplant centers. Patients with unresectable hilar tumors are candidates for palliative biliary drainage to prevent the development of cholangitis and hepatic failure. Without treatment, death from liver failure generally occurs within 3 to 6 months from initial clinical presentation.

Incidence

Extrahepatic bile duct cancers are relatively rare tumors with an incidence of 0.01% to 0.2% in large autopsy series [8]. The reported incidence

---

* Corresponding author.
E-mail address: roger.l.jenkins@lahey.org (R. Jenkins).

in the United States is about 1 to 2 cases per 100,000 patients [9]. The disease is more frequently diagnosed in the fifth and sixth decade of life, and there is a slight male predominance [10].

Etiology

Although the etiology of cholangiocarcinoma is obscure, it has been suggested that chronic inflammation of the biliary system or exposure to toxic agents concentrated in bile might result in DNA damage in the biliary epithelial cells leading to malignant transformation. In a recent report, 94% of resected specimens from patients with cholangiocarcinoma stained positive for the tumor suppressor p53 gene, and 100% stained positive for proliferating cell nuclear antigen (PCNA) [11]. Moreover, K-ras proto-oncogene mutations were found in 75% of specimens from patients with cholangiocarcinoma [12].

Certain disorders have been associated with an increased incidence of cholangiocarcinoma. Primary sclerosing cholangitis (PSC), an autoimmune disease characterized by multifocal strictures of the intrahepatic and extrahepatic bile ducts, is known to be associated with an increased incidence of cholangiocarcinoma. Unlike most cases of sporadic cholangiocarcinoma of the extrahepatic biliary tree, patients who have PSC are at an increased risk of multifocal disease that may not be amenable to resection. The incidence of cholangiocarcinoma in patients with PSC is unknown, but incidental cholangiocarcinoma was found in 4% to 8.6% of liver explants of patients who underwent liver transplantation for PSC [13,14]. Choledochal cysts and Caroli's disease are congenital disorders that carry an increased risk of cholangiocarcinoma. The risk of malignant degeneration increases to 15% to 20% for patients not treated until adulthood. The reason for the increased risk of cholangiocarcinoma in patients with congenital biliary cysts is not clear but is thought to be related to the abnormal entry of the pancreatic duct into the bile duct, resulting in reflux of pancreatic juice into the biliary tree. The resulting chronic inflammation may predispose to the development of cholangiocarcinoma. Bile stasis and chronic inflammation within the cyst may also be a predisposing factor [15–17].

Cholangiocarcinoma is more prevalent in Southeast Asia than anywhere else in the world. This prevalence is thought to be related to parasitic infection with the liver flukes Clonorchis sinensis and Opisthorchis viverrini. These liver flukes gain entry to the host through the duodenum and reside in the bile ducts. The resulting chronic biliary obstruction leading to stricture formation and chronic inflammation is thought to predispose to cancer [18]. Oriental cholangiohepatitis, which is prevalent in Japan and parts of Southeast Asia, is characterized by chronic portal bacteremia leading to sepsis and pigment stone formation. Chronic cholangitis and stricture formation have been thought to be predisposing factors for cholangiocarcinoma, which is present in 10% of patients with oriental cholangiohepatitis [19].

Associations with some chemical carcinogens or drugs have been reported, such as oral contraceptives [20], methyldopa [21], isoniazid [22], and asbestos [23].

Pathology

Three distinct macroscopic subtypes of cholangiocarcinoma have been described: sclerosing, nodular, and papillary [24]. The sclerosing variety is the most common and causes annular thickening of the bile duct with infiltration and fibrosis of adjacent tissues. These tumors are locally invasive and tend to invade periductal neural tissues as well as major vascular structures of the hilum. The nodular variety is characterized by irregular intraluminal nodules. When both features are present, the tumor is described as nodular-sclerosing. The papillary variant, which accounts for 10% of cases, is a soft and often friable tumor. These tumors are less likely to cause periductal fibrosis or invade adjacent structures, and they have a more favorable outcome than other variants.

Microscopically, more than 95% of tumors are adenocarcinomas ranging from well to poorly differentiated varieties [9,25]. Cholangiocarcinomas are mucin-secreting adenocarcinomas, and intracellular mucin can often be demonstrated. Immunohistochemical staining for epithelial membrane antigen and tissue polypeptide antigen may be useful in confirming the diagnosis of cholangiocarcinoma. Submucosal tumor spread is an important feature of cholangiocarcinoma. This subepithelial spread beyond the obvious tumor emphasizes the importance of wider resections and confirmation of negative margins by frozen section during the resection operation. Other histologic types such as squamous, leiomyosarcoma, rhabdomyosarcoma, and cystadenocarcinoma are rare.

Hilar cholangiocarcinoma is often slow growing; however, rapid progression has been seen in some patients. Spread by direct invasion to periductal hilar tissues with invasion of portal vein branches as well as hepatic arterial branches is a common feature of hilar cholangiocarcinoma. Direct invasion of adjacent liver tissue is also common. Regional lymph node involvement is present in 30% to 50% of cases, whereas blood-borne metastasis to the lungs, kidneys, bones, or brain is rare [24].

Clinical presentation

The clinical presentation of hilar cholangiocarcinoma varies with the site of origin but most commonly begins with painless jaundice. Intense generalized pruritus may develop months before the onset of jaundice when the site of tumor origin is in the main left or right hepatic duct. It has long been recognized that unilateral obstruction of the bile ducts results in atrophy of the corresponding lobe and compensatory hypertrophy of the contralateral lobe (Fig. 1) [26]. The ability of the contralateral lobe of the liver to

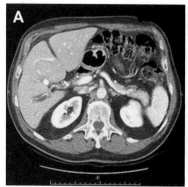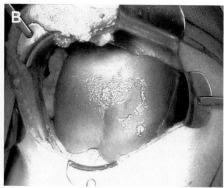

Fig. 1. (*A*) CT scan of a patient with hilar cholangiocarcinoma and long-standing right ductal obstruction resulting in atrophy of the right lobe and compensatory hypertrophy of the left lobe. (*B*) Findings at exploration showing sharply demarcated atrophic right lobe.

hypertrophy in the presence of complete biliary obstruction often delays the development of symptoms. Anorexia and fatigue are nonspecific symptoms that develop in the majority of patients; constant pain is an ominous sign that often (but not always) portends metastatic spread to surrounding tissues. Fever is unusual in the absence of instrumentation of an intact biliary tree despite a 30% incidence of bacterobilia [27]. Most patients have few symptoms and come to attention when they become jaundiced or when they are found to have abnormal liver function tests. Apart from jaundice and skin excoriation in patients with pruritus, physical examination is generally unremarkable.

Total serum bilirubin is elevated in most patients with hilar cholangiocarcinoma at presentation and is usually greater than 10 mg/dL. Alanine aminotransferase and aspartate aminotransferase are usually mildly elevated. Serum alkaline phosphatase and gammaglutamyl transferase are elevated in 90% of patients with cholangiocarcinoma even in the absence of hyperbilirubinemia [28]. In contrast to hepatocellular carcinoma, alphafetoprotein is rarely elevated in patients with cholangiocarcinoma. The level of carcinoembryonic antigen (CEA) is elevated in 40% to 60% of patients and carbohydrate antigen 19-9 in 80% [29].

Radiologic evaluation

Once a patient is diagnosed with obstructive jaundice based on clinical and laboratory data, the initial radiologic modalities are abdominal ultrasonography and abdominal CT scan. Ultrasonography is useful in differentiating hilar obstruction from other causes of obstructive jaundice, such as carcinoma of the head of the pancreas, ampullary tumors, gallbladder carcinoma, and choledocholithiasis. In patients with hilar cholangiocarcinoma, ultrasound often demonstrates a dilated intrahepatic biliary tree and a collapsed common bile duct and gallbladder. The gallbladder may be distended if the lesion extends distally to occlude the cystic duct orifice. In specialized centers, ultrasonography can identify with reasonable accuracy the presence of a mass and can delineate the extent of the tumor. It can also assess hepatic artery and portal vein patency through Doppler flow imaging [30].

Corporal imaging by CT or MRI scanning is essential in further evaluation of the patient and ideally should be performed before endoscopic retrograde cholangiopancreatography (ERCP) or percutaneous transhepatic cholangiography (PTC). The modality used is dependant on the quality of imaging available at a particular institution. In many centers, magnetic resonant cholangiopancreatography (MRCP) (Fig. 2) has become an invaluable tool in preoperative assessment of patients with hilar cholangiocarcinoma and has almost replaced endoscopic and percutaneous cholangiography [31,32]. MRCP is helpful in staging cholangiocarcinoma and determining resectability by providing information regarding tumor size, the extent of bile duct involvement, vascular invasion, extrahepatic extension, nodal or distant metastases, and the presence of lobar atrophy. The accuracy of MRCP for the assessment of tumor status, periductal infiltration, and lymph node metastases is 90%, 87%, and 66%, respectively [33]. The triphasic CT scan performed in a high-speed scanner is currently the authors' preferred modality for hepatic imaging (Fig. 3). When properly timed, this study can give accurate imaging of hilar vascular anatomy in conjunction with changes in subsegmental hepatic anatomy. Such images can be enhanced to provide three-dimensional mapping of projected surgical planes by providing accurate information about the relationship between the tumor and the adjacent vascular structures (Fig. 4) [34].

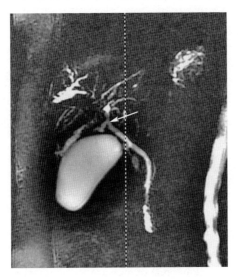

Fig. 2. MRCP of a patient with malignant hilar stricture (*arrow*).

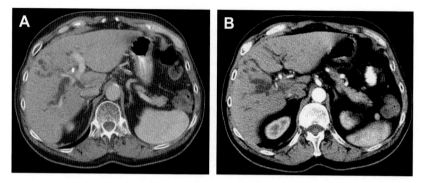

Fig. 3. Triphasic CT scan of a patient with hilar cholangiocarcinoma showing dilatation of the intrahepatic biliary tree. (*A*) Arterial phase. (*B*) Portal venous phase.

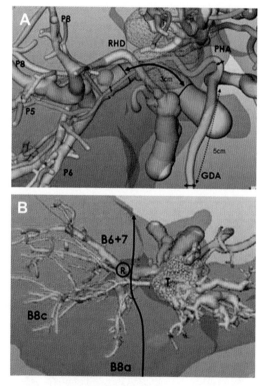

Fig. 4. (*A*) Three-dimensional image reveals narrowing of the portal vein. Resection of a 3-cm segment is required (*long thick line*). The right hepatic artery is also involved by tumor. The lines of transection of the proper hepatic artery and right hepatic artery are planned (*small arrows*). (*B*) Three-dimensional image in the cranial projection. Arrowed line indicates the planned line of resection, just to the left side of the R-point. (*From* Endo I, Shimada H, Sugita M, et al. Role of three-dimensional imaging in operative planning for hilar cholangiocarcinoma. Surgery 2007;142(5):672; with permission.)

Despite the emergence of newer imaging modalities as tools for the evaluation of proximal biliary strictures, cholangiography remains an important diagnostic modality after corporal imaging in many centers. It demonstrates the location and extent of the tumor and delineates the segmental biliary anatomy, which is helpful in planning the hepatic resection. Cholangiography allows both identification and drainage of obstructed ducts. Both ERCP (Fig. 5) and PTC (Fig. 6) have been used with success for preoperative tumor assessment as well as biliary drainage. In operable patients, the authors prefer ERCP with drainage of the uninvolved lobe. ERCP can be difficult to perform in patients with hilar cholangiocarcinoma and carries the risk of cholangitis and post procedure pancreatitis; however, in specialized large-volume centers, ERCP can be performed with a high success rate and low morbidity [35,36]. Despite the tightly obstructing nature of proximal hilar tumors, an experienced endoscopist can often demonstrate the proximal biliary anatomy and establish biliary drainage of the obstructed lobe or lobes. Close communication between the endoscopist and surgeon is vital to adequately delineate the tumor extent and to establish appropriate drainage of the obstructed segments. If endoscopic drainage is not successful or if jaundice persists despite adequate drainage, the authors perform unilateral or bilateral PTC to establish drainage to obstructed segments.

The 18F-fluorodeoxyglucose positron emission tomography (PET) scan is currently being used with increasing frequency to assist with the diagnosis of hilar cholangiocarcinoma [37]. Currently, the PET scan is not used routinely to diagnose hilar cholangiocarcinoma but has been used in patients with PSC, in whom it can be extremely difficult to identify a malignant

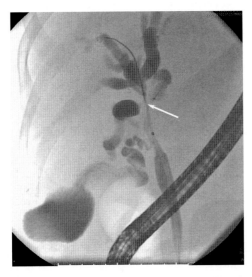

Fig. 5. ERCP of a patient with hilar cholangiocarcinoma showing dilatation of the intrahepatic bile ducts. The arrow points to the stricture.

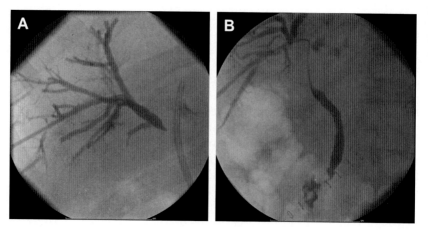

Fig. 6. (*A*) PTC in a patient with hilar cholangiocarcinoma and jaundice not relieved by ERCP stenting of the left hepatic duct. (*B*) The guidewire is passed through the stricture into the common bile duct.

stricture in the background of chronic widespread intrahepatic biliary strictures [38]. It is also being used to confirm recurrent cancer after resection. In a recent study evaluating the use of the PET scan in patients with biliary cancer, it identified occult metastatic disease and changed management in 24% of patients [39].

If patients are surgical candidates, efforts to establish preoperative tissue diagnosis by examining bile cytology, brush cytology, or endoscopic ultrasound–guided fine-needle aspiration are not essential. The sensitivity of bile cytology is only 24% and that of brush cytology 59% [40]. A negative cytology report in the presence of a hilar stricture should never dissuade the clinician from treating the stricture as a malignancy in the appropriate clinical setting. Endoscopic biliary brushings for cytology are only important when the patient is not a surgical candidate.

Preoperative biliary drainage

The value of preoperative biliary drainage for malignant obstructive jaundice remains controversial. Several prospective randomized studies have found no benefit from preoperative biliary drainage in malignant obstructive jaundice from all causes [41–43]. Moreover, a recent meta-analysis found that preoperative biliary drainage did not reduce operative morbidity or mortality in patients with malignant obstructive jaundice [44]; however, most of these studies lacked uniformity and included predominantly patients with distal bile duct obstruction from pancreatic cancer, ampullary tumors, or distal cholangiocarcinoma. In these studies, patients with proximal bile duct malignancy comprised only 12.1%. To date there are no prospective randomized studies examining the efficacy of preoperative biliary drainage in patients with proximal bile duct tumors; however, several retrospective reports support its use [45–47]. Proximal bile duct tumors comprise a different group because, unlike for distal malignant bile duct obstruction, major hepatic resection constitutes a major component of the resection operation. Extended hepatic resection in patients with complete obstructive jaundice and cholangitis carries a risk of bleeding, sepsis, and severe postoperative hepatic failure [48,49]. Preoperative drainage of obstructed yet salvageable hepatic segments allows resolution of the induration and cholestasis of the involved hepatic parenchyma with more prompt bile excretion in the postoperative period. Results of Japanese series show that preoperative biliary drainage increases resectability and tolerance after major hepatectomy [7,50].

The authors routinely perform preoperative percutaneous or endoscopic biliary drainage of the obstructed lobes or segments if they are anticipated to be important salvageable segments of hepatic parenchyma. To reduce the risk of postoperative hepatic failure, surgery is usually delayed until the total bilirubin levels fall below 2.5 to 3.0 mg/dL.

Patient selection and assessment of resectability

Preoperative staging and assessment of resectability are accomplished by radiologic studies with the goal of identifying potential candidates for surgery and planning the extent of resection. The currently widely used Bismuth-Corlette classification allows comparative stratification of tumor spread along the bile ducts but does not address portal vein or hepatic artery involvement. The classification is useful in operative planning but does not predict resectability or survival [51]. Many patients with types I and II spread may achieve better outcomes with wider resections including hepatectomy [4–7,45,46]. A new preoperative staging system developed by Burke and colleagues [52] stratifies patients according to the degree of biliary involvement, hepatic lobar atrophy, and ipsilateral or bilateral portal vein involvement (Table 1). This staging system has been reported to have better correlation with resectability than the Bismuth classification. Findings of bilobar peripheral hepatic metastasis or extrahepatic disease preclude resection, as does bilateral duct involvement up to the secondary biliary radicals. Unilateral involvement of the portal vein or hepatic artery is treated by ipsilateral hepatic lobectomy and is not a contraindication to resection. More advanced tumors with bilateral vascular involvement need careful preoperative assessment and planning because they may require more advanced vascular techniques with portal vein and hepatic arterial reconstruction and represent relative contraindications.

The overall general medical condition and fitness of the patient for operation, which usually includes major hepatectomy, should be carefully evaluated. Preoperative assessment should include evaluation of the cardiac risk,

Table 1
Proposed T stage criteria for hilar cholangiocarcinoma

Stage	Criteria
T1	Tumor confined to confluence and/or right or left hepatic duct without portal vein involvement or liver atrophy
T2	Tumor confined to confluence and/or right or left hepatic duct with ipsilateral liver atrophy No portal vein involvement demonstrated
T3	Tumor confined to confluence and/or right or left hepatic duct with ipsilateral portal venous branch involvement with/without associated ipsilateral lobar liver atrophy. No main portal vein involvement (occlusion, invasion, or encasement)
T4	Any of the following: (1) tumor involving both right and left hepatic ducts up to the secondary radicals bilaterally, or (2) main portal vein encasement

From Burke EC, Jarnagin WR, et al. Hilar cholangiocarcinoma: patterns of spread, the importance of hepatic resection for curative operation, and a presurgical clinical staging system. Ann Surg 1998;228(3):385–94; with permission.

pulmonary status, and liver and renal function. Nutritional status is generally assessed and nutritional support initiated as indicated. Coagulopathy should be corrected with the administration of vitamin K. Cholangitis should promptly be controlled with the appropriate antibiotics.

Treatment

Resection of hilar malignancies remains one of the most difficult operations in surgery and is heavily dependent on the experience and expertise of the operating surgeon. Nevertheless, surgical resection represents the only successful treatment for cure or significant prolongation of life. The nature of the surgery is determined by the proximal and distal extent of the tumor as defined by preoperative imaging and the anatomic characteristics of the neighboring vascular inflow. The surgical goal is resection of all regional nodal tissue and the common bile duct (and gallbladder) en bloc with the requisite portion of liver to achieve negative microscopic margins.

The authors perform diagnostic laparoscopy at the initiation of the surgical procedure to exclude patients with unrecognized metastases from major laparotomy. A right subcostal incision is used with upward midline extension to the xiphoid to provide exposure for resection. The peritoneal cavity is again inspected for evidence of regional or distant metastasis, and the liver is examined for evidence of metastasis not recognized by preoperative radiologic studies. The duodenum is kocherized to begin resection of the lymphoid tissue lateral and posterior to the common bile duct. We begin dissecting the lymphatic and neural tissue at the level of the celiac artery and proceed to skeletonize the common hepatic artery and its branches. The common bile duct is transected at the superior edge of the pancreas, and all lymphatic and neural tissue lateral and posterior to the bile duct is mobilized en block, skeletonizing the proper hepatic artery as well as the portal vein (Fig. 7). Dissection is carried cephalad including

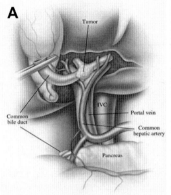
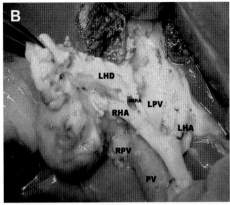

Fig. 7. (*A, B*) Skeletonization of the portal vein and hepatic artery. IVC, inferior vena cava; LHA, left hepatic artery; LHD, left hepatic duct; MHA, segment IV artery; PV, portal vein; RHA, right hepatic artery; RPV, right portal vein.

the gallbladder in the specimen. As more proximal mobilization of the bile duct continues, assessment of involvement of the hepatic artery and portal vein branches allows the operator to determine the need for vascular resection and reconstruction. The bile ducts are eventually divided at the secondary biliary radicals on the hepatic segments to be retained. This maneuver usually entails dividing the duct above the juncture of the right anterior and posterior branches on the right for left side dominant tumors or the segmental branches on the left for right side dominant tumors. The inflow and outflow vasculature of the hepatic lobe to be removed with the specimen is then divided, and the parenchyma transaction is performed using a combination of finger and instrument fracture. The resected liver lobe is removed in continuity with the specimen.

Extended right or left hepatectomies are sometimes necessary to achieve negative margins [4–7,45,46,52–54]. Biliary branches from the caudate lobe can represent an unsuspected repository of residual tumor after bile duct resection for cancer; therefore, most authorities advocate en bloc resection of the caudate lobe with bile duct tumors [45,55,56].

Because of the proximity of the tumor to the major vascular structures in the hilum of the liver, vascular invasion is common. Unilateral involvement is treated by ipsilateral hepatic lobectomy. More advanced vascular techniques with portal vein and hepatic arterial reconstruction are required to resect more advanced tumors with bilateral vascular involvement. The authors' approach to these complex advanced tumors is to completely excise the tumor and re-establish vascular inflow (portal vein and hepatic artery) to the remaining hepatic lobe. This task sometimes requires resection of the portal vein at the bifurcation and anastomosis of the main portal vein to the right or left portal vein. Similarly, arterial reconstruction might be required using microvascular techniques (Figs. 8, 9). Many of these more

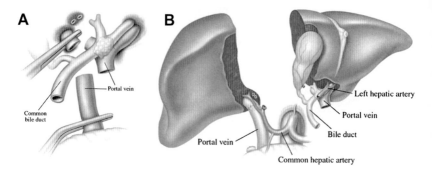

Fig. 8. (*A*) Hilar cholangiocarcinoma involving the portal vein bifurcation requiring resection of the portal vein. (*B*) Blood flow to the remnant lobe is re-established by anastomosing the main portal vein to the right portal vein.

advanced techniques have evolved directly as a result of our growing experience with living donor liver transplantation. Many reports have shown that this aggressive surgical approach increases the number of patients in whom complete excision of the tumor with negative margins can be achieved with acceptable morbidity and mortality [50,57–59].

Reconstruction of the biliary tree with a Roux-en-Y limb of jejunum completes the procedure. Frequently, with high resection into the secondary biliary radicals, multiple bile ducts require proper drainage after removal of the specimen. This drainage can be simplified by converting two or three neighboring ducts into a single orifice by dividing the septum between them and suturing the adjacent walls together. The anastomosis is performed using 5-0 polydioxanone sutures by laying the posterior layer first and completing the anterior layer over a pediatric feeding tube passed through the proximal end of the roux as a biliary stent. The biliary stents allow easy access for postoperative radiologic confirmation of biliary

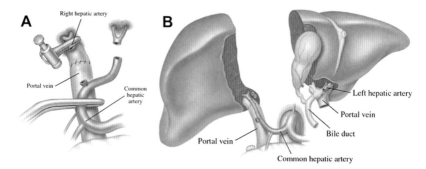

Fig. 9. (*A*) Bilateral involvement of the hepatic artery and portal vein requiring resection of the portal vein bifurcation and both right and left hepatic arteries involved with tumor. (*B*) Flow to the remnant lobe is established by sewing the main portal vein to the right portal vein and the proper hepatic artery to the right hepatic artery using microvascular techniques.

anatomy and are removed 3 to 4 weeks after discharge. Closed suction drainage is routinely performed.

Adjuvant therapy

Currently, there are no data supporting the routine use of adjuvant or neoadjuvant therapy in patients with hilar cholangiocarcinoma. Radiotherapy using external beam radiation delivering doses of up to 60 Gy with duodenal protection has been used as an adjunct to surgical resection in patients with positive surgical margins. In a prospective study, Pitt and colleagues [60] found that adjuvant radiotherapy had no effect on overall survival. Percutaneous and endoscopic endoluminal radiation techniques as well as radioimmunotherapy with ^{131}I-anti-CEA have also been used in combination with systemic chemotherapy in patients with cholangiocarcinoma with little benefit. Nevertheless, some retrospective studies have shown some survival advantage with adjuvant radiotherapy [61,62]. These studies were nonrandomized and included a heterogeneous group of patients. Moreover, many multivariate analyses looking at neoadjuvant therapy among other factors have identified resection with negative histologic margins as the only factor associated with prolonged survival [4–6,45]. Similarly, single agent or combination chemotherapy has failed to show efficacy. Drugs such as 5-fluorouracil (5-FU), methansulfon, cisplatin, mitomycin C, paclitaxel, and gemcitabine have shown little efficacy, with response rates ranging from 0% to 9% and median survivals between 2 and 12 months [63]. A prospective randomized trial comparing oral 5-FU with oral 5-FU plus streptozotocin and oral 5-FU plus methyl-CCNU in patients with unresectable cholangiocarcinoma demonstrated a response rate of only 9% [64]. Presently, there are no data to support the routine use of adjuvant chemoradiation, except in controlled trials. Despite the lack of evidence, adjuvant chemoradiation is used at the many centers around the world. The authors reserve the use of adjuvant chemoradiation for patients with positive nodal status or microscopically positive bile duct margins.

Results

Long-term survival can be achieved with acceptable morbidity and mortality. The perioperative mortality rate ranges from 1.3% to 11%, and morbidity rates range from 35% to 50% [4–7,45,46,65–67]. The presence or absence of positive histologic margins in the resected specimen is an important determinant of disease recurrence and patient survival [4–6,46,68,69]. The early experience with local hilar resection was associated with a high incidence of positive margins and poor long-term survival [2]. With growing experience in the management of hilar cholangiocarcinoma, the number of patients undergoing hepatic resection has increased steadily. Moreover, the addition of sophisticated vascular reconstructions to the surgical armamentarium has led to an increase in the number of patients undergoing R0 resection. This aggressive surgical approach has increased the number of patients undergoing curative resections and has been associated with improved patient survival. Five-year survival rates as high as 59% have been reported [70]; however, the 5-year survival rates in most recent reports range from 20% to 45% [4–7,45,46,65–67,71,72].

Combining hepatic resection with portal vein resection for locally advanced tumors has increased the resectability rate with acceptable morbidity and mortality. These complex vascular resections are technically difficult and may increase the risk of the procedure. Some authorities have reported worse 5-year survival in patients who undergo portal vein resection [50], whereas others have reported a similar outcome to those without portal vein resection [57,73].

The Lahey Clinic experience

The authors' program started in 1985 at the former New England Deaconess Hospital and moved to the Lahey Clinic in 1999. From 1985 to 2007, 124 patients with hilar cholangiocarcinoma underwent resection with curative intent. As our experience evolved, we adopted a more radical aggressive surgical approach with the addition of hepatectomy and complex vascular reconstruction to achieve negative surgical margins. When comparing our earlier experience between 1985 and 1999 (period 1) [74] with that between 1999 and 2007 (period 2) (Mohamed Akoad, MD, FACS, unpublished data, 2008), local and hepatic resection was performed in 75.9% of patients in period 2 as compared with 48.6% in period 1. Combined vascular resection was performed in 17 patients (3 in period 1 and 14 in period 2). Portal vein resection only was performed in 13 patients, hepatic artery resection only in 2, and both hepatic artery and portal vein resection in 2. Negative margins were achieved in 86.8% in period 2 compared with 50% in period 1($P<.05$). The perioperative mortality rate was 6% in period 1 and 5% in period 2. The 1-, 3-, and 5-year survival rates in period 1 were 83.1%, 56.1%, and 13.6%, respectively, as compared with 89.1%, 56%, and 32.5%, respectively, in period 2 ($P = .007$). The overall 1-, 3-, and 5-year survival rates in patients with R0 resection were 92.9%, 67.5%, and 38.3%, respectively, compared with 72%, 3.5%, and 0%, respectively, for R1 resections. Clearly, the improvement in survival is a result of the application of wider resections with the addition of partial hepatectomy and vascular resections.

Palliation

Extensive surgical resection should only be carried out with the goal of achieving complete tumor removal and negative histologic margins. In patients who are not candidates for surgical resection due to bilateral extensive biliary involvement, bilateral vascular invasion not amenable to reconstruction, or extensive regional spread, management options include adequate biliary drainage and preventing infectious complications.

The relief of jaundice can be achieved by surgical or nonsurgical means. To date, randomized studies comparing surgical palliation with nonoperative biliary drainage have demonstrated no difference in survival time, complication rates, or the relief of jaundice; therefore, surgical bypass should only be considered in patients who are found to be unresectable at operation. Because most of these patients have preoperative biliary drainage, surgical bypass is rarely indicated [75–77]. If surgical bypass is considered, we prefer to perform hepaticojejunostomy to bile ducts far away from the upper extent of the tumor to prevent obstruction from rapid tumor growth. Only one lobe of the liver needs to be bypassed to maintain adequate function. Traditionally, anastomosis to the segment III bile duct at the base of the round ligament has been the most common drainage option. Bypass of an atrophic lobe or a lobe heavily involved with tumor is generally ineffective.

Nonoperative biliary drainage can be accomplished by an endoscopic or percutaneous approach. In patients with advanced tumor, the endoscopic approach has a high failure rate. Percutaneous biliary drainage and subsequent placement of biliary stents can be performed in most patients with hilar cholangiocarcinoma. The self-expandable metallic wall stents provide a more durable option (Fig. 10) [78,79]. Regardless of whether an endoscopic or percutaneous approach is used, the presence of an atrophic lobe is an important factor to be considered before the drainage procedure. Drainage of an atrophic lobe does not provide relief of jaundice and should be avoided. Sometimes multiple stents may be required to adequately drain the obstructed segments and provide palliation. Recurrent jaundice after

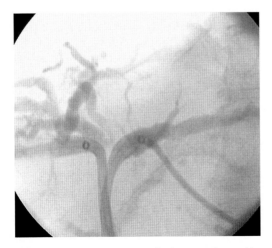

Fig. 10. Metal wall stents placed percutaneously in a patient with unresectable hilar cholangiocarcinoma.

wall stent placement occurs in approximately 18% to 28% of patients because of tumor growth through the mesh of the wall stent or beyond the proximal or distal margins of the stent [79,80]. Biliary drainage can be re-established by adding a longer stent place inside the existing stent. Jaundice that fails to subside after adequately draining all of the segments is likely due to hepatic dysfunction from prolonged obstruction or vascular compromise from tumor invasion and is not likely to be corrected with drainage procedures.

Liver transplantation

Logic would suggest that total hepatectomy and liver transplantation would be the best treatment option because adequate margins are more easily obtained; however, the initial experience with liver transplantation for hilar cholangiocarcinoma has been plagued by early mortality, high recurrence rates, and poor survival. The Cincinnati Transplant Tumor Registry reported a 5-year survival rate of 28% with a 51% tumor recurrence rate [81]. Most patients who underwent liver transplantation for cholangiocarcinoma died within 1 to 2 years due to rapid aggressive disease recurrence [82,83]. More aggressive regional resections, including bile duct resection and pancreaticodudenectomy to eradicate the entire biliary tree and achieve a wide margin, followed by liver replacement and upper abdominal exenteration with subsequent cluster transplantation (liver, pancreas, duodenum, and variable amounts of jejunum) have not demonstrated any added benefit, with few long-term survivors [84,85]. These results have led many centers to abandon liver transplantation for cholangiocarcinoma to avoid wasting the scarce donor organ, and cholangiocarcinoma has become an exclusion criterion for liver transplant.

Recently, a protocol combining radiotherapy, chemosensitization, and liver transplantation has resulted in a dramatic improvement in outcome, with 1-, 3-, and 5-year survival rates of 92%, 82%, and 82%, respectively [86–88]. These results were significantly better than those of resection alone; however, comparing the results between these two groups was difficult, because the medical selection criteria were more stringent for the transplant group, and patients were significantly younger and with higher incidences of PSC than the resection group. Nevertheless, this approach provides the most promising and encouraging treatment strategy for hilar cholangiocarcinoma and is worth further evaluation.

Summary

Hilar cholangiocarcinoma is a rare malignancy that occurs at the bifurcation of the bile ducts. Complete surgical excision with negative histologic margins remains the only hope for cure or long-term survival. Because of its location and proximity to the vascular inflow of the liver, surgical resection is technically difficult and may require advanced vascular reconstructions to achieve complete excision. Despite advances in surgical techniques, the 5-year survival rate in most recent reports ranges from 20% to 45%. The role of neoadjuvant therapy and liver transplantation in the management of hilar cholangiocarcinoma remains to be defined in light of recent promising results. Patients with advanced unresectable tumors and patients who are not candidates for surgical resection because of other comorbidities are candidates for palliative biliary drainage.

References

[1] Anthony PP. Tumours and tumour like lesions of the liver and biliary tract. In: MacSween RNM, Anthony PP, Scheuer PJ, editors. Pathology of the liver. 2nd edition. Edinburg (UK): Churchill Livingstone; 1987. p. 574.

[2] Nakeeb A, Pitt HA, Sohn TA, et al. Cholangiocarcinoma: a spectrum of intrahepatic, perihilar, and distal tumors. Ann Surg 1996;224:463–75.

[3] Klatskin G. Adenocarcinoma of the hepatic duct at its bifurcation within the porta hepatis. Am J Med 1965;38:241–56.

[4] Kosuge T, Yamamoto J, Shimada K, et al. Improved surgical results for hilar cholangiocarcinoma with procedures including major hepatic resections. Ann Surg 1999;230:663–71.

[5] Lee SG, Lee YJ, Park KM, et al. One hundred and eleven liver resections for hilar bile duct cancer. J Hepatobiliary Pancreat Surg 2000;7(2):135–41.

[6] Jarnagin WR, Fong Y, DeMatteo RP, et al. Staging, resectability, and outcome in 225 patients with hilar cholangiocarcinoma. Ann Surg 2001;234(4):507–17.

[7] Seyama Y, Kubota K, Sano K, et al. Long-term outcome of extended hemihepatectomy for hilar bile duct cancer with no mortality and high survival rate. Ann Surg 2003;238:73–83.

[8] Kuwayti K, Baggenstoss AH, Stauffer MH, et al. Carcinoma of the major intrahepatic and the extrahepatic bile ducts exclusive of the papilla of Vater. Surg Gynecol Obstet 1957;104: 357–66.

[9] Carriaga MT, Henson DE. Liver, gallbladder, extrahepatic bile ducts, and pancreas. Cancer 1995;75:171–90.

[10] Broe PJ, Cameron JL. The management of proximal biliary tract tumors. Adv Surg 1981;15: 47–91.

[11] Batheja N, Suriawinata A, Saxena R, et al. Expression of p53 and PCNA in cholangiocarcinoma and primary sclerosing cholangitis. Mod Pathol 2000;13(12):1265–8.

[12] Isa T, Tomita S, Nakachi A, et al. Analysis of microsatellite instability, K-ras gene mutation and p53 protein overexpression in intrahepatic cholangiocarcinoma. Hepatogastroenterology 2002;49(45):604–8.

[13] Goss JA, Shackleton CR, Farmer DG, et al. Orthotopic liver transplantation for primary sclerosing cholangitis: a 12-year single center experience. Ann Surg 1997;225(5):472–81.

[14] Graziadei IW, Wiesner RH, Marotta PJ, et al. Long-term results of patients undergoing liver transplantation for primary sclerosing cholangitis. Hepatology 1999;30(5):1121 7.

[15] Tsuchiya R, Harada N, Ito T, et al. Malignant tumors in choledochal cysts. Ann Surg 1977; 186(1):22–8.

[16] Todani T, Watanabe Y, Narusue M, et al. Congenital bile duct cysts: classification, operative procedures, and review of thirty-seven cases including cancer arising from choledochal cyst. Am J Surg 1977;134(2):263–9.

[17] Flanigan DP. Biliary carcinoma associated with biliary cysts. Cancer 1977;40(2):880–3.

[18] Kurathong S, Lerdverasirikul P, Wongpaitoon V, et al. *Opisthorchis viverrini* infection and cholangiocarcinoma: a prospective, case-controlled study. Gastroenterology 1985;89(1): 151–6.

[19] Kubo S, Kinoshita H, Hirohashi K, et al. Hepatolithiasis associated with cholangiocarcinoma. World J Surg 1995;19:637–41.

[20] Littlewood ER, Barrison IG, Murray-Lyon IM, et al. Cholangiocarcinoma and oral contraceptives. Lancet 1980;1(8163):310–1.

[21] Brodén G, Bengtsson L. Biliary carcinoma associated with methyldopa therapy. Acta Chir Scand Suppl 1980;500:7–12.

[22] Lowenfels AB, Norman J. Isoniazid and bile duct cancer. JAMA 1978;240(5):434–5.

[23] Szendröi M, Németh L, Vajta G. Asbestos bodies in a bile duct cancer after occupational exposure. Environ Res 1983;30(2):270–80.

[24] Weinbren K, Mutum SS. Pathologic aspects of cholangiocarcinoma. Am J Pathol 1983;139:217–38.

[25] Rodgers CM, Adams JT, Schwartz SI. Carcinoma of the extrahepatic bile ducts. Surgery 1981;90:596–601.

[26] Hadjis NS, Blumgart LH. Role of liver atrophy, hepatic resection and hepatocyte hyperplasia in the development of portal hypertension in biliary disease. Gut 1987;28:1022–8.

[27] Hochwald SN, Burke EC, Jarnagin WR, et al. Association of preoperative biliary stenting with increased postoperative infectious complications in proximal cholangiocarcinoma. Arch Surg 1999;134:261–6.

[28] Thuluvath PJ, Rai R, Venbrux AC, et al. Cholangiocarcinoma: a review. Gastroenterologist 1997;5:306–15.

[29] Jalanko H, Kuusela P, Roberts P, et al. Comparison of a new tumor marker, CA19-9T with α-fetoprotein and carcinoembryonic antigen in patients with upper gastrointestinal disease. J Clin Pathol 1984;37:218–22.

[30] Hann LE, Greatrex KV, Bach AM, et al. Cholangiocarcinoma at the hepatic hilus: sonographic findings. AJR Am J Roentgenol 1997;168(4):985–9.

[31] Guthrie JA, Ward J, Robinson PJ. Hilar cholangiocarcinomas: T2-weighted spin-echo and gadolinium-enhanced FLASH MR imaging. Radiology 1996;201(2):347–51.

[32] Vanderveen KA, Hussain HK. Magnetic resonance imaging of cholangiocarcinoma. Cancer Imaging 2004;4(2):104–15.

[33] Hänninen EL, Pech M, Jonas S, et al. Magnetic resonance imaging including magnetic resonance cholangiopancreatography for tumor localization and therapy planning in malignant hilar obstructions. Acta Radiol 2005;46(5):462–70.

[34] Endo I, Shimada H, Sugita M, et al. Role of three-dimensional imaging in operative planning for hilar cholangiocarcinoma. Surgery 2007;142(5):666–75.

[35] Soehendra N, Grimm H, Berger B, et al. Malignant jaundice: results of diagnostic and therapeutic endoscopy. World J Surg 1989;13(2):171–7.

[36] Rerknimitr R, Kladcharoen N, Mahachai V, et al. Result of endoscopic biliary drainage in hilar cholangiocarcinoma. J Clin Gastroenterol 2004;38(6):518–23.

[37] Petrowsky H, Wildbrett P, Husarik DB, et al. Impact of integrated positron emission tomography and computed tomography on staging and management of gallbladder cancer and cholangiocarcinoma. J Hepatol 2006;45(1):43–50.

[38] Keiding S, Hansen SB, Rasmussen HH, et al. Detection of cholangiocarcinoma in primary sclerosing cholangitis by positron emission tomography. Hepatology 1998;28(3):700–6.

[39] Corvera CU, Blumgart LH, Akhurst T, et al. 18F-fluorodeoxyglucose positron emission tomography influences management decisions in patients with biliary cancer. J Am Coll Surg 2008;206(1):57–65.

[40] Kurzawinski T, Deery A, Dooley J, et al. A prospective controlled study comparing brush and bile exfoliative cytology for diagnosing bile duct strictures. Gut 1992;33(12):1675–7.

[41] Pitt HA, Dooley W, Yeo C, et al. Does preoperative percutaneous biliary drainage reduce operative risk or increase hospital cost? Ann Surg 1985;201:545–52.

[42] McPherson GA, Benjamin IS, Hodgson HJ, et al. Preoperative percutaneous transhepatic biliary drainage: the results of a controlled trial. Br J Surg 1984;71(5):371–5.

[43] Hatfield AR, Tobias R, Terblanche J, et al. Preoperative external biliary drainage in obstructive jaundice: a prospective controlled clinical trial. Lancet 1982;2(8304):896–9.

[44] Sewnath ME, Karsten TM, Prins MH, et al. A meta-analysis on the efficacy of preoperative biliary drainage for tumors causing obstructive jaundice. Ann Surg 2002;236(1):17–27.

[45] Nimura Y, Kamiya J, Kondo S, et al. Aggressive preoperative management and extended surgery for hilar cholangiocarcinoma: Nagoya experience. J Hepatobiliary Pancreat Surg 2000;7:155–62.

[46] Kawasaki S, Imamura H, Kobayashi A, et al. Results of surgical resection for patients with hilar bile duct cancer: application of extended hepatectomy after biliary drainage and hemihepatic portal vein embolization. Ann Surg 2003;238(1):84–92.

[47] Kawarada Y, Higashiguchi T, Yokoi H, et al. Preoperative biliary drainage in obstructive jaundice. Hepatogastroenterology 1995;42(4):300–7.

[48] Cherqui D, Benoist S, Malassagne B, et al. Major liver resection for carcinoma in jaundiced patients without preoperative biliary drainage. Arch Surg 2000;135:302–8.

[49] Belghiti J, Hiramatsu K, Benoist S, et al. Seven hundred forty-seven hepatectomies in the 1990s: an update to evaluate the actual risk of liver resection. J Am Coll Surg 2000;191(1): 38–46.

[50] Ebata T, Nagino M, Kamiya J, et al. Hepatectomy with portal vein resection for hilar cholangiocarcinoma: audit of 52 consecutive cases. Ann Surg 2003;238:720–7.

[51] Weber A, Landrock S, Schneider J, et al. Long-term outcome and prognostic factors of patients with hilar cholangiocarcinoma. World J Gastroenterol 2007;13(9):1422–6.

[52] Burke EC, Jarnagin WR, Hochwald SN, et al. Hilar cholangiocarcinoma: patterns of spread, the importance of hepatic resection for curative operation, and a presurgical clinical staging system. Ann Surg 1998;228(3):385–94.

[53] Capussotti L, Muratore A, Polastri R, et al. Liver resection for hilar cholangiocarcinoma: in-hospital mortality and long term survival. J Am Coll Surg 2002;195:641.

[54] Neuhaus P, Jonas S, Settmacher U, et al. Surgical management of proximal bile duct cancer: extended right lobe resection increases resectability and radicality. Langenbecks Arch Surg 2003;388(3):194–200.

[55] Mizumoto R, Suzuki H. Surgical anatomy of the hepatic hilum with special reference to the caudate lobe. World J Surg 1988;12(1):2–10.

[56] Nimura Y, Hayakawa N, Kamiya J, et al. Hepatic segmentectomy with caudate lobe resection for bile duct carcinoma of the hepatic hilus. World J Surg 1990;14(4):535–43.

[57] Hemming AW, Kim RD, Mekeel KL, et al. Portal vein resection for hilar cholangiocarcinoma. Am Surg 2006;72(7):599–604.

[58] Miyazaki M, Kato A, Ito H, et al. Combined vascular resection in operative resection for hilar cholangiocarcinoma: does it work or not? Surgery 2007;141(5):581–8.

[59] Muñoz L, Roayaie S, Maman D, et al. Hilar cholangiocarcinoma involving the portal vein bifurcation: long-term results after resection. J Hepatobiliary Pancreat Surg 2002;9(2): 237–41.

[60] Pitt HA, Nakeeb A, Abrams RA, et al. Perihilar cholangiocarcinoma: postoperative radiotherapy does not improve survival. Ann Surg 1995;221:788–97.

[61] Todoroki T, Ohara K, Kawamoto T, et al. Benefits of adjuvant radiotherapy after radical resection of locally advanced main hepatic duct carcinoma. Int J Radiat Oncol Biol Phys 2000;46:581–7.

[62] Gerhards MF, van Gulik TM, Gonzalez D, et al. Results of postoperative radiotherapy for resectable hilar cholangiocarcinoma. World J Surg 2003;27:173–9.

[63] Todoroki T. Chemotherapy for bile duct carcinoma in the light of adjuvant chemotherapy to surgery. Hepatogastroenterology 2000;47:644–9.

[64] Falkson G, MacIntyre JM, Moertel CG. Eastern Cooperative Oncology Group experience with chemotherapy for inoperable gallbladder and bile duct cancer. Cancer 1984;54:965–9.

[65] Nagino M, Nimura Y, Kamiya J, et al. Segmental liver resections for hilar cholangiocarcinoma. Hepatogastroenterology 1998;45(19):7–13.

[66] Todoroki T, Kawamoto T, Koike N. Radical resection of hilar bile duct carcinoma and predictors of survival. Br J Surg 2000;87(3):306–13.

[67] Hemming AW, Reed AI, Fujita S, et al. Surgical management of hilar cholangiocarcinoma. Ann Surg 2005;241(5):693–9.

[68] Pichlmayr R, Weimann A, Klempnauer J, et al. Surgical treatment in proximal bile duct cancer: a single-center experience. Ann Surg 1996;224(5):628–38.

[69] Klempnauer J, Ridder GJ, von Wasielewski R, et al. Resectional surgery of hilar cholangiocarcinoma: a multivariate analysis of prognostic factors. J Clin Oncol 1997;15(3):947–54.

[70] Neuhaus P, Jonas S. Surgery for hilar cholangiocarcinoma–the German experience. J Hepatobiliary Pancreat Surg 2000;7(2):142–7.

[71] Silva MA, Tekin K, Aytekin F, et al. Surgery for hilar cholangiocarcinoma: a 10-year experience of a tertiary referral centre in the UK. Eur J Surg Oncol 2005;31(5):533–9.

[72] Hasegawa S, Ikai I, Fujii H, et al. Surgical resection of hilar cholangiocarcinoma: analysis of survival and postoperative complications. World J Surg 2007;31(6):1256–63.

[73] Launois B, Terblanche J, Lakehal M, et al. Proximal bile duct cancer: high respectability rate and 5-year survival. Ann Surg 1999;230:266–75.

[74] Washburn W, Lewis D, Jenkins R. Aggressive surgical resection for cholangiocarcinoma. Arch Surg 1995;130:270–6.

[75] Andersen JR, Sørensen SM, Kruse A, et al. Randomised trial of endoscopic endoprosthesis versus operative bypass in malignant obstructive jaundice. Gut 1989;30(8):1132–5.

[76] Magistrelli P, Masetti R, Coppola R, et al. Changing attitudes in the palliation of proximal malignant biliary obstruction. J Surg Oncol Suppl 1993;3:151–3.

[77] Shepherd HA, Royle G, Ross AP, et al. Endoscopic biliary endoprosthesis in the palliation of malignant obstruction of the distal common bile duct: a randomized trial. Br J Surg 1988; 75(12):1166–8.

[78] Pappas P, Leonardou P, Kurkuni A, et al. Percutaneous insertion of metallic endoprostheses in the biliary tree in 66 patients: relief of the obstruction. Abdom Imaging 2003;28(5):678–83.

[79] Inal M, Akgül E, Aksungur E, et al. Percutaneous self-expandable uncovered metallic stents in malignant biliary obstruction: complications, follow-up and reintervention in 154 patients. Acta Radiol 2003;44(2):139–46.

[80] Laméris JS, Stoker J, Nijs HG, et al. Malignant biliary obstruction: percutaneous use of self-expandable stents. Radiology 1991;179(3):703–7.

[81] Meyer CG, Penn I, James L. Liver transplantation for cholangiocarcinoma: results in 207 patients. Transplantation 2000;69:1633–7.

[82] Goldstein RM, Stone M, Tillery GW, et al. Is liver transplantation indicated for cholangiocarcinoma? Am J Surg 1993;166:768–71.

[83] Shimoda M, Farmer DG, Colquhoun SD, et al. Liver transplantation for cholangiocellular carcinoma: analysis of a single-center experience and review of the literature. Liver Transplant 2001;7:1023–33.

[84] Cherqui D, Alon R, Piedbois P, et al. Combined liver transplantation and pancreatoduodenectomy for irresectable hilar bile duct carcinoma. Br J Surg 1995;82:397–8.

[85] Alessiani M, Tzakis A, Todo S, et al. Assessment of five-year experience with abdominal organ cluster transplantation. J Am Coll Surg 1995;180:1–9.

[86] Heimbach JK, Gores GJ, Haddock MG, et al. Liver transplantation for unresectable perihilar cholangiocarcinoma. Semin Liver Dis 2004;24:201–7.

[87] Rea JG, Heimbach JK, Rosen CB, et al. Liver transplantation with neoadjuvant chemoradiation is more effective than resection for hilar cholangiocarcinoma. Ann Surg 2005;242: 451–8.

[88] Heimbach JK, Gores GJ, Haddock MG, et al. Predictors of disease recurrence following neoadjuvant chemoradiotherapy and liver transplantation for unresectable perihilar cholangiocarcinoma. Transplantation 2006;82(12):1703–7.

SURGICAL
CLINICS OF
NORTH AMERICA

Surg Clin N Am 88 (2008) 1429–1447

Distal Biliary Malignancy

Gregory Veillette, MD*,
Carlos Fernández-del Castillo, MD

*Department of Surgery, Massachusetts General Hospital, 55 Fruit Street,
Boston, MA 02114, USA*

Distal biliary malignancy (cholangiocarcinoma) remains a rare diagnosis with a dismal prognosis. The vast majority of these cancers are adenocarcinomas that preferentially invade adjacent structures and drain to local lymph nodes. Given the small diameter of the common bile duct, early tumor detection with current imaging is not possible. Consequently, these patients typically present with symptoms and most with advanced disease. These cancers tend to grow perpendicularly to, and horizontally along, the bile duct, and therefore tumors that are detected by imaging tend to be underestimated and are often more extensive on surgical exploration. The anatomic relationship of the distal bile duct to the pancreas, duodenum, portal vein, and hepatic artery can also make removal of these tumors technically challenging.

Classification

Cholangiocarcinoma is traditionally classified anatomically as intrahepatic or extrahepatic, with extrahepatic disease further classified as proximal (hilar) or distal. The original report by Klatskin in 1965 [1] described cancer of the perihilar region, which currently accounts for about 60% to 80% of all cholangiocarcinomas. Subsequently, hilar malignancies have been further classified based on the Bismuth-Corlette system, which includes all extrahepatic disease down to the confluence of the cystic and common hepatic ducts [2]. Cholangiocarcinoma of the common bile duct (CBD) down to the level of the ampulla is considered distal disease, and is the

* Corresponding author. Department of Surgery, Massachusetts General Hospital, 15 Parkman Street, Wang Ambulatory Care Center Suite 460, Boston, MA 02114.
E-mail address: gveillette@partners.org (G. Veillette).

doi:10.1016/j.suc.2008.07.003
surgical.theclinics.com

type discussed in this article. Some of the early studies [3,4] made a distinction between lesions in the middle third (below the cystic duct but not intrapancreatic) and lower third (the intrapancreatic portion) of the bile duct. Because malignancies in the middle third of the extrahepatic bile duct are distinctly rare, more recent reports favor the classification of middle third lesions as distal disease [5].

Epidemiology

Cholangiocarcinoma, as a whole, accounts for approximately 3% of all gastrointestinal cancers, with distal bile duct cancer accounting for about 20% to 30% of all cholangiocarcinomas [5,6]. The likelihood of developing distal cholangiocarcinoma increases with age, with a peak in the seventh decade. There also tends to be a slight male predominance for these lesions. The overall incidence of extrahepatic cholangiocarcinoma seems to be declining [6]. The large, population-based statistics are difficult to interpret for two reasons, however. First, hilar and distal cholangiocarcinomas are analyzed together as extrahepatic disease, and second, gallbladder cancer is usually combined with extrahepatic cholangiocarcinoma in these reports [6,7].

Pathology

Microscopically, the vast majority (95% to 97%) of bile duct malignancies are adenocarcinomas (Fig. 1). They are typically well-differentiated, mucin-positive lesions that have a propensity to extend submucosally along the bile ducts. Cholangiocarcinomas also tend to have a strong desmoplastic stroma, invasive perineural spread, and, like many adenocarcinomas, they preferentially spread to regional lymph nodes [8,9].

Macroscopically, these lesions are divided into three types: sclerosing, nodular, and papillary. The sclerosing lesions appear as diffusely firm and tend to circumferentially occlude the lumen of the duct. The nodular type appears as a firm mass projecting into the duct lumen with the base continuous with the duct wall. Large, nodular lesions may look circumferential, however, and have features of the sclerosing type (nodular-sclerosing). The papillary subtype grows as a friable, polypoid mass that can have accompanying ductal sclerosis but tends to extend into surrounding structures. In a sentinel paper on the pathology of cholangiocarcinoma [8], 33 gross specimens were evaluated. Of these, 22 were of the sclerosing type and involved the proximal ducts or hilum. There were 8 papillary lesions, 7 of which involved the distal bile duct, and 3 nodular lesions, 1 involving the suprapancreatic CBD and two involving the intra-pancreatic distal CBD.

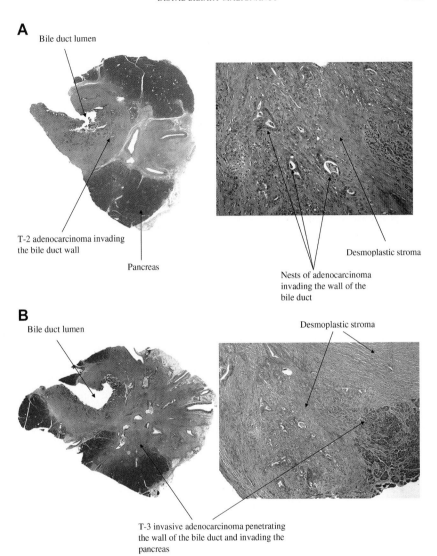

Fig. 1. (A) Histology demonstrating low- and high-power views of a T-2 distal bile duct adeno-carcinoma. The cancer extends beyond the wall of the duct, but does not invade the surrounding pancreas. (B) Low- and high-power views of a T-3 cancer demonstrating tumor infiltration of the pancreas. In both, there is a strong desmoplastic stroma surrounding the malignant cells.

Risk factors

Like in other carcinomas, cholangiocarcinoma is associated with conditions that directly injure or lead to longstanding inflammation of the bile duct epithelium, which leads to a compensatory increase in the mitotic activity of the cholangiocytes and the consequent increase in the likelihood of mutation and error. Although most cases are sporadic and without an identifiable cause, the biliary epithelium can suffer several different forms of injury that may initiate the development of cholangiocarcinoma. Broadly, these injury patterns include acquired (primary sclerosing cholangitis [PSC], chronic stone disease), congenital (choledochal cysts, Caroli disease), infectious (*Salmonella typhi*, *Clonorchis sinensis*, *Opisthorchis viverrini*, hepatitis C) or chemical (smoking, thorotrast, dioxin).

Primary sclerosing cholangitis

PSC is a chronic, autoimmune inflammatory disease that results in multifocal strictures and fibrosis of the intrahepatic and extrahepatic biliary tree. Roughly 80% of patients who have PSC have associated inflammatory bowel disease (usually ulcerative colitis); however, few patients who have inflammatory bowel disease go on to develop PSC [10,11].

Although the natural history of PSC is variable, it is clear that these patients have an increased risk for cholangiocarcinoma. Although colectomy in the setting of ulcerative colitis does remove the risk for colon cancer, it does not affect the incidence or severity of sclerosing cholangitis [12,13]. The true overall risk for the development of cholangiocarcinoma in the setting of PSC is difficult to define because a large percentage of patients die of their disease and do not undergo autopsy. From the available natural history data, roughly 6% to 14% of patients who have PSC will have a cholangiocarcinoma diagnosed during their lifetime [10,12,14], although the true incidence (including autopsy diagnosed) of cholangiocarcinoma in this population is estimated to be as high as 30% to 40%. Although cholangiocarcinoma of the distal bile duct is uncommon in the setting of PSC, it does occur. In one report, it accounted for 13% of all PSC-associated cholangiocarcinomas [15].

Nearly half of these cholangiocarcinomas are diagnosed within 1 year of the initial diagnosis of PSC, suggesting subclinical inflammation and subsequent malignant degeneration, typically heralded by abdominal pain and jaundice. Furthermore, given the multifocal nature of PSC, the diagnosis of cholangiocarcinoma may be delayed, resulting in a higher percentage of unresectable tumors [10,12,14].

Choledochal cystic disease

There is a well-described 10% to 15% lifetime risk for cholangiocarcinoma in patients who have choledochal cysts. The development of these cysts is likely a consequence of pancreaticobiliary ductal malunion, in which the pancreatic duct joins the common bile duct proximal to the sphincter complex. It is believed that this abnormal junction of the pancreatic duct allows reflux of pancreatic enzymes proximally up the bile duct. This reflux not only injures the biliary epithelium but also increases the intraductal flow, and consequently pressure, leading to dilation (cyst formation) of the bile ducts. Once formed, there is biliary stasis and chronic inflammation within the cyst [16,17]. If excised early in life, the risk for malignant degeneration is minimal. If allowed to persist into adulthood, however, the lifetime risk for cholangiocarcinoma in these patients can be as high as 30% [18].

Liver fluke infection

The ingestion of undercooked fish can result in infection with the hepatobiliary flukes *O viverrini* and *C sinensis*. These parasites are particularly common in Thailand, which has the highest incidence of cholangiocarcinoma in the world. The flukes gain entry to the biliary tree through the ampulla of Vater, and the subsequent infestation leads to a localized chronic inflammatory state that is strongly associated with the development of cholangiocarcinoma. The chronic inflammation results in not only biliary ductal hyperplasia but also increased production of nitric oxide and N-nitroso compounds that cause DNA damage [19].

Hepatolithiasis

Cholelithiasis is seen in up to 30% of patients who have cholangiocarcinoma. Although it is clear that gallstones increase the likelihood of gallbladder adenocarcinoma, the incidence of gallstones in patients who have cholangiocarcinoma approaches that of the general population [11]. It has been suggested in a case report [20] that cholelithiasis with associated choledocholithiasis increases the risk for distal bile duct adenocarcinoma; however, this relationship has not been proved. In contrast, the presence of chronic biliary stone disease (hepatolithiasis, Oriental cholangiohepatitis, or recurrent pyogenic cholangiohepatitis) significantly increases the risk for biliary ductal malignancy [21,22]. The consequences of biliary stones are obstruction of the intrahepatic ducts, recurrent cholangitis, stricture formation, and bile stasis, all of which contribute to chronic inflammation and subsequent malignancy.

Toxins

The prototype chemical associated with cholangiocarcinoma is thorotrast. This radiologic contrast agent was banned in the 1950s when its carcinogenic potential was realized. The development of cholangiocarcinoma is greatly increased in patients who received thorotrast, and these malignancies typically develop decades (up to 48 years in one report) after exposure [23]. Other chemical exposures implicated in cholangiocarcinoma development are alcohol, dioxin, nitrosamines, and smoking [24].

Biliary papillomatosis

Biliary papillomatosis is a rare, premalignant lesion characterized by multiple papillary adenomas distributed along the bile ducts. These tumors can be mucin or non–mucin secreting and typically present with repeated episodes of right upper quadrant pain, jaundice, or cholangitis. One of the largest published series of biliary papillomatosis [25] reports that 83% of papillary adenomas contain carcinoma.

Other

Other risk factors implicated in the development of cholangiocarcinoma, but with less well-established cause–effect relationships, include hepatitis B, hepatitis C, cirrhosis, HIV infection, and diabetes.

Clinical presentation

The clinical difference between intra- and extrahepatic disease is based on biliary occlusion and local invasion. In general, the more distal the tumor the sooner clinical symptoms suggestive of biliary obstruction are present. Intrahepatic cholangiocarcinoma tends to present later in its course given the multiple drainage options around the tumor and atrophy of the obstructed liver parenchyma. Conversely, extrahepatic disease tends to present much earlier with painless jaundice, pruritus, dark urine, light stools, and fat malabsorption from bile acid deficiency. These patients can also experience abdominal fullness, early satiety, nausea, vague abdominal discomfort, malaise, fevers, night sweats, and weight loss. Given the proximity to the portal vein, hepatic artery, duodenum, and pancreas, distal cholangiocarcinomas quickly become locally invasive and ultimately metastatic. Rarely, distal bile duct malignancy is suspected incidentally when right upper quadrant ultrasound or computed tomographic scans are done for other reasons. Suggestive findings here include biliary ductal dilation, distension of the gallbladder, or a small mass.

All patients suspected of having a cholangiocarcinoma should have routine laboratory tests, including complete blood counts, electrolytes, liver chemistries, and liver function tests. Patients who have distal biliary obstruction are expected to have a direct hyperbilirubinemia and elevated alkaline phosphatase. Depending on the duration and severity of the obstruction, other liver function tests (serum albumin, prothrombin time, transaminases) may be normal. In those patients who have an incidentally discovered elevation in alkaline phosphatase, gamma-glutamyl transferase (GGT) levels should be checked. If the GGT is elevated in the setting of an elevated alkaline phosphatase, biliary etiology is likely and should prompt further investigation.

Molecular pathogenesis

The molecular pathogenesis of biliary malignancy consists of multiple alterations in normal cholangiocyte homeostasis. Although many cases of cholangiocarcinoma have no clear identifiable cause, there is typically some inciting damage to the biliary epithelium [26]. At the cellular level, malignant transformation proceeds by several mechanisms, including cell-cycle dysregulation/autonomous growth (cyclin D, K-ras, IL-6, COX-2), inactivation of tumor suppressor genes (p53, p16), enhanced antiapoptotic factors (bcl-2, Mcl-1), angiogenesis (VEGF), and invasion/metastases (E-cadherin, α-catenin) [27–29].

In states of chronic inflammation (eg, PSC, liver fluke infection, hepatolithiasis) there is up-regulation of IL-6 and iNOS. The subsequent increase in nitric oxide not only potentiates DNA oxidative damage but also promotes cell growth by inhibiting apoptosis. Biliary inflammation also induces cyclooxygenase -2 (COX-2), which results in cell growth and survival by way of prostaglandin synthesis [27].

The group from Memorial Sloan-Kettering [30] has recently demonstrated a differential expression of various cell-cycle regulatory proteins based on the location of cholangiocarcinoma. Using tissue microarrays, they showed a progressive decline in the expression of p27 from intrahepatic to distal malignancies. Intrahepatic tumors were more likely to have overexpression of cyclin D1 and bcl-2 compared with hilar, gallbladder, and distal tumors. Conversely, distal tumors had overexpression of the tumor suppressor p53 when compared with the more proximal lesions.

Tumor markers

The two most widely used serum markers for cholangiocarcinoma are carbohydrate antigen (CA) 19-9 and carcinoembryonic antigen (CEA). Much of the literature on the relationship between these tumor markers and cholangiocarcinoma is in patients who had underlying PSC. CA 19-9 is an antibody directed at circulating glycoproteins that are coated with sialylated blood group antigens. The level depends on the blood Lewis phenotype and therefore is undetectable in about 7% of the population [31]. Using a cutoff value of 100 U/mL, the reported sensitivity and specificity of CA 19-9 for detecting cholangiocarcinoma ranges from 53% to 89% and 80% to 91%, respectively [31–35]. The diagnostic accuracy is not improved by using higher cutoff values, for example, 180 U/mL [36]. CA 19-9 levels can be elevated not only in other malignancies (ovarian, stomach, pancreas, and colon) but also in any condition leading to dilation or inflammation of the bile ducts (benign stricture, cholangitis, and cholestasis).

CEA levels are even less accurate than CA 19-9 for diagnosing cholangiocarcinoma. CEA is an oncofetal glycoprotein that is most useful in detecting recurrences of colorectal cancers. It has also been shown to have some diagnostic usefulness in cholangiocarcinoma, however. Using a cutoff value of 5 ng/mL, the reported sensitivity and specificity are 33% to 68% and 82% to 95%, respectively [31,32,36,37]. Because CEA is often monitored together with CA 19-9, a scoring system (the Ramage score) was developed that combines these markers in an attempt to raise the diagnostic accuracy of each individually. In the original study [38] a score (CA19-9 + [CEA × 40]) of greater than 400 had a reported sensitivity and specificity of 66% and 100%, respectively, in patients who had PSC. In a study performed by Lindberg and colleagues [32], the sensitivity and specificity for the Ramage score in identifying cholangiocarcinoma in patients who had endoscopic retrograde cholangiopancreatography (ERCP)–confirmed strictures was only 43% and 89%, respectively. In those patients who had underlying PSC, however, the sensitivity and specificity went up to 71% and 91%, respectively.

It is clear that CA 19-9 or CEA in isolation are not accurate in making the diagnosis of cholangiocarcinoma. In the appropriate clinical setting and with a high suspicion, however, these tests may aid in the diagnosis. More importantly, these markers should be followed closely in patients after surgical resection and if increasing should prompt aggressive imaging to search for recurrence or metastatic disease.

Other novel molecular tests used for the diagnosis of cholangiocarcinoma include digitized image analysis (DIA) and fluorescent in situ hybridization (FISH). These assays require biliary ductal brushing/aspirate samples collected during ERCP. The DIA allows computer analysis of the cell nucleus and quantification of DNA [39], whereas the FISH assay labels cholangiocyte DNA to detect specific chromosomal abnormalities [26]. In one study, a FISH assay using probes to chromosomes 3, 7, 9, and 17 had a superior sensitivity to routine cytology for the detection of malignancy in patients who had biliary strictures [40].

Staging

The most recent staging guidelines for extrahepatic bile duct cancers (6th edition) from the American Joint Committee on Cancer were published in 2002 and are shown in Table 1 [41]. The major difference from the 5th edition (published in 1997) was in the tumor (T) classification. In the earlier edition, a T-3 lesion was defined as tumor invading the liver, pancreas, gallbladder, duodenum, and stomach, whereas in the recent 6th edition, T-3 lesions do not invade the duodenum, stomach, or colon. This change reflects the concept of local invasion following an anatomic pattern and suggests that duodenal invasion portends a worse prognosis than pancreatic invasion alone. Given that these lesions are treated with pancreaticoduodenectomy, some have questioned the idea of duodenal invasion conferring a worse outcome. In a recent study from Japan, 95 patients underwent pancreaticoduodenectomy for distal cholangiocarcinoma. There was no difference in survival between those patients who had T-3 (N = 32) and T-4 lesions (N = 30). There was a clear difference, however, between those who had T-1 or T-2 cancers and those who had T-3 or T-4 cancers [42]. These data suggest that tumor extension outside the wall of the bile duct (whether into the pancreas, duodenum, or both) is a key step in the

Table 1
Staging guidelines for extrahepatic bile duct cancers from the American Joint Committee on Cancer 6th edition

Primary tumor (T)
  T-0 No evidence of tumor
  T-is Carcinoma in situ
  T-1 Tumor confined to the bile duct
  T-2 Tumor invades beyond the wall of the bile duct
  T-3 Tumor invades the liver, gallbladder, pancreas, or right or left branches of portal vein
    or hepatic artery
  T-4 Tumor invades main portal vein or both right and left branches, common hepatic
    artery, or other adjacent structures, such as colon, stomach, duodenum, or abdominal
    wall
Regional lymph node status (N)
  N-0 No regional lymph node metastasis
  N-1 Regional lymph node metastasis (hilar, celiac, periduodenal, peripancreatic,
    and superior mesenteric artery groups)
Distant metastasis (M)
  M-0 No distant metastasis
  M-1 Distant metastasis present

Stage	T	N	M
0	T-is	N-0	M-0
1-A	T-1	N-0	M-0
1-B	T-2	N-0	M-0
2-A	T-3	N-0	M-0
2-B	T-1 to T-3	N-1	M-0
3	T4	Any N	M-0
4	Any T	Any N	M-1

natural history of distal cholangiocarcinoma. Furthermore, the likelihood of nodal spread is much higher once tumor has extended beyond the wall of the bile duct, and numerous studies have shown significantly reduced survival in patients who had node-positive disease.

Diagnostic imaging

The ideal diagnostic imaging modality for distal bile duct cancer is one that is easy to perform, is capable of diagnosing disease at an early stage, is without complications, and is able to detect any metastatic disease that may be present. Unfortunately, none of our current imaging modalities are capable of all of these. A combination of multiple complimentary imaging modalities is often required to not only make the correct diagnosis of a distal cholangiocarcinoma but also to adequately stage the patient.

The initial diagnostic modality for evaluating distal bile duct malignancy is based on the clinical presentation, with essentially two possibilities. First are those who undergo abdominal imaging for some other reason (eg, appendicitis, diverticulitis) and are incidentally found to have either a visible mass or irregularity, or biliary ductal dilation. The second and much more common group of patients present with symptoms in some way related to the cancer (pain, jaundice). Ultrasound is typically performed in anyone presenting with right upper quadrant pain and jaundice. This modality may be helpful in detecting ductal dilation and, possibly, the level of obstruction. It will rarely visualize a tumor, however. CT is therefore essential if there is concern for the possibility of a distal malignancy (Figs. 2 and 3). A contrast-enhanced CT scan allows visualization of the ductal anatomy and most metastatic disease. More importantly, the arterial and portal-venous phases are separated allowing accurate assessment of the relationship between the cancer and the vascular structures [43], which is essential for proper assessment of resectability.

Computed tomography can provide a large amount of information, but it can underestimate the extent of tumor spread along the ducts and within the peritoneum. Further imaging is typically required before surgical intervention. The most useful tests after CT scan are magnetic resonance cholangiopancreatography (MRCP) and ERCP (Fig. 4). Each modality allows accurate visualization of the biliary tree. ERCP (Fig. 5) has the additional advantage of allowing preoperative biliary drainage and brush cytology to aid in the confirmation of cholangiocarcinoma. Although CT and ERCP are essential for the initial work-up of distal bile duct malignancies, the addition of endoscopic ultrasound (EUS) with fine-needle aspiration can be considered if the diagnosis is still in question (Fig. 6) [44,45].

Management

Surgery remains the mainstay of treatment of cholangiocarcinoma and up to 10% of all pancreaticoduodenectomies done for cancer are performed for distal bile duct malignancy [46–48]. Unfortunately, many patients present with advanced, unresectable disease and can only be offered palliative

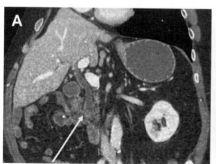
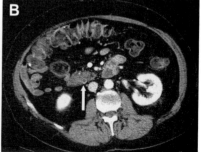

Fig. 2. Coronal reformatted CT image demonstrating a transition point near the pancreatic head with dilation of the common bile duct (*A*). Axial images confirm an enhancing mass within the wall of the distal common bile duct (*B*).

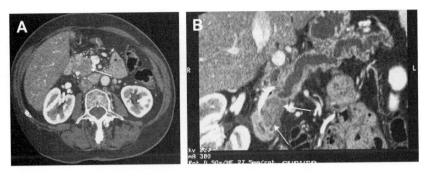

Fig. 3. Low (A) and magnified (B) CT images demonstrating a mass in the head of the pancreas. These were taken from a 75-year-old woman who presented with painless jaundice. She underwent pancreaticoduodenectomy and was found to have a T-3 N-1 distal cholangiocarcinoma.

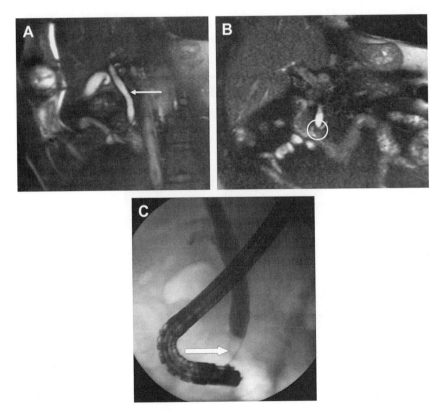

Fig. 4. Coronal MRCP image demonstrating mild dilation of the common bile duct up to the distal portion (A) with a T-2 dark lesion at the level of the transition point (B). Subsequent ERCP demonstrates a stricture in the distal CBD with proximal dilation (C).

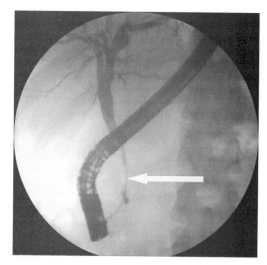

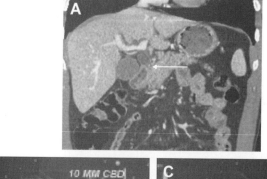

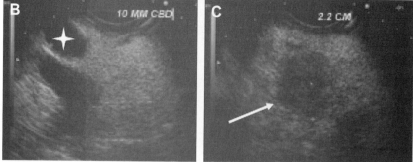

Fig. 5. ERCP performed in a 53-year-old male who had nausea, pruritus, and a 20-pound weight loss. The patient initially underwent a CT scan that showed some mild ductal dilatation. Subsequently, this ERCP confirmed a distal bile duct stricture. He underwent pancreaticoduodenectomy and the final histology revealed a T-3 lesion with pancreatic and perineural invasion.

Fig. 6. Coronal reformatted computed tomographic image showing a transition point in the distal CBD (*A*). Subsequent EUS demonstrated dilation of the CBD (*B*) and a mass (*C*). The star indicates the dilated CBD and the arrow points to the mass.

measures. In those who do present with nonmetastatic disease, surgery is the only chance for prolonged survival and, possibly, cure.

In 1975, Dr. Warren [49] at the Lahey clinic published his series on the radical resection for periampullary cancer over the preceding 30 years. Between 1942 and 1971, he performed 348 pancreaticoduodenectomies, 47 of which (13.5%) were for distal bile duct malignancy. The operative mortality for all pancreaticoduodenectomies was 15%, and 21% after Whipple for distal bile duct cancer. This series was the first to analyze long-term outcomes after resection for these cancers. The overall 5-year survival for those patients who underwent resection was 25%, not much different from current reports. Furthermore, there was a distinct difference in the outcomes of patients who did or did not have lymph node metastases.

Over the past 30 years, there have been multiple reports in the literature on outcomes for distal bile duct cancer [3,5,42,49–58]. From these, it is clear that surgery remains the cornerstone of treatment (Table 2). These papers demonstrate that R-0 resection confers a survival advantage and that the prognosis for those who have unresectable disease is dismal. They also show that nodal status is the most important prognostic factor in those who undergo resection. Although the average overall 5-year survival for all patients undergoing resection is 24% (range 0%–44%), this goes up to 39% (range 22%–61%) in those who have R-0 resection and node-negative disease. Conversely, the average 5-year survival after resection with positive nodes is only 8.7% (range 0%–21%) and the median survival for palliated disease is months.

The largest series in the literature comes from the group at Johns Hopkins. They initially reported their experience with all histologically confirmed cholangiocarcinomas (N = 294) between January 1973 and December 1995 [5]. They subsequently combined this with data collected between January 1995 and March 2004 to give a total of 564 patients [58]. Over the 31-year period, 239 (42%) distal lesions were reported. During the early period, 27% (N = 80) of cholangiocarcinomas were distal cancers, whereas in the later period, 59% (N = 159) were distal cancers. This high proportion of distal lesions during the later period likely reflects referral patterns. In those who underwent surgery for a distal cholangiocarcinoma, 96% were resected (91% in the early period and 98% in the late period). The overall 5-year survival for distal lesions was 23% with a median of 18 months, and patients who had positive margins or nodes had significantly lower survival.

Since Whipple's [59] description of pancreaticoduodenectomy in 1935, it remains the operation of choice for distal biliary malignancies. Pancreatico-duodenectomy is now a safer procedure, with current operative mortality rates of less than 5% (see Table 2). At our institution, we prefer a standard Whipple (with antrectomy) and we routinely perform a stented end-to-side pancreaticojejunostomy. The surgical outcomes after Whipple are improved when this procedure is performed at experienced centers. Despite great

Table 2
Available published series on distal cholangiocarcinoma

Reference	Institution	Year	Total number of distal bile duct cancers	Number of resections for distal bile duct cancers (%)	Survival, all resections (%)				Survival, node negative (%)			Survival, node positive (%)			Operative mortality for distal bile duct cancer resection (%)	Operative mortality for all Whipples (%)
					1-y	3-y	5-y	Median (mo)	1-y	3-y	5-y	1-y	3-y	5-y		
Warren, et al [49]	Lahey Clinic	1975	—	47	76.3	32.3	25	—	75.7	35.4	27.5	80	0	0	21	15
Nakase, et al [50]	Kyoto University (Japan)	1977	309	161 (52)	38	8	5	—	—	—	—	—	—	—	22.3	20.8
Tompkins, [3] et al	UCLA	1981	18	12 (67)	63	28	28	21	—	—	—	—	—	—	8	8
Lerut, et al [51]	University of Louvain (Belgium)	1984	—	5	40	20	0	—	—	—	—	—	—	—	—	10.6
Fong, et al [52]	Memorial-Sloan Kettering	1996	104	45 (43)	79	46	27	33	—	—	54	—	—	0	4.4	—
Nakeeb, et al [5]	Johns Hopkins	1996	—	73	70	31	28	22	89	38	30	50[a]	8[a]	8[a]	0	—
Wade, et al [53]	VA Medical Center, St. Louis	1997	156	34 (22)	69[a]	18[a]	14	15[a]	—	—	22	—	0	0	11	—
Bortolasi, et al [54]	Mayo Clinic	2000	—	15	—	—	20	21	—	—	33	—	—	0	0	—

Study	Institution	Year															
Yoshida, et al [55]	Nakatsu Municipal Hospital (Japan)	2002	—	27	65	37	37	20.5	91	61	61	47	20	20	3.7	—
Murakami, et al [56]	Hiroshima University (Japan)	2007	—	43	72	53	44	26	94[a]	76[a]	58	40[a]	21[a]	21	0	—
Ebata, et al [42]	Nagoya University (Japan)	2007	—	100	75	47	35	30	86	60	46	57	25	19	5	—
Cheng, et al [57]	Second Military Medical University (China)	2007	131	116 (89)	86	51	25	35.5	94	62	30	56	12	4	3.4	—
DeOliveira, et al [58]	Johns Hopkins	2007	—	229	—	—	23	18	—	—	30[a]	—	—	15[a]	3	—

[a] Estimated from survival curve.

improvements in overall operative mortality, morbidity remains high. The most common complication after Whipple procedure is a pancreatic fistula, with leak rates ranging from 11% to 30% depending on the definition [60–63]. Although overall operative mortality may be as low as 1%, the mortality associated with pancreatic fistula after pancreaticoduodenectomy is significant. Moreover, these deaths may not occur within the first 30 days of surgery or during the same hospitalization. Typically, mortality from pancreatic fistula is from bleeding pseudoaneurysms or intra-abdominal sepsis [64].

Palliation

Unfortunately, not all patients who have distal bile duct malignancy present at a resectable stage. The reported resectability rates range from 22% to 89% [3,50,52,53,57]. Because there is no good evidence to support the use of chemotherapy or radiation, palliative measures should be offered. The goals of palliative management for distal cholangiocarcinoma are threefold. First is the alleviation of biliary obstruction. This alleviation can be accomplished surgically (hepaticojejunostomy or choledochojejunostomy) or endoscopically (plastic or metal stenting). Our general approach is to place a plastic stent at the initial ERCP if clinically indicated (complete obstruction with severe hyperbilirubinemia) or if surgical intervention will be delayed. Because most pancreaticoduodenectomies are performed at large academic centers, it is a common scenario for patients to receive a stent at the outside institution to allow time for transfer and appropriate work-up at the tertiary center. Metal stents are placed if it is clear that a patient has unresectable disease or if the patient had a plastic stent placed initially, but is subsequently found to have unresectable disease.

The second goal of palliative care is the relief of duodenal obstruction. Although this represents a premorbid state, obstruction of the duodenum must be treated in a way to minimize time in the hospital. Endoscopic duodenal stenting offers a relatively easy method of relieving obstruction with minimal risk for postprocedure complications.

Finally, all patients should have adequate pain control. Because these tumors have a tendency for perineural invasion, they can become painful. If pain is uncontrollable with oral narcotics, patients should be offered hospice care with intravenous narcotics, antiemetics, and other medications as needed.

Other biliary malignancies

Aside from cholangiocarcinoma, some other malignant neoplasms of the distal bile duct include carcinoid, other neuroendocrine tumors, lymphoma, squamous cell carcinoma, and undifferentiated tumors. These malignancies are rare, however, representing less than 3% to 5% of tumors in this location [11,58], with most descriptions of these tumors in case reports [65–67].

Summary

Cancer of the distal bile duct remains a diagnosis with a dismal outlook. Despite great advances in diagnostic imaging, molecular pathogenesis, and surgical outcomes, the 5-year overall survival remains poor. A pancreaticoduodenectomy with an R-0 resection gives the best likelihood of prolonged survival.

References

[1] Klatskin G. Adenocarcinoma of the hepatic duct at its bifurcation within the porta hepatis. An unusual tumor with distinctive clinical and pathological features. Am J Med 1965;38: 241–56.

[2] Bismuth H, Nakache R, Diomond T. Management strategies in resection for hilar cholangiocarcinoma. Ann Surg 1992;215(1):31–8.

[3] Tompkins RK, Thomas D, Wile A, et al. Prognostic factors in bile duct carcinoma. Analysis of 96 cases. Ann Surg 1981;194:447–57.

[4] Reding R, Buard JL, Lebeau G, et al. Surgical management of 552 carcinomas of the extrahepatic bile ducts (gallbladder and periampullary tumors excluded): results of the French Surgical Association survey. Ann Surg 1991;213(3):236–41.

[5] Nakeeb A, Pitt HA, Sohn TA, et al. Cholangiocarcinoma: a spectrum of intrahepatic, perihilar, and distal tumors. Ann Surg 1996;224:463–73 [discussion: 473–5].

[6] Shaib Y, El-Serag HB. The epidemiology of cholangiocarcinoma. Semin Liver Dis 2004;24: 115–25.

[7] Khan SA, Taylor-Robinson SD, Toledano MB, et al. Changing international trends in mortality rates for liver, biliary and pancreatic tumors. J Hepatol 2002;37:806–13.

[8] Weinbren K, Mutum SS. Pathological aspects of cholangiocarcinoma. J Pathol 1983;139: 217–38.

[9] Kozuka S, Tsubone M, Hachisuka K. Evolution of carcinoma in the extrahepatic bile ducts. Cancer 1984;54:65–72.

[10] Fevery J, Verslype C, Lai G, et al. Incidence, diagnosis, and therapy of cholangiocarcinoma in patients with primary sclerosing cholangitis. Dig Dis Sci 2007;52:3123–35.

[11] Ahrendt SA, Nakeeb A, Pitt HA. Cholangiocarcinoma. Clin Liver Dis 2001;5(1):191–218.

[12] Broome U, Olsson R, Loof L, et al. Natural history and prognostic factors in 305 Swedish patients with primary sclerosing cholangitis. Gut 1996;38(4):610–5.

[13] Jarnagin WR. Cholangiocarcinoma of the extrahepatic bile ducts. Semin Surg Oncol 2000; 19:156–76.

[14] Bergquist A, Ekbom A, Olsson R, et al. Hepatic and extrahepatic malignancies in primary sclerosing cholangitis. J Hepatol 2002;36:321–7.

[15] Rosen CB, Nagorney DM, Wiesner RH, et al. Cholangiocarcinoma complicating primary sclerosing cholangitis. Ann Surg 1991;213(1):21–5.

[16] Iwai N, Yanagihara J, Tokiwa K, et al. Congenital choledochal dilatation with emphasis on pathophysiology of the biliary tract. Ann Surg 1992;215(1):27–30.

[17] Stain SC, Guthrie CR, Yellin AE, et al. Choledochal cyst in the adult. Ann Surg 1995;222(2): 128–33.

[18] Liu CL, Fan ST, Lo CM, et al. Choledochal cysts in adults. Arch Surg 2002;137:465–8.

[19] Watanapa P, Watanapa WB. Liver fluke-associated cholangiocarcinoma. Br J Surg 2002;89:962–70.

[20] Nishimura M, Naka S, Hanazawa K, et al. Cholangiocarcinoma in the distal bile duct: a probable etiologic association with choledocholithiasis. Dig Dis Sci 2005;50(11):2153–8.

[21] Sheen-Chen SM, Chou FF, Eng HL. Intrahepatic cholangiocarcinoma in hepatolithiasis: a frequently overlooked disease. J Surg Oncol 1991;47(2):131–5.

[22] Chen PH, Lo HW, Wang CS, et al. Cholangiocarcinoma in hepatolithiasis. J Clin Gastroenterol 1984;6(6):539–47.

[23] Sahani D, Prasad SR, Tanabe KK, et al. Thorotrast-induced cholangiocarcinoma: case report. Abdom Imaging 2003;28:72–4.

[24] Khan SA, Thomas HC, Davidson BR, et al. Cholangiocarcinoma. Lancet 2005;366:1303–14.

[25] Lee SS, Kim MH, Lee SK, et al. Clinicopathologic review of 58 patients with biliary papillomatosis. Cancer 2004;100(4):783–93.

[26] Lazaridis KN, Gores GJ. Cholangiocarcinoma. Gastroenterology 2005;128:1655–67.

[27] Sirica AE. Cholangiocarcinoma: molecular targeting strategies for chemoprevention and therapy. Hepatology 2005;41(1):5–15.

[28] Malhi H, Gores GJ. Cholangiocarcinoma: modern advances in understanding a deadly old disease. J Hepatol 2006;45:856–67.

[29] Berthiaume EP, Wands J. The molecular pathogenesis of cholangiocarcinoma. Semin Liver Dis 2004;24(2):127–37.

[30] Jarnagin WR, Klimstra DS, Hezel M, et al. Differential cell cycle-regulatory protein expression in biliary tract adenocarcinoma: correlation with anatomic site, pathologic variables, and clinical outcome. J Clin Oncol 2006;24(7):1152–60.

[31] Nehls O, Gregor M, Klump B. Serum and bile markers for cholangiocarcinoma. Semin Liver Dis 2004;24(2):139–54.

[32] Lindberg B, Arnelo U, Bergquist A, et al. Diagnosis of biliary strictures in conjunction with endoscopic retrograde cholangiopancreatography, with special reference to patients with primary sclerosing cholangitis. Endoscopy 2002;34:909–16.

[33] Chalasani N, Baluyut A, Ismail A, et al. Cholangiocarcinoma in patients with primary sclerosing cholangitis: a multicenter case-control study. Hepatology 2000;31(1):7–11.

[34] Nichols JC, Gores GJ, LaRusso NF, et al. Diagnostic role of serum CA 19-9 for cholangiocarcinoma in patients with primary sclerosing cholangitis. Mayo Clin Proc 1993;68(9):874–9.

[35] Patel AH, Harnois DM, Klee GG, et al. The utility of CA 19-9 in the diagnosis of cholangiocarcinoma in patients without primary sclerosing cholangitis. Am J Gastroenterol 2000;95(1):204–7.

[36] Siqueira E, Schoen R, Silverman W, et al. Detecting cholangiocarcinoma in patients with primary sclerosing cholangitis. Gastrointest Endosc 2002;56(1):40–7.

[37] Bjornsson E, Kilander A, Olsson R. CA 19-9 and CEA are unreliable markers for cholangiocarcinoma in patients with primary sclerosing cholangitis. Liver 1999;19(6):501–8.

[38] Ramage JK, Donaghy A, Farrant JM, et al. Serum tumor markers for the diagnosis of cholangiocarcinoma in primary sclerosing cholangitis. Gastroenterology 1995;108:865–9.

[39] Rumalla A, Baron TH, Leontovich O, et al. Improved diagnostic yield of endoscopic biliary brush cytology by digital image analysis. Mayo Clin Proc 2001;76(1):29–33.

[40] Kipp BR, Stadheim LM, Halling SA, et al. A comparison of routine cytology and fluorescence in situ hybridization for the detection of malignant bile duct strictures. Am J Gastroenterol 2004;99:1675–81.

[41] American Joint Committee on Cancer. AJCC cancer staging. New York: Springer-Verlag; 2005, p. 1–150.

[42] Ebata T, Nagino M, Nishio H, et al. Pancreatic and duodenal invasion in distal bile duct cancer: paradox in the tumor classification of the American joint committee on cancer. World J Surg 2007;31:2008–15.

[43] Slattery JM, Sahani DV. What is the current state-of-the-art imaging for detection and staging of cholangiocarcinoma? Oncologist 2006;11:913–22.

[44] Walsh RM, Connelly M, Baker M. Imaging for the diagnosis and staging of periampullary carcinomas. Surg Endosc 2003;17:1514–20.

[45] Eloubeidi MA, Chen VK, Jhala NC, et al. Endoscopic ultrasound-guided fine needle aspiration biopsy of suspected cholangiocarcinoma. Clin Gastroenterol Hepatol 2004;2:209–13.

[46] Aranha GV, Aaron JM, Shoup M, et al. Current management of pancreatic fistula after pancreaticoduodenectomy. Surgery 2006;140:561–9.

[47] Muscari F, Suc B, Kirzin S, et al. Risk factors for mortality and intra-abdominal complications after pancreaticoduodenectomy: multivariate analysis in 300 patients. Surgery 2005; 139:591–8.

[48] Yeo CJ, Cameron JL, Sohn TA, et al. Six hundred fifty consecutive pancreaticoduodenectomies in the 1990s: pathology, complications, and outcomes. Ann Surg 1997;226:248–57.

[49] Warren KW, Choe DS, Plaza J, et al. Results of radical resection for periampullary cancer. Ann Surg 1975;181:534–40.

[50] Nakase A, Matsumoto Y, Uchida K, et al. Surgical treatment of cancer of the pancreas and the periampullary region: cumulative results in 57 institutions in Japan. Ann Surg 1977;185:52–7.

[51] Lerut JP, Gianello PR, Otte JB, et al. Pancreaticoduodenal resection. Surgical experience and evaluation of risk factors in 103 patients. Ann Surg 1984;199:432–7.

[52] Fong Y, Blumgart LH, Lin E, et al. Outcome of treatment for distal bile duct cancer. Br J Surg 1996;83(12):1712–5.

[53] Wade TP, Prasad CN, Virgo KS, et al. Experience with distal bile duct cancers in U.S. veterans affairs hospitals: 1987–1991. J Surg Oncol 1997;64:242–5.

[54] Bortolasi L, Burgart LJ, Tsiotos GG, et al. Adenocarcinoma of the distal bile duct: a clinicopathologic outcome analysis after curative resection. Dig Surg 2000;17:36–41.

[55] Yoshida T, Matsumoto T, Sasaki A, et al. Prognostic factors after pancreaticoduodenectomy with extended lymphadenectomy for distal bile duct cancer. Arch Surg 2002;137:69–73.

[56] Murakami Y, Uemura K, Hayashidani Y, et al. Prognostic significance of lymph node metastasis and surgical margin status for distal cholangiocarcinoma. J Surg Oncol 2007;95:207–12.

[57] Cheng Q, Luo X, Zhang B, et al. Distal bile duct carcinoma: prognostic factors after curative surgery. A series of 112 cases. Ann Surg Oncol 2007;14(3):1212–9.

[58] DeOliveira ML, Cunningham SC, Cameron JL, et al. Cholangiocarcinoma: thirty-one year experience with 564 patients at a single institution. Ann Surg 2007;245(5):755–62.

[59] Whipple AO, Parsons WB, Mullins CR. Treatment of carcinoma of the ampulla of Vater. Ann Surg 1935;102(4):763–79.

[60] Balcom JH, Rattner DW, Warshaw AL, et al. Ten-year experience with 733 pancreatic resections: changing indications, older patients, and decreasing length of hospitalization. Arch Surg 2001;136:391–8.

[61] Yeo CJ, Cameron JL, Maher MM, et al. A prospective randomized trial of pancreaticogastrostomy versus pancreaticojejunostomy after pancreaticoduodenectomy. Ann Surg 1995; 222:580–8.

[62] Pratt WB, Maithel SK, Vanounou T, et al. Clinical and economic validation of the International Study Group of Pancreatic Fistula (ISGPF) classification scheme. Ann Surg 2007;245: 443–51.

[63] Kazanjian KK, Hines OJ, Eibl G, et al. Management of pancreatic fistulas after pancreaticoduodenectomy: results in 437 consecutive patients. Arch Surg 2005;140:849–55.

[64] Veillette GR, Dominguez I, Ferrone C, et al. Implications and management of pancreatic fistulas following pancreaticoduodenectomy: the MGH experience. Arch Surg 2008; 143(5):476–81.

[65] Sewkani A, Kapoor S, Sharma S, et al. Squamous cell carcinoma of the distal common bile duct. JOP 2005;6(2):162–5.

[66] Podnos YD, Jimenez JC, Zainabadi K, et al. Carcinoid tumors of the common bile duct: report of two cases. Surg Today 2003;33(7):553–5.

[67] Nagai E, Shinohara M, Yonemasu H, et al. Undifferentiated carcinoma of the common bile duct: case report and review of the literature. J Hepatobiliary Pancreat Surg 2002;9:627–31.

ELSEVIER
SAUNDERS

SURGICAL
CLINICS OF
NORTH AMERICA

Surg Clin N Am 88 (2008) 1449–1455

Index

Note: Page numbers of article titles are in **boldface** type.

A

Acute acalculous cholecystitis, 1246–1248.
See also *Cholecystitis, acute acalculous.*

Acute calculous cholecystitis, 1242–1246.
See also *Cholecystitis, acute calculous.*

Acute cholecystitis, laparoscopic
cholecystectomy for, 1300–1303,
1308–1310

Age, cholesterol stones related to, 1184

B

Barium cholangiography, 1195, 1202–1203

Benign biliary strictures, endoscopic
evaluation and treatment of,
1227–1231

Bile
composition of, 1176–1178
flow through biliary system, 1253
production of, 1176–1178

Bile acid synthesis, 1178–1179

Bile duct(s)
caudate lobe, anatomy of, 1166–1168
common, anatomy of, 1168–1170
confluence of, 1168
extrahepatic, relationship to vascular
structures, 1172
left lobe, anatomy of, 1163–1166
malignant strictures of, endoscopic
evaluation and treatment of,
1231–1232
right lobe, anatomy of, 1161–1163

Bile duct cysts, **1369–1384**
cancer and, 1378–1379
causes of, 1369–1371
classifications of, 1371–1375
clinical presentation of, 1369,
1375–1377
diagnostic imaging of, 1377–1378
epidemiology of, 1369
incidence of, 1369
surgical management of, 1379–1382

Bile duct stricture, proximal, endoscopic
evaluation and treatment of,
1233–1234

Bile metabolism, **1176–1181**

Biliary disorders, endoscopic evaluation and
treatment of, **1221–1240**
benign biliary strictures, 1227–1231
biliary leaks, 1229–1230
choledocholithiasis, 1224–1227
described, 1221–1222
distal common bile duct stricture,
1232–1233
malignant strictures, 1231–1232
proximal bile duct stricture, 1233–1234
sclerosing cholangitis, 1230–1231
sphincter of Oddi dysfunction,
1235–1236
stricture secondary to chronic
pancreatitis, 1228–1229

Biliary dyskinesia, **1253–1272**
types of, 1253

Biliary imaging
current techniques, overview of,
1195–1197
update on, **1195–1220**

Biliary injuries
classification of, 1330–1334
iatrogenic, **1329–1343**
identification of, 1335–1337
management of, 1337–1339
initial, 1337–1338
outcomes following, 1339–1340
surgical, 1338–1339
mechanism of, 1334–1335

Biliary leaks, biliary stricture secondary to,
1229–1230

Biliary papillomatosis, distal biliary
malignancy related to, 1433–1434

Biliary sampling, in suspected gallbladder
dyskinesia evaluation, 1256

Biliary sludge, cholesterol stones and,
1183–1184

doi:10.1016/S0039-6109(08)00169-2

Moving?

Make sure your subscription moves with you!

To notify us of your new address, find your **Clinics Account Number** (located on your mailing label above your name), and contact customer service at:

E-mail: elspcs@elsevier.com

800-654-2452 (subscribers in the U.S. & Canada)
314-453-7041 (subscribers outside of the U.S. & Canada)

Fax number: 314-523-5170

Elsevier Periodicals Customer Service
11830 Westline Industrial Drive
St. Louis, MO 63146

*To ensure uninterrupted delivery of your subscription, please notify us at least 4 weeks in advance of move.